Nelson Yuan-sheng Liang

Sense Organs

Sense Organs

General Editors

M. S. LAVERACK
B.Sc., Ph.D., F.I.Biol., F.R.S.E.
Gatty Marine Laboratory, University of St Andrews

and

D. J. COSENS
B.Sc., Ph.D.
Department of Zoology, University of Edinburgh

Blackie

Glasgow and London

Blackie & Son Limited
Bishopbriggs
Glasgow G64 2NZ

Furnival House
14–18 High Holborn
London WC1V 6BX

First published 1981

British Library Cataloguing in Publication Data

Sense organs.
1. Sense organs
I. Laverack, Michael Stuart
II. Cosens, D J
591.1′82   QP431

ISBN 0–216–91094–3

Filmset by Advanced Filmsetters (Glasgow) Ltd.
Printed by Thomson Litho, East Kilbride, Scotland

Contributors

Professor H. Autrum, Zoologisches Institut der Universität München, 8 München 2, Luisenstrasse 14, West Germany.

Dr. F. G. Barth, Fachbereich Biologie/Zoologie, J. W. Goethe–Universität, 6000 Frankfurt am Main, Siesmayerstrasse 70, West Germany.

Dr. J. Boeckh, Fachbereich Biologie, Universität Regensburg, 8400 Regensburg, Universitätsstrasse 31, West Germany.

Dr. F. A. Brown, Jr., Marine Biological Laboratory, Woods Hole, Mass. 02543, U.S.A.

Professor T. H. Bullock, Department of Neurosciences, University of California, San Diego, La Jolla, California 92093, U.S.A.

Dr. C. Den Otter, Groningen State University, 9750 AA Haren, The Netherlands.

Professor C. J. Duncan, University of Liverpool, Department of Zoology, P.O. Box 147, Liverpool L69 3BX, U.K.

Professor R. L. Gregory, University of Bristol, Department of Anatomy, University Walk, Bristol BS8 1TD, U.K.

Dr. A. Hawkins, Department of Agriculture and Fisheries for Scotland, Marine Laboratory, P.O. Box 101, Victoria Road, Aberdeen AB9 8DB, U.K.

Dr. K. Horner, Department of Agriculture and Fisheries for Scotland, Marine Laboratory, P.O. Box 101, Victoria Road, Aberdeen AB9 8DB, U.K.

Professor A. Iggo, Department of Veterinary Physiology, Royal (Dick) School of Veterinary Studies, Summerhall, Edinburgh EH9 1QH, U.K.

Professor K. Kirschfeld, Max-Planck-Institut für Biologische Kybernetik, 7400 Tübingen, Spemannstrasse 38, West Germany.

Dr. M. Land, University of Sussex, Ethology & Neurophysiology Group, School of Biological Sciences, Brighton, Sussex BN1 9QG, U.K.

Professor M. S. Laverack, Gatty Marine Laboratory, University of St. Andrews, Fife KY16 8LB, U.K.

Professor M. Lindauer, Zoologisches Institut II, Universität Würzburg, D-8700 Würzburg, Röntgenring 10, West Germany.

Professor O. Lowenstein, University of Birmingham, Neurocommunications Research Unit, The Medical School, Birmingham B15 2TJ, U.K.

Professor H. Martin, Zoologisches Institut II, Universität Würzburg, D-8700 Würzburg, Röntgenring 10, West Germany.

Dr. I. Russell, University of Sussex, Ethology & Neurophysiology Group, School of Biological Sciences, Brighton, Sussex BN1 9QG, U.K.

Dr. D. C. Sandeman, Australian National University, Department of Neurobiology, Box 4 P.O., Canberra A.C.T. 2601, Australia.

Dr. J. H. Scholes, MRC Cell Biophysics Unit, 26–29 Drury Lane, London WC2B 5RL, U.K.

Professor H. Stieve, KFA, Institut für Neurobiologie, Postfach 1913, D-5170 Jülich 1, West Germany.

Dr. T. Szabo, C.N.R.S.—L.P.N.3, 91190 Gif-sur-Yvette, France.

Dr. S. Young, University of London, Department of Zoology, Imperial College, London SW7 2AZ, U.K.

Preface

To make sense of sense organs and to understand how biological transducers work is a major interest of biologists and physiologists. This book is intended as a review of current and recent activity in the field of sense organs. It is not intended as a textbook, but rather a set of stimulating contributions covering what is known about how biological sensors work, their sensitivities, their ambiguities, their input to the central nervous system and the manner in which their signals are interpreted. This is a large canvas to cover, yet the attempt seems opportune, and we feel that the authors represented here will convey the fascination and excitement of the topic.

The arrangement of the chapters provides an introduction together with a general chapter which discusses the various environmental influences on organisms and the adaptive radiation of sensors to tap these energies. These set the scene for the more specific chapters that follow. The argument established is that the natural world is a continuum, and that the rather precise sensitivities determined for any one species do not necessarily indicate the sensitivities of others—one must expect the variety of animals to demonstrate a spectrum of sensitivities in a number of modalities.

These facilities are explored through the book by discussions of mechanical, chemical, photic, electrical and magnetic senses; this latter sense in particular being a topic only just emerging from folklore, yet undoubtedly significant in the lives of bacteria, bees and birds. Similarly man, through his own inexperience and naivety, has only recently recognised that electrical phenomena too are sensed and guide certain other organisms in their daily lives.

The chapters by Land, Young, Boeckh, Russell, Hawkins and Barth cover vision, chemoreception and mechanoreception in a style designed to review the structure of respective sense organs: their anatomy and disposition, as well as adaptation of morphology to endow greater or lesser sensitivity towards particular parameters of their special modality. Land's discussion of the crustacean eye reinvestigates the arguments over Exner's proposition regarding superposition and apposition eyes, in the knowledge of recent findings of light-guides, corneal nipple arrays and facet shapes; his conclusion that such matters may lead to a reclassification of the Crustacea is intriguing to both physiologists and zoologists. Young's discourse on the cladoceran *Daphnia* treats this pond-dwelling crustacean as a model of why an eye is as it is: even in such an apparently simple compound eye comprised of a small number of widely spaced individual receptors, there are adaptive differences, and receptor position in the eye is influential in determining spectral sensitivity and so has implications for behaviour and for feeding in particular. Feeding behaviour is also controlled by chemoreception, both distant (olfaction) and contact (gustation), and Boeckh provides a pithy summary of the characteristics of chemoreceptors in that best known group of animals for the purpose—the insects. Barth ranges across the Arthropoda, from arachnids and crustaceans to insects, in the search for common principles behind mechanoreceptor design. His chapter includes, to the biologist's great benefit, a discussion of engineering demands and the principles of stress, strain and displacement, and their focal localization at certain points in a skeleton, which govern distribution, properties and mechanism of mechanoreceptors. Russell and Hawkins deal with the particular case of mechanoreception in auditory organs of vertebrates.

The initial steps in the transduction of environmental energies into meaningful bioelectric signals, introduced by Duncan, are only beginning to be understood. The location of sensors at some advantageous point on the body surface would be worthless if the cell (receptor) membrane and its component molecules were not exquisitely tuned to, and able to absorb, some external energy, and if the transmembrane potential were not modified by alterations of the membrane properties in response to that absorbed energy. How the energy is absorbed, and the events that occur at the receptor membrane (possibly internally as well in some cases), are discussed by Kirschfeld and Stieve for photoreceptors, which are the best investigated sensors, and by Den Otter for chemoreceptors. Only the complexity of the molecular events is clear—understanding is in the realm of conjecture because much remains to be discovered. For the intending sensory physiologist, the elucidation of transduction is the great challenge of the field.

The arrangement of sense organs into *systems* is dealt with by Lowenstein in a general introduction, and thence by Scholes for the eye in a masterly discussion of the reason for inversion, the existence of an optic chiasm and how the brain sorts out the message received from the eye in vertebrates (and also the octopus), which has long been a puzzle. Sandeman reveals the procedures undertaken to ensure correct orientation in space by arthropods, through from primary receptors to the unscrambling of the message in the central nervous system. Szabo does likewise for the electroreceptors of fish, and Bullock provides an excellent review of the principles of sensory systems, using electrosensory and octavolateralis organs as examples.

The book concludes with chapters on less easily characterized senses which deserve lengthy treatment—but argument, scepticism and doubt still remain as potent stimulants to stringent experimentation in search of understanding. Iggo carefully goes through the evidence for skin receptors that respond to such stimuli as vibration, temperature, and chemicals, and of which some mediate in the sensation of pain. The characterization of nociception, which can be indicated by vocal animals, is difficult, yet is of great importance to man and his subjective view of the environment. For non-vocal animals the field is less amenable to definition and becomes a question of thresholds and interpretation—identification of 'noxious' stimuli is fraught with uncertainty.

The uncertainty principle has also been the concern of Brown's work of a lifetime with "unusual senses"—including, for example, magnetism, barometric pressure and cosmic influences. There is now little doubt that magnetism in some form has a profound influence on the behaviour of some organisms (perhaps more subtly on others?), and it is possible that other minute energy sources may also affect animals. A specific case is given for bees by Martin and Lindauer, together with a theoretical interpretation.

Gregory provides a view of how an animal interprets the information it acquires from environmental cues. If sensation is a reflection of sense, then interpretation of the incoming electrical signals in the sensory nerves by the central nervous system is of paramount importance. Mistakes at the periphery may be overcome by numerous parallel inputs providing many sources of reference; but mistakes at the centre may lead to gross errors of behaviour. That such mistakes occur is evident from such phenomena as optical illusions engendered by very simple patterns seen by the photoreceptors, but giving wrong impressions in the brain. How many octopus and crabs have been misled by illusions generated by waving seaweeds?

The book is completed by an epilogue by that doyen of sensory physiologists Otto Lowenstein, whose cutting edge has lost none of its sharpness and whose incisive analysis of problems points the way to new endeavours.

The Scottish Electrophysiological Society held its third International Symposium in Edinburgh in April 1980. This book is based on the meeting and the contributions of its participants.

M.S.L.
D.J.C.

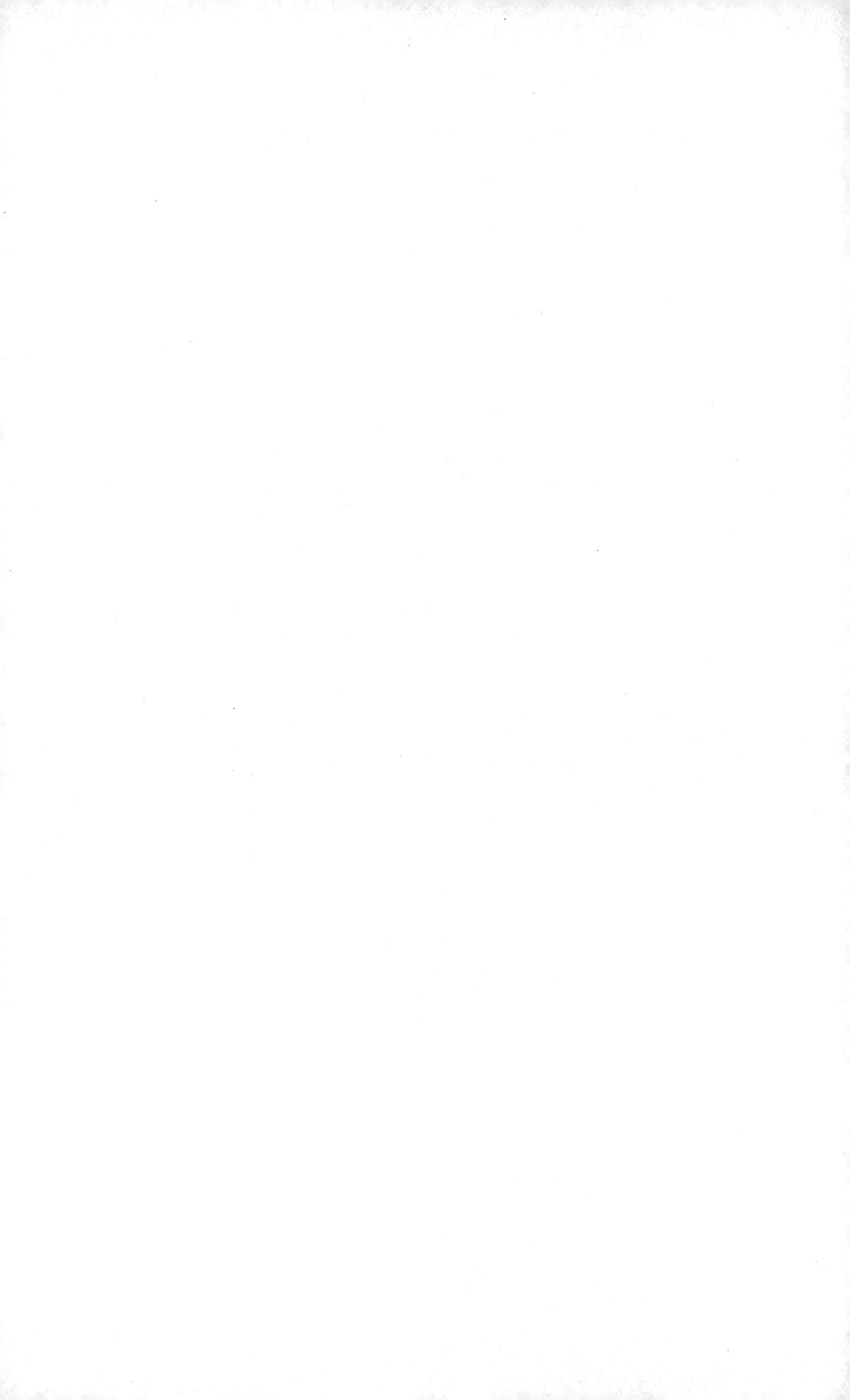

Contents

Abbreviations

cAMP	cyclic 3,5-adenosine monophosphate
ccw	counterclockwise
CDR	Ca^{2+}-dependent regulator
cGMP	cyclic 3,5-guanosine monophosphate
CM	cochlear microphonic
CNS	central nervous system
cw	clockwise
dB	decibel
DUM	dorsal unpaired median
EDTA	ethylene diamine tetra-acetic acid
EGTA	ethylene glycol-bis (β-amino ethylether)-N,N′-tetra-acetic acid
EMF	earth's magnetic field
EOD	electric organ discharge
epsp	excitatory post-synaptic potential
HRP	horseradish peroxidase
Hz	hertz
I	intensity
IMP	intramembranous particles
IR	infrared
LLL	lateral line lobe
LRP	late receptor potential
ms	millisecond
P	permeability
PDA	prolonged depolarizing afterpotential
ROS	retinal outer segment
SAR	structure-activity relationship
SDS	sodium dodecyl sulphate
SPL	sound pressure level
SR	sarcoplasmic reticulum
TEP	transepithelial potential
UV	ultraviolet
W	watt

Part 1

STRUCTURE AND FUNCTION OF SENSE ORGANS

CHAPTER ONE
INTRODUCTION

H. AUTRUM

There is fascination in the study of sense organs, for we are so often confronted with unexpected and astonishing results that open new insights into nature. And there is fascination, too, in the hope that what we learn will bring us closer to an understanding (or at least the beginning of an understanding) of the sense of life in general. As far as ultimate meanings are concerned, of course, we can be well content to leave such questions to philosophers. If they are honest they will say that they have no answer either, and that all the philosophy in the world never will provide an answer. An answer to this question would mean the end of philosophy; we would have no further need of it.

We sensory physiologists have a more modest goal. We are asking about the sense—the significance—of sense organs. And here the answer seems trivial. Sense organs make possible two kinds of achievement. First, they allow man and animal to find their way around their environment. Second, they underlie the homeostasis of organisms, of the individual, of the society, and in the last analysis of the biotope, of what today is generally called the "ecological equilibrium".

To find the way in an environment, in the extreme case, requires no sense organs at all. Consider an object—a boulder rounded in a glacier, or the perhaps more familiar present-day sight, a lump of oil or tar in the sea, a gluey mass of sponge spicules and hairs, rounded by the constant movement of the water. Such an object arrives at its destination entirely by the laws of physics. The boulder rolls down the slope; the ball of debris is cast on to the beach by the waves. Each has reached a "goal". But neither will ever, of its own accord, climb back up the mountain or roll back into the ocean. In theory, of course, statistical mechanics allows that a stone might one day move upward from the ground. Indeed, rumour has it that bricklayers work so slowly because they are waiting for this (physically possible, after all) event to occur!

Such a process, in which the entropy of a closed physical system increases, requires a Maxwell's Demon. The living organism, on the other hand, has no such requirement. It *can* climb from the valley to the peak; to do so, it uses energy, and thus itself obeys the law of physics. However, man and animal require more than simple physical energy to find the way upward. They need, for example, gravity receptors. Receptors of this sort take many different forms and are found in animals ranging from protozoans to humans. By means of these, organisms can make efficient use of the energy they consume.

The relationships of organisms to their environment and the maintenance of homeostasis are central to our understanding of sense organs. Both systems are exceedingly complex, and there must be a corresponding complexity in the sensory systems. The word "system", in this context, must be taken seriously. The environment is a system, not a sum of more or less numerous individual entities. It is a sum of entities *plus* the spatial, temporal, causal and random relationships among them. The whole is more than the sum of its parts—but not more than the parts plus the relationships and interactions among them. The same is true of an organism. The environment is one system, the animal another. This notion is an old one, but only recently have mathematical and cybernetic methods been developed to analyse such systems (see, e.g., Reichardt and Poggio, 1976; Poggio and Reichardt, 1976; Reichardt, 1978).

Still more complex than these systems themselves are the relationships between them. These are usually nonlinear, and involve reciprocal influences. In biology, then, we are dealing with three systems: (1) the environment, (2) the organism, and (3) the environment-organism system. The analysis of this third system proceeds on two levels. First, behaviour is studied under controlled conditions, with no explicit treatment of the organization and function of the sensory system (this is phenomenological analysis). Second, a search is made for the microsystems (receptors and their special properties, neurone groups of increasing complexity) that make these phenomenologically specified behaviour patterns possible and determine their nature. This line of research can lead far—as, for example, Reichardt and Poggio (1976) and Poggio and Reichardt (1976) have shown. Such studies can provide information about the function and the necessary number of neural microsystems, and can raise questions subject to investigation not only in the laboratory, but under natural conditions as well. An excellent example of the latter is given in the papers by Collett and Land (1975*a*,*b*).

Even without direct monitoring of the neuronal processes themselves, one can learn a good deal. For example, it turns out that although the Reafference Principle of Mittelstaedt and von Holst (for a review see Mittelstaedt, 1971) is a valuable heuristic which helps to interpret such complicated events as orienting behaviour, figure recognition and figure-ground recognition, it is not an absolute prerequisite for complex behaviour (Reichardt and Poggio, 1976).

Sense organs often comprise not only receptors, but second- and higher-order neurones as well; these also belong to the sensory system. In these areas of research, morphological analysis has far outstripped physiological (and biochemical) analysis (see, e.g., Braitenberg and Burkhardt, 1976). The proven classical methods of electrophysiology and biochemistry have recently been supplemented, with some success, by genetic methods. Morphologically defective mutants have become a familiar tool, and recently Greenspan, for example, has studied mutants with defective transmitters (Greenspan, 1980).

To understand sense organs, we need to do more than study neuronal networks and microstructures, however ingenious our approach. Sense organs have a long history, going back more than three billion years. To understand the structure, the limitations, the tasks and the meaning of sense organs, we must look into their past. Eyes for instance have arisen independently more than 40 times in evolution (Salvini-Plaven and Mayr, 1977). In few if any of these cases have we an idea of the factors that led to the particular direction of development. We do not even know all the sense organs that once existed. Wehner, in his 1980 review, refers to the so-called schizochroal eyes of the now extinct trilobites. Clarkson and Levi-Setti (1975) made thin sections through the fossil lenses of these eyes. They concluded that

> the trilobites had exploited Huygens' principle of an aspherical aplanatic lens by using a specifically shaped optical correcting interface between the outer and the inner part of the lens. Provided that the refractive indices of the inner and outer parts of the lens were properly adjusted, imaging as well as light collecting capacities would have been maximized in this remarkable type of eye.

If we want to make any progress in studying the evolutionary aspects of sense organs, we must be able to relate environmental factors and ecological conditions to the performance and structure of sense organs. In other words: we must examine system relationships not only in the area of microstructures and behaviour, but also in the context of the ecological-historical system. First steps in the direction of such sensory ecology have been made by many workers; see, for example, the review of Crescitelli (1977), and the symposium "Sensory Ecology", edited by Ali (1978).

You will no doubt ask, "Who can be expected to comprehend all this? Who is going to unite all the different approaches into a single picture that gives us a sense of sense organs in their entirety?" We ought not to despair of success. It is true that the mass of facts is steadily increasing. The data are like drops in the ocean, which—as in the old tale—we must drink up in order to gain the paradise of simple, easily surveyed theories. But this is not an impossible task. The facts that establish the theory of evolution fill large libraries; the pure theory of evolution can today be presented on a few pages.

The following quotations seem particularly appropriate. First a word from Sir Karl Popper (1979).

> As far as the natural sciences are concerned, in my opinion it would be a sin to regard them, with Francis Bacon, essentially as a means to increase our power. The best antidote to this temptation is to keep on reminding ourselves how little we know. The significance of our highest intellectual achievements does not lie in their extension of our range of knowledge; I believe it is of still greater significance that they have opened up new regions of our ignorance, and will continue to do so.

And second: we should not forget how much joy there is in exploring living nature. When Karl von Frisch received the Nobel Prize, a reporter asked him what his feelings were. Professor von Frisch's answer was, "The buzzing of a bee in the garden gives me more pleasure than the Nobel Prize."

REFERENCES

Ali, M.A. (ed.) (1978) *Sensory Ecology: Review and Perspectives* Plenum, New York, London, Washington, Boston.

Braitenberg, V. and Burkhardt, W. (1976) "Beyond the wiring diagram of the lamina ganglionaris of the fly" in *Neural Principles in Vision* (ed. Zettler, F., Weiler, R.) Springer, Berlin-Heidelberg-New York, 238–244.

Clarkson, E. N. K. and Levi-Setti, R. (1975) Trilobite eyes and the optics of Descartes and Huygens *Nature*, **254**, 663–667.

Collett, T. S. and Land, M. F. (1975*a*) Visual control of flight behavior in the hoverfly, *Syritta pipiens J. Comp. Physiol.*, **99**, 1–66.

Collett, T. S. and Land, M. F. (1975*b*) Visual spatial memory in a hoverfly *J. Comp. Physiol.*, **100**, 59–84.

Crescitelli, F. (ed.) (1977) *The Visual System in Vertebrates* (Handbook of Sensory Physiology, Vol. **VII**/5) Springer, Berlin-Heidelberg-New York.

Greenspan, R. J. (1980) Mutations of choline acetyltransferase and associated neural defects in *Drosophila melanogaster J. Comp. Physiol.* (in press).

Mittelstaedt, H. (1971) "Reafferenzprinzip—Analogie und Kritik" in *Vorträge der Erlanger Physiologentagung* (eds. Keidel, W. D., Plattig, K.-H.) Springer, Berlin-Heidelberg-New York.

Poggio, T. and Reichardt, W. (1976) Visual control of orientation behaviour in the fly. II. Towards the underlying neural interactions *Quart. Rev. Biophysics*, **9**, 377–438.

Popper, K. (1979) "Die moralische Verantwortlichkeit des Wissenschaftlers" in *Forum Heute*, **2** Bibliographisches Institut, Mannheim-Wien-Zürich, 210–214.

Reichardt, W. (1978) "Figure-ground discrimination by the visual system of the fly" in *Lecture Notes in Biomathematics* 21*: theoretical approaches to complex systems* (eds. Heim, R., Palm, G.) Springer, Berlin-Heidelberg-New York, 117–146.

Reichardt, W. and Poggio, T. (1976) Visual control of orientation behaviour in the fly. I. A quantitative analysis *Quart. Rev. Biophysics*, **9**, 311–375.

Salvini-Plaven, L. v. and Mayr, E. (1977) "On the evolution of photoreceptors and eyes" in *Evolutionary Biology*, Vol. **10** (eds. Hecht, W. C., Steere, B., Wallace, B.) Plenum, New York, 207–283.

CHAPTER TWO

THE ADAPTIVE RADIATION OF SENSE ORGANS

M. LAVERACK

Introduction

This chapter is concerned with the evolution and adaptive radiation of sense organs. It will attempt to say something about the many types of sensors so far discovered in animals, not forgetting that there may well be some we do not yet suspect, let alone know anything about.

In such a discussion it is necessary to step outside oneself. One cannot understand alien phenomena if one takes only an anthropocentric standpoint. In many ways the best start for a sensory investigation is that of natural history. The well-known folklore phenomena of horses, sheep, and cattle "knowing" when the weather is about to change, or when an earthquake is about to occur, indicate sensitivities well beyond that of human perception. Animal migrations, mate finding, site and prey selection all suggest sensitivity to modalities available to man only through instruments, and possibly not even then.

The design of appropriate experiments requires the availability of instruments and the application of thought based on thorough knowledge of the animal and its capabilities. Conceptual difficulties abound, for it is not always easy to put oneself in the place of a planktonic copepod or a parasitic helminth to determine what stimuli are of adaptive (survival) significance to it and its offspring.

The environment as a continuum

The major events that govern the behaviour of animals fall within the physical and chemical attributes of the environment. It is not very helpful to attempt a classification of sensors without some realization of what the external parameters are that may influence the living organism.

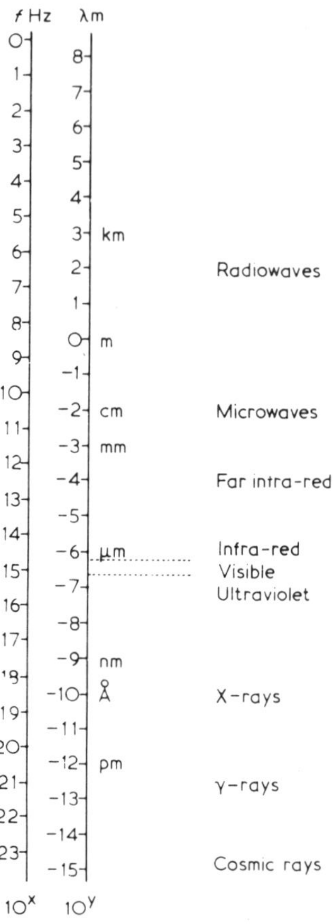

Figure 1 The electromagnetic radiation spectrum. This figure shows radiation at different frequencies and different wavelengths. Terminology on the right indicates the radiation identified and characterized by man as measurable phenomena. Note that light visible to man encompasses a very small range of the whole, and that infra-red (heat) and ultra-violet (insect vision) extend the overall range to some extent. Mechanical agitation may be a function of heat as well as other movements. Magnetism also covers a considerable range (from White, 1974).

For this reason it seems appropriate to illustrate very simply the range of physical events that may be of significance. Fig. 1 (from White, 1974) is the standard linear arrangement of electromagnetic radiation phenomena demonstrating the enormous span of known examples measured in a variety of ways by instruments. It is conventional to include a bracket that indicates the rather narrow portion for which we have some personal obvious evidence in the form of sensitivity, namely in heat and light (infra-red through the visible spectrum). It is nonetheless obvious that the physical environment is a continuum leading from very short to ultra-

Table 1 This table separates scalar from vector quantities. Scalar events are those of magnitude only, and are not usually involved in sensory perception, whilst vector quantities of magnitude plus direction often are (from White, 1974).

Scalar quantities	*Vector quantities*
distance	displacement
speed	velocity
time	acceleration
mass	force
area	electric current
volume	electrostatic field
frequency	electromagnetic field
viscosity	momentum
energy	torque
work	
moment of inertia	

long wavelength and of very low to very high frequency oscillation. The apparent sensitivity of animals has always been accepted as falling within a very narrow range, but the recent discoveries in ultra-sound, in electric organs, and in the magnetic sensitivity of organisms as well as the rather better known ultraviolet sensitivity of the insect eye seem to show that it is necessary to maintain a healthy scepticism that we have reached the limit of surprise.

Table 1 indicates that it is insufficient to think just of the magnitude of an event. Scale is not in itself the most important feature of a stimulus; it is influential certainly and affects the gross response, but is secondary in significance to the vector and directional components of the stimulus. An assessment of viscosity might be difficult to achieve although of paramount importance to many minute organisms such as tiny flying insects and feeding copepods. So it is not just the quality of the stimulus but the manner in which it is delivered that governs sensory activity, albeit through the medium of structural adaptation (taken in its widest sense to include animal morphology, detailed anatomy, ultrastructural disposition and even biochemical and molecular arrangements). However, these distinctions differ subtly in importance. Morphology is an indication of actual position, and hence of great significance for directionality (right and left sidedness, anterior-posterior positions, dorsal-ventral attitudes); anatomy of individual sense organs determines how much stimulus energy is accepted through orientation and development of accessory structures; the ultrastructure is much more concerned with the acceptance of the stimulus energy since here we deal with single cellular entities which do not discriminate between possible directions and angles, only with the delivery of a stimulus, its quality, and its quantitative value; and at the biochemical level (virtually unknown in many types of sensory systems) the changes are solely concerned with presence or absence of a physical event within a very precise range (hence the subdivision of many sensory labours amongst the component cells of the organ as a whole).

The way in which a sensor is approached therefore varies profoundly according to the attitude and vision of the questioner. On one hand one asks information of the whole, and is concerned largely with vectors and directions; on the other, one asks about the nature of the basic event, and looks at transduction mechanisms which are molecular and scalar.

The term "receptor" might be applied to a sensor or a sense organ and this is a description frequently used. On the other hand, the site of transduction also deserves the title, as it is here that the actual event takes place, and by analogy with, say, chemical transmitting synapses, an acceptor molecule is involved.

A classification of senses

Any attempt to categorize the senses will probably fail in one way or another, but it is useful to have some guidelines and the following is intended to provide some assistance. It represents the range of functional adaptations exhibited by sensors.

Mechanical sense

This is a basic property of all animals, and represented in simple situations as well as highly sophisticated versions. Mechanical events such as stretch, compression, touch and deformation are significant. It is represented in many different ways, such as:

(i) ciliary beat alterations due to particle impingements (Strathmann, Jahn and Fonseca, 1972);

(ii) deformation of soft areas (e.g. leech body wall, Nicholls and Baylor, 1968; crustacean cuticle, Wales, Clarac and Laverack, 1971);

(iii) deflection of setae, hairs, cupulae and statoliths (on body surfaces, lateral lines, and in statocysts);

(iv) proprioception via skeletal elements (chordotonal organs in arthropods; muscle spindles in vertebrates);

(v) changes in volume of gas-filled spaces generating information in another modality by its mechanical influence (e.g. heat detectors in rattlesnakes, Bullock and Diecke, 1956; swimbladder pressure detection, Qutob, 1962);

(vi) gravity and acceleration in equilibrium (such as vestibular) systems (middle ear, cephalopod statocysts).

Photic sense

A very primitive function of living organisms, since the capture of photons by pigments is well established in the lowliest photosynthetic organisms. If animals arose from protists by becoming autotrophs rather than photosynthetic, they did not at the same time lose all light sensitivity. General light sense (often known as the dermal light sense) is a property of non-specific areas, whilst specific light sensors, eyes and ocelli, are located in particular areas and are specialized in structure for light capture.

Chemical sense

An appreciation of chemical properties of materials is vital to life, for instance in regulation of internal homeostasis, detection of food, seeking of mates, sperm approaching the egg, or larva seeking a settlement site.

Categories erected on chemical attributes alone, such as carbohydrates, amines and salts, are no more helpful than the subjective classes: salt, bitter, sour, and sweet. These areas may more usefully be divided into:

(i) distant, low concentration, receptors; i.e. olfaction or smell;

(ii) contact, high concentration, receptors; i.e. gustation or taste, regardless of class of compound. We might, however, recognize that some receptors are stimulus specific within chemical classes, whilst others are more generally stimulated.

Electric sense

This represents a genuine category, the perception of electrical events in the environment, appropriate to aquatic animals, particularly fish.

Thermal sense

Changes in environmental temperature influence activity in certain specialized cells (Schmidt, 1978) but such receptors are virtually unknown outside the vertebrates.

Magnetic sense

Recent discoveries of the presence of magnetite in the heads of insects (bees), and of pigeons (and of the responses of marine animals to magnetic fields), bring the likelihood of magnetic sensitivity closer to our understanding, although the mechanism is not yet clear (Walcott and Green, 1974; Gould, 1979).

Unusual senses

Whilst the majority of animals possess mechanical, photic and chemical senses, few have electrical and magnetic sensitivity so far as we know.

Various other possibilities exist such as X-rays or barometric pressure, and Brown (this volume) has been involved many times in efforts to elucidate these.

Nociceptors. Nociceptors, or receptors adapted to the reception of noxious stimuli, are probably the most notoriously difficult to categorize. The problem is one of distinguishing noxious events. Most authors presumably mean events that are considered extreme, or outside the normal environmental range of the animal. These are somewhat ill-defined; for example, Nicholls and Baylor (1968) consider 1 g to be a touch stimulus, 7 g a pressure stimulus, whilst 21 g is noxious to a leech; hence the T, P, N cell system classification now firmly in the literature. The same arrangement has been adopted by Martin and Wickelgren (1971) and Matthews and Wickelgren (1978) in their consideration of lamprey sensors (threshold for N cells being 1–9 g, though in some cases the probe punctured the skin).

Such classifications are nonetheless subjective and should be accepted with caution, but may indicate that all classes of known receptors deserve an "extreme" category. Those described above are for mechanoreceptors; Necker and Reiner (1980) have produced examples for thermoreceptors in pigeons where receptor firing does not commence until a temperature of about 42°C is reached, and then increases to 48°, eventually reaching a maximum at 52°, stopping after 30 s.

No doubt similar events can be, and have been, described for photo-receptors (a punch in the eye), chemoreceptors (nasty smells) and so on. Pain undoubtedly distinguishes a whole class of receptors, but their definition in many animals should not be just a whim of the investigator.

Three examples will now be examined more closely to indicate the overall range displayed by adaptations of sense organs.

Mechanical sensitivity

The frequency range demonstrated for sensitivities in the mechanical mode falls into a number of optimal areas.

For a number of marine invertebrates, the appropriate level of frequency lies at the very lowest periodicity, around 1–100 Hz. This has been shown for Crustacea (Laverack, 1963; Mellon, 1963), Bryozoa (Thorpe *et al.*, 1975), Ctenophora (Horridge, 1966), Chaetognatha (Horridge and Boulton, 1967; Bone and Pulsford, 1978) and perhaps Urochordata (Bone and Ryan, 1979). The power required also very often falls within the near-field region of a vibrating source, and the far-field propagated pressure wave may be of less significance. Hearing has been difficult to demonstrate unequivocally in groups such as molluscs and Crustacea, but this possibly depends more on semantic definitions than on physical realities.

Amongst vertebrates, the development of the acoustico-lateralis system certainly encompasses hearing as a function of the well-developed organ complex, but there is also a low frequency component in the lateral line response that mimics the situation elsewhere in aquatic animals. This naturally vanishes in the more advanced vertebrates where the lateral line no longer exists. The frequency range in this mechanoreceptor assemblage is considerable, running from the lowest up to about 20 kHz (in terrestrial vertebrates such as man).

Beyond this are those animals that produce, utilize and perceive high frequency sound (bats, birds, edentates, cetaceans) though this may be pulsed so as to provide a low frequency and a high frequency range. This is modified by the environment, so that information about its characteristics is gained. Some insects have evolved counteracting mechanisms that rely on analysis of the bat's pulse by sensory cells (Roeder, 1975). It is possible that some fish may show similar characteristics with regard to predatory marine mammal signals.

The highest frequency range utilized seems to be in the 50–60 kHz bandwidth, but whether or not this is due to the mechanical difficulty of producing the sound pulse, or some other attribute, remains to be determined.

Nonetheless we can erect a series of optimal curves that fall in distinct bands (Fig. 2), but what is perhaps more interesting is that across the whole sound spectrum from 1 Hz–60 kHz animals have evolved responsive mechanisms. Each animal has its own specific range, there is environmental range fractionation as it were, and the ranges specify the animal, its sensory capacity and its vocal or sound productive area.

Chemical sensitivity

It could be argued that all exchanges of chemicals across membranes constitute a form of chemoreception, but this seems such an all-embracing idea as to be worthless in a sensory concept. The movement of ions such as Na^+, K^+ and Ca^{2+}, or Cl^- into and out of nerve cells might be the concomitant of stimulation, but following rather than leading in the response. Even so, the very nature of "saltiness" and the discrimination of various salts is marked in some cases, and evidently does represent a real sensory modality. Insect studies on responses to sodium chloride and other similar chemicals show that there are real differences in stimulatory value. When coupled with evident behavioural effects on oviposition, feeding and so on, the salts are undoubtedly important.

More often, however, chemoreception, though analogous to nerve cell transmission, is usually separated from it. But the apparent similarity of stimulation is notable, and indeed even involves some similar compounds and chemical groupings. Thus, glutamate is known as a stimulant of external receptors (Case, 1964), and also as a nerve transmitter (in insects especially; Usherwood, 1971; Piggott, Kerkut and Walker, 1975). No doubt the membranes involved are closely related in structure. The amine moiety (NH_2 radical) is implicated both in feeding responses and in nerve transmission. The carrier portion of the molecule may differ markedly, but the amine moiety is its significant feature. Over the last fifteen years or so the anthropocentric classification of "taste" into salty, bitter, acid and sweet, has been shown to be altogether too narrow a view of chemosensation. Bitters like quinine, and sugars and sugar-like molecules do not seem to have much value to aquatic animals, whilst "meaty" flavours and substances such as amines and perhaps polypeptides may act as valid clues for feeding. The list of stimulants, such as the common amino acids (Shepheard, 1974; Laverack, 1964; Case and Gwilliam, 1963) both alone and in combination (Shelton and Mackie, 1971) reveals distinct sensitivity ranges for single cells and for populations but extends the range of chemosensation markedly.

Added to this observation must be the knowledge that some large, long-chain molecules not only bring about chemical stimulation, but they do so specifically (isomeric specification) and evoke very precise responses; these are the pheromones, allomones, kairomones.

So in this category one can arrange hierarchies of stimulation which represent a "frequency" response for chemoreceptors (see also Hansen, 1978). Some appear commonly throughout the animal kingdom; some have specific importance for one part of the animal's overall behaviour such as feeding, and yet others have significance for just one precise item in the behavioural repertoire. The most widespread seems to be that of reproductive activity, although site selection by metamorphosing larvae may be equally precise. Scents, lures and attractants are often complex molecules and specific in effect, and are probably so throughout the animal kingdom.

Photoreceptors

Electromagnetic radiation, as we have seen (Fig. 1), is widespread and almost infinitely variable. It is a matter of common knowledge that portions of the range are detectable, and that this has led to the separation of distinct populations of sensors which are classified separately. Since man is a visual animal *par excellence*, photoreceptors receive a large share of attention in the sensory field, and are considered as a particular category.

If it is borne in mind, however, that we are considering a range of radiation that spans the very restricted region between 400 nm and 750 nm, and that this is extended very little by consideration of those allied wavelengths of the ultra-violet (valuable to insects) and the infrared (detectable as heat) then we realize that the classification is artificial. Nonetheless, because of the overriding influence of sight in our own lives it is accepted that photoreception constitutes a natural division and it is usually categorized alone. Reference to Fig. 2, however, puts it in its proper place, namely as a small portion of a very lengthy scale.

Of course within the very small portion of the electromagnetic scale that we care to label as visible light, and hence identify as involved in photoreception, there are further subdivisions, the colours. Although Newton firmly demonstrated that the visible spectrum is continuous and that in the natural world one colour grades imperceptibly into the next we still utilize the concept of primary colours for our classification. Red, yellow and blue are recognized as indivisible. We now have some indications that our photoreceptors are typically organized to be predominantly sensitive towards stimulation within the rather narrow range of radiation corresponding to what we recognize as colours. But might it not be worthwhile considering why these three colours? Why not three others with slightly different wavelengths? Is it just that these can be mixed to provide all the others, or is there some other fundamental property we have not recognized?

Could it be that adaptation has engineered our colour-receptive pigments for one scale, whilst it has arranged for insects to cover a different spectrum, not because of the indivisibility of the frequency of oscillation, but because of the biological necessity of these colours?

Should we really expect all animals to possess similar attributes? Why should some complex highly visual animals, e.g. *Octopus*, be colour-blind (Messenger, 1977) even though they live in an environment where at least some parts of the spectrum must be available? *Octopus* feeds on crustaceans and molluscs, which are relatively colourful in the normal environment, but the highly visual predator appears unable to utilize clues of stimulus wavelength. The inability of annelids and other invertebrates to respond to red light is well known, and often used in investigations of behaviour that requires no overt light stimulation for success. Does this mean that a restricted range of colour sensitivity is common to many animals, and that many animals really respond only to the presence or absence of light as such, and ignore all other parameters? Does it also mean that it is less easy to evolve a pigment responding to the longer wavelengths, than the short? If so, why? Extra-ocular photoreceptors may have sensitivities to different wavelengths than those of the eye.

Bowmaker (1980) has recently pointed out that some birds also have sensitivity to ultra-violet light. Indeed he has indicated another feature that is similar to the point I am trying to make here, namely that the ranges over which photochemical reactions occur are larger and more variable than is generally recognized. If the available energy lies between 300 nm and about 800 nm (being too small in value above and below

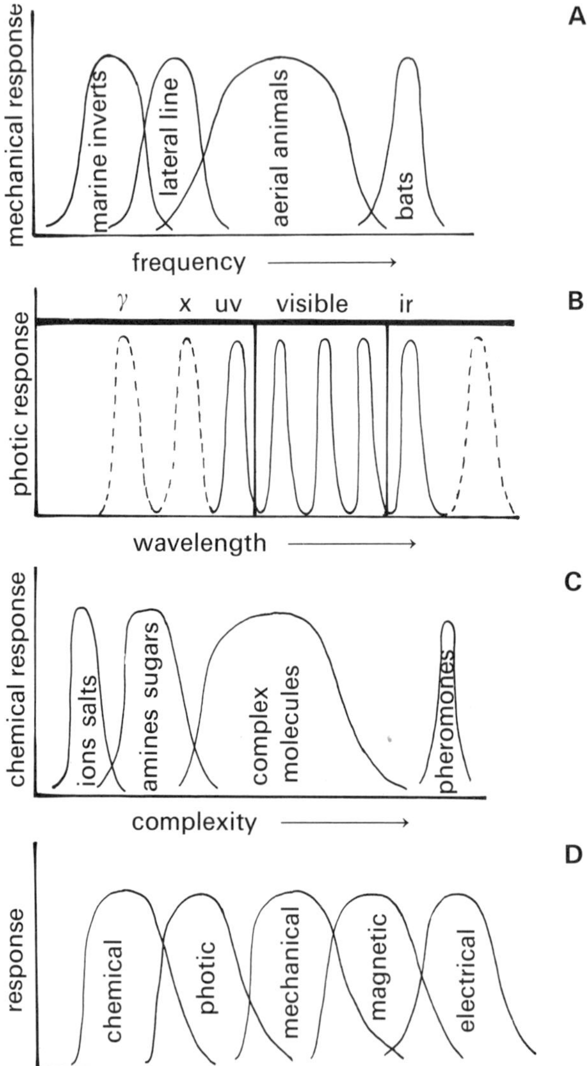

Figure 2 The range of sensory perception.
A: the mechanical sensitivities of animals fall into certain frequency bandwidths ranging from 1–100 Hz for marine invertebrates, 50–400 Hz for lateral line, 50–20 kHz for aerial animals, and 30–40 kHz for bats and cetaceans.
B: the visual spectrum also covers a number of bandwidths, very narrow for the three primary visible colour receptors, but with additional narrow ranges for UV and perhaps IR levels, and perhaps in other examples the possibility exists for wider range still.
C: in the field of chemical sensation ranges may encompass small molecules such as NaCl, and ions, followed by the more complex levels of amines and sugars, a wide range of complex molecules and a very narrow ultra-sophisticated system of pheromones.
D: taken together and with additions such as magnetism and electrical phenomena the sensory abilities of animals cover a continuum over a considerable range of natural phenomena.

these figures to be of much value (caution!)) then it is not surprising if the examples known fall in a range across the scale. Thus the human "blue" pigment absorbs maximally at 415–420 nm, but due to filtering by the lens the effective optimal wavelength is 440 nm, and there is a marked cut-off at 400 nm. Overlapping with this range the birds have receptors with maximum sensitivity at 400–415 nm, but also possess pigments responding at around 370 nm.

The proposition that the range demonstrated by man is probably very misleading, and that considering the natural world as a whole the possibilities existing are continuous, seems well supported by this evidence. More information on fish, reptile and invertebrate eyes would be of considerable value.

The biological significance of these phenomena must be profound, as also is the influence of polarization of the plane of light. This property again seems to be of more significance to other groups of organisms than man. The fish, crustaceans and insects have all been demonstrated to possess this attribute.

Fig. 2 summarizes the viewpoint taken here, namely that the natural world is a continuum, and that the stimuli it provides are broad spectra which overlap. Sensory mechanisms have adapted to enable signals of all types to be detected. Fertile areas to examine in the future may prove to be where no pertinent example has so far been described, though natural signals must be involved. The portions of the figure show (A) mechanical events, with a number of ranges well represented over a broad frequency band, low frequencies being well detected by aquatic invertebrates and vertebrates (lateral line in fish) with optima at about 50–60 Hz and 100–150 Hz. Above this is found the middle frequency range from 100 Hz to about 10–15 kHz as observed in man and lastly the high-frequency band of 40–60 kHz typical of bats and other animals utilizing pulsed signals.

(B) indicates a similar set of curves for the chemical senses with a narrow band (i) for sensitivity to ions and salts, (ii) a broader band for slightly more complex substances such as amines and sugars, (iii) a peak for many complex substances, polypeptides, proteins, starches, and so on and lastly (iv) a very narrow peak for complex molecules of great specificity such as pheromones.

(C) is the electromagnetic series encompassing the visible light range (with three peaks for the prime receptors), and the extra-visible extensions of ultra-violet and infra-red. Beyond these lie the less obvious peaks of X-rays (no known cases) and γ-rays (see Brown, this volume) and magnetism proper (Gould, 1979; Walcott and Green, 1974; Blakemore, 1975).

(D) gives envelopes for each of these categories to try to indicate that there is an all-embracing sequence of sensitivities represented in the animal kingdom.

Origin of sense organs and their relationship to the nervous system

Sensitivity towards external influences is now well established as a component of the lives of even the lowliest organisms. The directed movement of bacteria towards a chemical source has been demonstrated (see Springer, Goy and Adler, 1979) and indicates that such prokaryotes possess sensitivity towards a particular modality. The flagellum of the bacterium rotates either clockwise or counterclockwise and determines whether the cell swims smoothly or erratically.

Chemoreception therefore is an early and important feature in sensory mechanisms. Such reactions may be described for many protists, many gametes (Miller, 1978), lowly larval forms and so on. The level of morphological complexity necessary is not great, and may take place in the absence of a specific *known* transmission or conduction system (nervous system).

The transformation of a surface membrane by the impact of molecules, photons, thermal agitation, or mechanical effects requires only a fairly

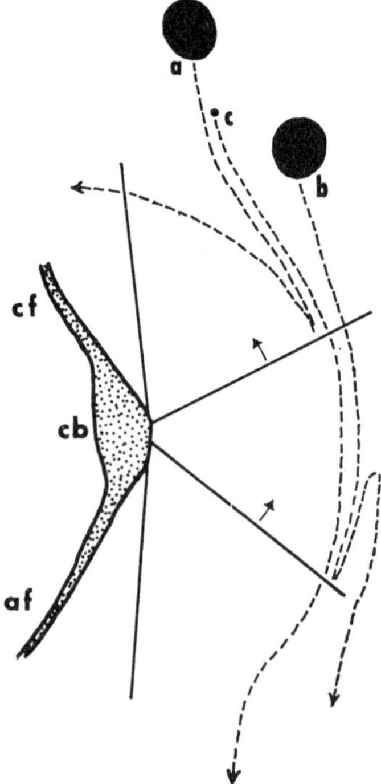

Figure 3 Investigation of the ciliary beat of the pluteus larva of an echinoderm reveals that impingement of particles of given size leads to a reversal of the beat of a cilium. This is an immediate effect, and indicates a change in behaviour of the cilium. The effect on the animal is one of rejection or acceptance of food (from Strathmann, Jahn and Fonseca, 1972).

small modification of the membrane. It may therefore occur in non-complex organisms. The whole organism is not required to respond, only some particular site. Thus the bacterium may well have specific sites on its surface that respond as does the protozoan *Didinium* (Hara and Asai, 1980), photic effects may take place through a special region (e.g. *Euglena*) and mechanical effects through a specially placed cilium (Tucker, 1968, in *Nassarius*). Strathmann, Jahn and Fonseca (1972) demonstrated an immediate mechanical effect on cilia in the feeding apparatus of the echinoderm pluteus larva in which cilia reverse the beat when encountering a solid particle (Fig. 3). These units are "normal" cilia used rapidly in a beating sequence, yet they respond as independent units and change their behaviour when a mechanical stimulus of appropriate size hits them. They are acting as single receptor/effector units and the resulting behaviour is simple but powerfully effective: the animal either feeds or it does not! This finding correlates well with the work of Thurm (1968) who experimentally demonstrated mechanical sensitivity of the frontal cilia of the gill of the mussel (*Mytilus*). Mechanical sensitivity thus seems a commonplace event in cilia, and makes them prime candidates for further refinement into sensors as well as effectors. The variability of structure of cilia and its value in systematics has been noted by Tyler (1979). Adaptation is thus shown even at this level in lowly animals. It is only in somewhat more advanced organisms that the basic organelle or membrane system becomes sequestered into an individual, specially organized cell with a high sensitivity towards one stimulus modality or another.

Horridge (1968), in his essay on the origin of the nervous system, suggested that this step (of special sense cell formation) would have taken place late in the evolution of the nervous system as a whole, being required only after the appearance of a conducting system. The development of an independent sensory-cum-effector unit, capable of receiving stimuli and responding to them, does not occur often in the animal world, the prime example being perhaps the nematocyst of Cnidaria, which has trigger and response mechanism, but does not seemingly transfer information elsewhere.

This example leads me to suggest that in fact the nervous system may have originated in a different way to that proposed earlier, and that the sense organ is a basic and initial requirement for development. Horridge's scheme (1968) postulated a conducting epithelium leading to an effector as a prime step in developing a nervous system (Fig. 4). The work of Bone and Mackie (1975), Warner (1975), Roberts (1975), McFarlane (1976) and others suggests that in such disparate groups as coelenterates and vertebrates, conducting epithelia do exist, and that stimulation gives rise to impulses that travel over considerable distances to some end-organ or effector.

The *stimulus*, however, is essential. It does not affect the argument that

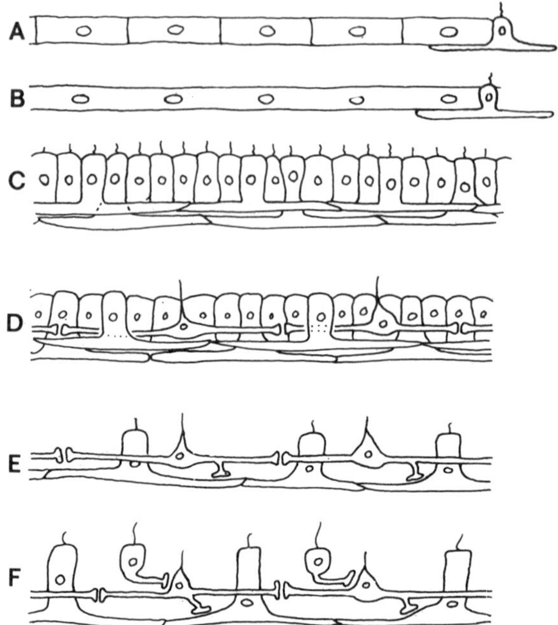

Figure 4 The origin of the nervous system (from Horridge, 1968).
A. A conducting epithelium leads to a musculo-epithelial cell.
B. A syncytial epithelial system.
C. Muscle cells are connected by their contractile tails.
D. Epithelial cells connect only with each other and travel some distance as axons.
E. Such cells connect to muscle cells, and
F. sensory cells appear, but only after the appearance of the conducting system (see also Horridge, 1966).

all cells may be equally sensitive and hence provide input points to the system. Radial symmetry may necessitate multiple sensory inputs that are later restricted in the process of cephalization. Wherever polarization of the body occurs there will develop *specific* sites. It seems more logical perhaps to look for a system in which a sensor feeds information into a conducting epithelium.

Fig. 5 summarizes the hypothesis advanced here. In the first instance a unicellular organism (prokaryote, protist) is both sensor and effector in total behaviour (Fig. 5A). If the ciliated cell is incorporated into an epithelial layer it may still respond individually (Strathmann, Jahn and Fonseca, 1972) although adjoining other cells (Fig. 5B). More dramatic events may take place in receptor/effector cells such as nematocysts (Fig. 5C) which are also included in epithelial layers. If now, however, the sensor transmits information through a conducting epithelium (Fig. 5D) more cells, and distant effectors, will be influenced. Such a phenomenon is

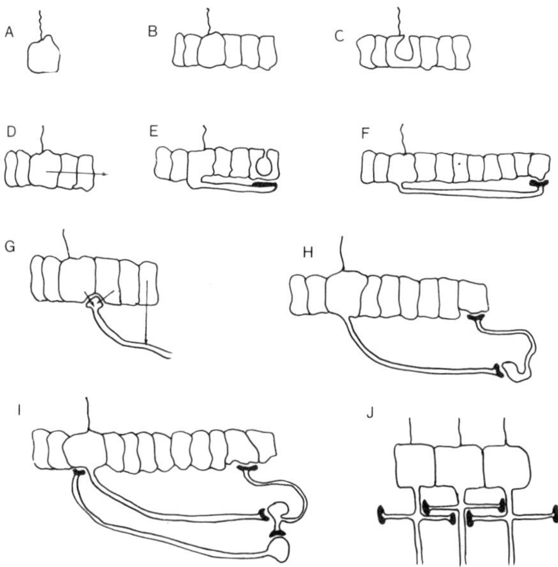

Figure 5 The derivation and interactions of sensory cells.

A. The single organism concept in which the whole cell acts as receptor and effector. The receptor may be a cilium, or some portion of a cilium (e.g. bacteria, spirochaetes, protozoa).

B. The simple receptor/effector as part of a more complex organism. The cilium responds directly to a stimulus, and the whole animal (larva) changes its behaviour in some way (e.g. pluteus larva, after Strathmann *et al*., 1972) through the change of ciliary beat.

C. The receptor/effector as a unit in which some portion of the cell surface (e.g. cnidocil) triggers a cellular response (e.g. nematocyst discharge) without external interaction.

D. The inclusion of a receptor cell as part of an epithelial layer. Any response of the receptor does not influence its own activity as an effector, but information spreads electrically through the surrounding epithelium (e.g. Cnidaria, after McFarlane, 1976; chordate tadpoles, Roberts, 1975).

E. The receptor cell becomes not only a sensor but a neurone of sorts by extending to an effector, thus by-passing the epithelial cells and transmitting directly to the effector (e.g. *Aplysia*, Coggeshall, 1971; possibly also echinoderm pedicellariae).

F. An extension of this argument would place the effector further and further away from the sensor thus extending the transmission lines.

G. A receptor cell associated with a conducting epithelium, but with both systems evidently affecting a separate neurone. Stimulation of both systems leads to modulation of the same neuronal activity in the CNS (after Bone and Ryan, 1979).

H. A simple reflex arc of receptor to motor fibre to effector cell but without an interneurone.

I. The influence of the receptor on the motor fibre may also be returned as feedback to the sense cell, leading to modulation, biasing or central control.

J. As sense organs grow more complex and involve more cells so the interactions between them become more variable, but direct interaction such as lateral inhibition becomes possible (e.g. *Limulus* eye, Hartline and Ratliffe, 1958).

unpolarized and spreads generally around the organism (e.g. coelenterates), and more specific pathways may appear via the development of local, short, axonal effects of sensor on a separate effector (Fig. 5E, as in *Aplysia*, Coggeshall, 1971). It is then but a short step to lengthen the axon in such a way that the effector cell is at a considerable distance from the receptor (Fig. 5F).

The likelihood of direct interaction between sensor and effector seems probable in a number of larvae, although at present we have little direct information. Many invertebrate phyla possess planktonic motile larvae. The swimming as well as feeding of the larva is a function of the prototroch ring of cilia (Carter, 1926; Koshtoyants *et al.*, 1961). Classical descriptions of the larvae of annelids, molluscs, sipunculids, echiuroids and bryozoans all feature an apical tuft of cilia, the function of which remains obscure yet could be implicated here.

Recent work using the transmission electron microscope suggests that there is direct interaction between the apical organ ciliated tuft, and the prototroch motile cilia (e.g. Bonar, 1978; Wollacott and Zimmer, 1978; Holborow and Laverack, unpublished). Further analysis is required, but the evidence so far leads one to the conclusion that the apical cells may be chemosensory and/or mechanosensory, and that they may connect directly with the motile cilia which could conceivably either be inhibited as in metamorphosis, or stimulated to further swimming activity by recognition of undesirable surroundings (Chia and Rice, 1978), or lack of suitable food.

Complexity may arise if both epithelial conduction and sensory individuality occur, and both influence a third entity, namely an axon (Fig. 5G); a situation noted in the larvacean *Oikopleura* (Bone and Ryan, 1979). Subsequent developments incorporate more elements in the transmission pathway, leading to integration, smoothing and biasing (Fig. 5H, 5I). In receptors where populations of cells lie aggregated together, close interaction may be noted through the development of synaptic spurs and inhibitory contacts (Fig. 5J).

An interesting example of "mosaic" evolution is shown by *Oikopleura*, a larvacean ascidian, which has a skin that conducts action potentials (Bone and Mackie, 1975) as also does the ascidian tadpole (Mackie and Bone, 1976). For a long time *Oikopleura* has been known to possess what are called Langerhans receptors, a single pair of bristle-like organs located on the surface. Their structure appears to be that of a highly modified cilium suspended in a cup (Bone and Ryan, 1979). Skin impulses are set up by electrical or mechanical stimuli applied anywhere on the skin surface, and stimulation of the Langerhans receptor accomplishes the same result, namely a modification of the locomotor rhythm. At the base of the receptors and abutting against them via a gap junction is an axon, and transmission to the caudal ganglion is via this axon, regardless of the source of the signal. The electrical synapse postulated is crossed by both epithelial and receptor signals.

Thus we might summarize that the steps in sensory reception require that the surface be specially sensitive, that eventually it is advantageous to have such sensitivity located in one rather than in many cells, and hence there is a separation of sensors from others. This is followed by a sequence in which sensors transmit to the sheet of epithelial cells in which they are located, and thence to some other organ. An intermediate stage might consist of sensor and effector together.

These sensors associated with epithelia may then further develop into groups, perhaps each with slightly differing sensitivities, and located anteriorly (the process of cephalization) as animals became morphologically polarized.

The response of bacteria with which I started my argument depends upon an immediate response of the flagellar (ciliary) apparatus. This primitive condition no doubt exposes some portion of the cell surface to the environment, an area which might be quite small. It is more advantageous to expose a large surface or catchment area to the stimulus, and to achieve this the cell surface should be lengthened or folded in some characteristic manner. Any projection would be valuable, and under these circumstances cilia would be prime contenders for modification, since they form outstandingly long extensions of the surface. Other types of cell surface such as stereocilia or brush borders seem not to have been involved to the same degree, though they may be concerned in accessory structures. Sensory capability may therefore involve internal as well as surface structure.

The basic nature of the cilium and its implication in sense organs cannot be doubted although there are, of course, receptors lacking these attributes. The adaptable nature of the cilium is shown by its presence in sense organs in all phyla from Protozoa to Chordata. Even in those phyla where the surface is stiff and cuticulate (nematodes and arthropods), the cilium has been incorporated into sense organs (mechanoreceptors, photoreceptors and chemoreceptors).

Accessory structures

Cephalization or the development of a head is usually considered as a result of the polarization of the animal body (bilateral symmetry) with advancing complexity. Associated with this trend, the sense organs often become more pronounced in this area; but this is not, at least amongst invertebrates and lower vertebrates, an exclusive attribute. Whilst the development of eyes may become pronounced anteriorly, photosensitivity may nonetheless be distributed elsewhere, e.g. the 6th abdominal ganglion of the crayfish (Prosser, 1934) or the caudal eyespots of the polychaete *Fabricia sabella* (Irving and Laverack, personal observation). Taste buds and chemoreceptors are not all located on or near mouths or mouthparts. Instead they may be quite widely distributed on the body as is the case in crustaceans or fish (Bardach and Villars, 1974; Whitear, 1971). The gradual increase in complexity of sense organs, as opposed to sensors, has two causes. First there is the simple accumulation of numbers of sense cells. Several cells gathered together subserving the same modality form a sense organ. Within the group there may be subdivision of function, for example, not all cells have the same sensitivity. Secondly, there is the development of accessory structure.

In protozoa and sponges there are few possibilities for accessory structure appearance. A fusion of some surface structure, or the asymmetry of occurrence of an organelle, might be sufficient to impart an advantage to the sensor, but little else is feasible. The ubiquity of the cilium, however, has been remarked on elsewhere, and the flexibility of use of this remarkable structure allows an immediate improvement on sensitivity. There is now a large number of reports of (suspected) sensory cilia that are stiff. The basic flexible shaft cilium is supplanted by an organelle in which bending takes place occasionally and usually from or at the base only. The rigidity of the cilium confers mechanical advantage, and distortion at the base allows stimulation. The possibility of such arrangements exists in protozoa, although positive examples have not been described.

The stiff cilium then represents perhaps the simplest type of accessory structure available in a sensor; but many developments subsequently took place. The association with cuticular changes (bristles, setae, campaniform domes, depressions, slits, fans, flexible areas); with secreted cupulae surrounding the cilium (lateral lines); with enclosures in capsules, tunnels and canals for channelling of directional stimuli (statocysts, vestibular mechanisms); with loaded particles for gravity detection (statocysts), and localized patches of otherwise unspecialized epithelium can all be found in various phyla.

The cilium, however, is also remarkably adaptable in its own form and is implicated in other types of sense organs besides mechanoreceptors, notably in photoreceptors, and in chemoreceptors, not to mention neuromasts of the electroreceptor sense. In these cases accessory structures tend to reflect the nature of the stimulus, e.g. photoreceptors may be cilia surrounded by pigment cell cups, tapeta, and protective linings, and supplied with lenses of varying complexity and diaphragm devices such as the iris of the vertebrate eye. Chemoreceptors on the other hand (again not all necessarily ciliary in nature) tend to be associated with pores and channels, and may be subdivided to establish the largest number of sites possible for exposure to the environment. In this case the whole organ (antenna, tentacles) may be greatly expanded and divided to provide a large catchment area.

The impetus of adaptation in accessory structure provision then is a direct question of advantage, precision, catchment and focusing. That organs of different sensitivity have different appearances and arrange-

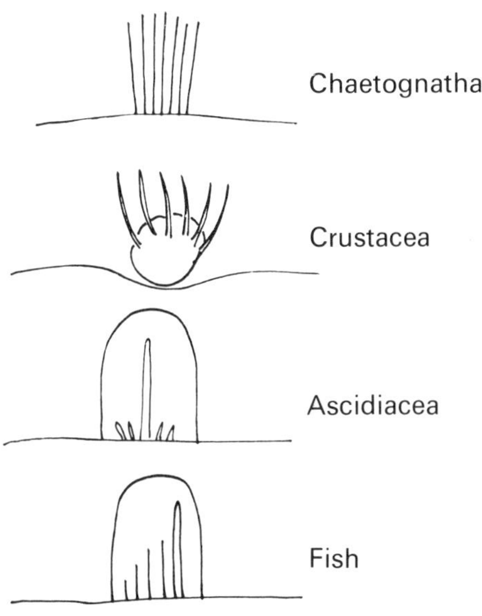

Figure 6 Convergent evolution in water-vibration detectors (top to bottom): Chaetognatha (Bone and Pulsford, 1978); Crustacea: Decapoda (Laverack, 1963); ascidian (Bone and Ryan, 1979); fish (after Flock, 1965).

ments should surprise no-one, but that the underlying organelle, the cilium, is of such widespread occurrence is remarkable.

Convergent evolution is a well-established principle amongst structural studies. It must be accepted as occurring amongst receptor structures as well as guts, body shapes, and behaviour. One example is the receptors involved in water vibration and movement detection in such different groups as arthropods, chaetognaths, ascidians and fish. All possess thin, large surface area superficial projections, hair fans in the case of crustacea, cupulae in ascidians and fish, and aggregated cilia in chaetognaths (Fig. 6). The nature of the end-organ is different (cuticular or gelatinous) in these cases, but the result is the same, sensitivity to vibrations of low frequency.

Adaptive radiation

Adaptive radiation indicates that advantage has been taken of every opportunity available to exploit a new environmental niche or opening. As described elsewhere in this paper, radiation can be accepted as the sensitivity to various modalities but may also be thought of as a refinement and sophistication of basic mechanisms.

The statocyst of invertebrates is a patch of sensory ciliated epithelium that becomes loaded with heavy particles such as sand grains or calcium carbonate concretions. This provides a weighted region sensitive to the

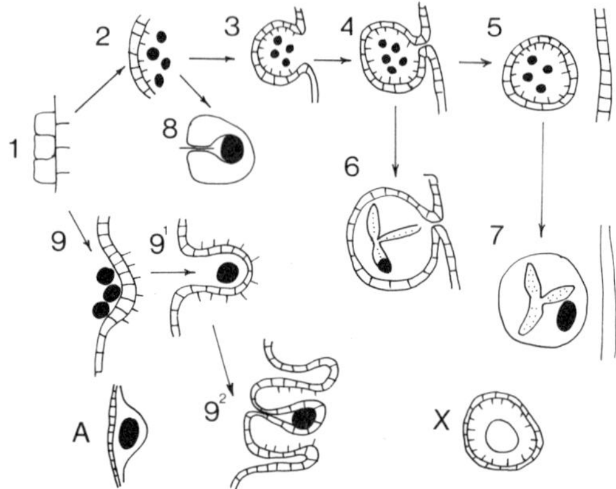

Figure 7 The evolution of the statocyst.

Mechanoreceptors collected into aggregations serve a number of purposes, but none is more significant than the statocyst in invertebrates. In this organ both gravity sense and acceleration sense are represented. Development seems to follow two distinct lines: the first where the statoliths (heavy particles that fall under the influence of gravity, and hence indicate its direction) are located outside the cells as sandgrains or calcium carbonate-secreted liths; the second incorporates the liths within the tissue of the animal.

(1) From a simple ciliated mechanosensory epithelium the first line leads to

(2) in which the epithelium becomes associated with weighted particles lying outside the body in a small cavity which becomes more pronounced

(3) as in annelids such as *Arenicola* and *Branchiomma* (Bullock and Horridge, 1965).

(4) The pinching off from the external surface is almost complete and little is left of a parent opening to the exterior, e.g. arthropod statocyst, and molluscs in which Kolliker's canal remains open.

(5) sees the complete enclosure of the organ and its removal from a surface site, e.g. most molluscs.

(6) is a special case of (4) in which a canal remains open but the sensory epithelium is no longer a complete lining to the lumen of the organ, but is restricted to patches along the three main axes of movement. The statolith may also be much reduced in size, and located in one position instead of being free falling, e.g. decapod crustaceans.

(7) The same kind of adaptation occurs in cephalopod molluscs in which the otolith is suspended on the macula (one sensory patch of epithelium) and the watery movements within the statocyst are monitored by three linear patches of sensory epithelium.

(8) is a peculiar arrangement found in urochordates (Dilly, 1962) where the weighted particle lies within a capsule, but is suspended from the end of a ciliary stalk. The weighted structure is thus still peripheral to the sense cell.

The second line is demonstrated by 9, 9^1 and 9^2; these are all special cases within medusae (Horridge, 1969). In these cases the statolith particles are located internally within the tissue of the animal, but become suspended on pendulous extensions that fall against an external sensory ciliated epithelium.

Two bizarre cases are shown in A and X. A is the situation in turbellarian helminthes (Ferrero, 1973) where the apparent statolith lies in a capsule attached to the brain, but has no sensory cells associated with it. Sensitivity seems to be a function of the adjacent nervous tissue in the brain. X is an enclosed capsule in which the statolith is a cell with a large vacuole containing a heavy density fluid rather than a calcareous structure (found in synaptid Holothuria, Laverack, unpublished).

influence of gravity. When orientation changes, the weighted particle falls and distorts some part of the sensory patch (Fig. 7; 9, 9^1 and 9^2) as in medusae (Horridge, 1969). Some specificity is conveyed by sequestering the apparatus in a capsule (ctenophore, Tamm, 1973; Chun, 1880); which may become totally isolated from the outside world (Fig. 7; 1, 2, 3, 4, 5, 6). Eventually the statolith becomes fixed in one place (e.g. on the macula in cephalopod molluscs, Budelmann, 1976; crab statocysts, Sandeman and Okajima, 1972) and is effective by shearing distortion of the underlying sensory cells. In this event movement, especially linear and angular acceleration, is monitored by fluid flows around the statocyst capsule particularly in the three prime axes of yaw, tilt and pitch. It is this aspect that is best developed in the most active animals, large crustaceans, cephalopods, fish, and other vertebrates.

Peculiarities of type also exist, e.g. helminths (Ferrero, 1973) and ascidian tadpoles (Dilly, 1962) but every generality has exceptions, and the biggest in this case is undoubtedly the insects. This group has no statocysts at all and gravity and acceleration must be detected in another fashion.

Implications and conclusion

The intention of this short review has been to attempt to show that the natural world is a continuum, and that the sensory adaptations of living organisms also form a continuum. The ability to respond to changing conditions is conferred by structure and by biochemical nature. For reasons of design, certain portions of the environment are discriminated and fall into certain distinct compartments (frequencies), but the animal population as a whole shows a very wide bandwidth and covers a considerable proportion of the known natural range. Man's inability to detect certain parameters except by instrumentation should not be allowed to distort the examination of sensory capacity in animals. On the other hand there is as yet little if any real evidence that some forms of radiation (X-rays, cosmic rays) are detected by animals, though man is instrumentally aware of such charged particles.

Future investigations for zoologists should be planned from an understanding of the lives of animals, from their natural history in fact since it is only understanding of the adaptations of the organism to the environment that will lead to sensible and meaningful investigations into the cues affecting the responses of the organism.

The recent work of zoologists and comparative physiologists has demonstrated that the sensory spectrum is as widespread and all-embracing as physicists' and chemists' view of the electromagnetic, mechanical and chemical spectrum of the environment; that we should not restrict our vision of the world to the blinkered attitude taken by our predecessors; and that the "if we cannot detect it then it isn't there" type of standpoint should be overthrown.

REFERENCES

Bardach, J. and Villars, T. (1974) "The chemical senses of fishes" in *Chemoreception by Marine Organisms* (eds. Grant, P., Mackie, A. M.) Academic Press, London and New York, 49–104.

Blakemore, R. (1975) Magnetotactic bacteria *Science*, **90**, 377–379.

Bonar, D. B. (1978) Ultrastructure of a cephalic sensory organ in larvae of the gastropod *Phestilla sibogae* (Aeolidacea, Nudibranchia) *Tissue & Cell*, **10**, 153–165.

Bone, Q. and Mackie, G. O. (1975) Skin impulses and locomotion in *Oikopleura* (Tunicata: Larvacea) *Biol. Bull.*, **149**, 267–286.

Bone, Q. and Pulsford, A. (1978) The arrangement of ciliated sensory cells in *Spadella* (Chaetognatha) *J. Mar. Biol.*, **58**, 565–570.

Bone, Q. and Ryan, K. P. (1979) The Langerhans receptor of *Oikopleura J. Mar. Biol. Ass. U.K.*, **59**, 69–76.

Bowmaker, J. K. (1980) Birds see ultraviolet light *Nature*, **284**, 306.

Budelmann, B-B. (1976) "Equilibrium receptor systems in molluscs" in *Structure and Function of Proprioceptors in the Invertebrates* (ed. Mill, P. J.) Chapman & Hall, London.

Bullock, T. H. and Diecke, F. P. J. (1956) Properties of an infra-red receptor *J. Physiol.*, **134**, 47–87.

Bullock, T. H. and Horridge, G. A. (1965) *Structure and Function in the Nervous Systems of Invertebrates* W. H. Freeman & Co., San Francisco and London.

Carter, G. S. (1926) On the nervous control of the velar cilia of the nudibranch veliger *J. exp. Biol.*, **4**, 1–26.

Case, J. (1964) Properties of the dactyl chemoreceptors of *Cancer antennarius* Stimpson and *C. productus* Randall *Biol. Bull.*, **127**, 428–446.

Case, J. and Gwilliam, G. F. (1963) Amino acid detection by marine invertebrates. Proc. XVI International Congress of Zoology, p. 47.

Chia, F-S. & Rice, M. E. (1978) *Settlement and metamorphosis of marine invertebrate larvae* Elsevier, New York and Oxford.

Chun, C. (1880) *Die Ctenophoren des Golfes von Neapel und der angrenzenden Meeres-Abschnitte* Engelmann, Leipzig.

Coggeshall, R. E. (1971) A possible sensory-motor neuron in *Aplysia californica Tissue & Cell*, **3**, 637–648.

Dilly, P. N. (1962) Studies on the receptors in the cerebral vesicle of the ascidian tadpole. 1. The otolith *Quart. J. micr. Sci.*, **103**. 393–398.

Ferrero, E. (1973) A fine structural analysis of the statocyst in turbellaria acoela *Zool. Scripta*, **2**, 5–16.

Flock, A. (1965) Transducing mechanisms in the lateral line canal organ receptors *Cold Spring Harbor Symp. Quant. Biology*, **30**, 133–151.

Gould, S. J. (1979) A natural precision designer *New Scientist*, **84**, 446–447.

Hansen, K. (1978) in *Insect Chemoreception in Taxis and Behaviour* (ed. Hazelbauer, G. L.) Chapman & Hall, London.

Hara, R. and Asai, H. (1980) Electrophysiological responses of *Didinium nasutum* to *Paramecium* capture and mechanical stimulation *Nature*, **283**, 869–870.

Hartline, H. K. and Ratliffe, F. (1958) Inhibitory interaction of receptor units in the eye of *Limulus J. Gen. Physiol.*, **41**, 1049–1066.

Home, E. M. (1972) Centrioles and associated structures in retinula cells of insect eyes *Tissue & Cell*, **4**, 227–234.

Horridge, G. A. (1966) Non-motile sensory cilia and neuromuscular junctions in a ctenophore independent effector organ *Proc. Roy. Soc. B*, **162**, 333–350.

Horridge, G. A. (1968) *Interneurones* W. H. Freeman & Co., London and San Francisco.

Horridge, G. A. (1969) Statocysts of medusae and evolution of stereocilia *Tissue & Cell*, **1**, 341–353.

Horridge, G. A. and Boulton, P. S. (1967) Prey detection by Chaetognatha via a vibration sense *Proc. Roy. Soc. B.*, **168**, 413–419.

Koshtoyants, K. S., Buznikov, G. A. and Manukhin, B. N. (1961) The possible role of 5-hydroxytryptamine in the motor activity of embryos of some marine gastropods *Comp. Biochem. Physiol.*, **3**, 20–26.

Laverack, M. S. (1963) Responses of cuticular sense organs of the lobster, *Homarus vulgaris* (Crustacea). III. Activity invoked in sense organs of the carapace *Comp. Biochem. Physiol.*, **10**, 261–272.

Laverack, M. S. (1964) The antennular sense organs of *Panulirus argus Comp. Biochem. Physiol.*, **13**, 301–321.

Mackie, G. O. and Bone, Q. (1976) Skin impulses and locomotion in ascidian tadpoles *J. Mar. Biol. Ass. U.K.*, **56**, 751–768.

Martin, A. R. and Wickelgren, W. O. (1971) Sensory cells in the spinal cord of the sea lamprey *J. Physiol.*, **212**, 65–83.

Matthews, G. and Wickelgren, W. O. (1978) Trigeminal sensory neurons of the sea lamprey *J. comp. Physiol.*, **123**, 329–334.

McFarlane, I. D. (1976) Two slow conduction systems co-ordinate shell-climbing behaviour in the sea anemone *Calliactis parasitica J. exp. Biol.*, **64**, 431–445.

Mellon, de F. (1963) Electrical responses from dually innervated tactile receptors on the thorax of the crayfish *J. exp. Biol.*, **40**, 137–148.

Messenger, J. (1977) Evidence that *Octopus* is colour blind *J. exp. Biol.*, **70**, 49–56.

Miller, R. L. (1978) Site-specific sperm agglutination and the timed release of a sperm chemo-attractant by the egg of the Leptomedusan *Orthopyxis caliculata J. exp. Zool.*, **205**, 385–392.

Necker, R. and Reiner, B. (1980) Temperature-sensitive mechanoreceptors, thermoreceptors and heat nociceptors in the feathered skin of pigeons *J. comp. Physiol.*, **135**, 201–207.

Nicholls, J. G. and Baylor, D. L. (1968) Specific modalities and receptive fields of sensory neurons in the C.N.S. of the leech *J. Neurophysiol.*, **31**, 740–756.

Piggott, S. M., Kerkut, G. A. and Walker, R. J. (1975) Structure-activity studies on glutamate receptor sites of three identifiable neurones in the sub-oesophageal ganglia of *Helix aspersa Comp. Biochem. Physiol.*, **51C**, 91–100.

Prosser, C. L. (1934) Action potentials in the nervous system of the crayfish. II. Responses to illumination of the eye and caudal ganglion *J. cell. comp. Physiol.*, **4**, 363–377.

Qutob, Z. (1962) The swimbladder of fishes as a pressure receptor *Acta Neerl. Zool.*, **15**, 1–67.

Roberts, A. (1975) "Some aspects of the development of membrane excitability, nervous system and behaviour in embryos" in *Simple Nervous Systems* (eds. Usherwood, P. N. R., Newth, D. R.) Edward Arnold, London.

Roeder, K. D. (1975) Neural factors and evitability in insect behaviour *J. exp. Zool.*, **194**, 75–88.

Sandeman, D. C. and Okajima, A. (1972) Statocyst-induced eye movements in the crab *Scylla serrata*. 1. The sensory input from the statocysts *J. exp. Biol.*, **57**, 187–204.

Schmidt, R. F. (1978) in *Fundamentals of Sensory Physiology* (ed. Schmidt, R. F.) Springer Verlag, New York, Berlin.

Shelton, R. G. J. and Mackie, A. M. (1971) Studies on the chemical preferences of the shore crab, *Carcinus maenas J. exp. mar. Biol. Ecol.*, **7**, 41–49.

Shepheard, P. (1974) Chemoreception in the antennule of the lobster, *Homarus americanus Mar. Behav. Physiol.*, **2**, 261–273.

Springer, M. S., Goy, M. F. and Adler, J. (1979) Protein methylation in behavioural control mechanisms and in signal transduction *Nature*, **280**, 279–284.

Strathmann, R. R., Jahn, T. L. and Fonseca, J. R. C. (1972) Suspension feeding by marine invertebrate larvae: clearance of particles by ciliated bands of a rotifer, pluteus, and trochophore *Biol. Bull.*, **142**, 505–519.

Tamm, S. L. (1973) and personal communication. Mechanisms of ciliary co-ordination in ctenophores *J. exp. Biol.*, **59**, 231–245.

Thorpe, J. P., Shelton, G. A. B. and Laverack, M. S. (1975) Electrophysiology and co-ordinated behavioural responses in the colonial Bryozoan, *Membranipora membranacea J. exp. Biol.*, **62**, 389–404.

Thurm, U. (1968) Steps in the transducer process of mechanoreceptors *Symp. Zoo. Soc. London*, **23**, 199–214.

Tucker, J. B. (1968) Fine structure and function of the cytopharyngeal basket in the ciliate *Nassula J. Cell Science*, **3**, 493–514.

Tyler, S. (1979) Distinctive features of cilia in metazoans and their significance for systematics *Tissue & Cell*, **11**, 385–400.

Usherwood, P. N. R. (1971) Evidence for release of glutamate from arthropod nerve endings *Proc. Int. Union Physiol. Sci.*, **8**, 251–252.

Walcott, C. L. and Green, R. P. (1974) Orientation of homing pigeons altered by a change in the direction of an applied magnetic field *Science*, **184**, 180–182.

Wales, W., Clarac, F. and Laverack, M. S. (1971) Stress detection at the autotomy plane in the decapod Crustacea *Z. vergl. Physiol.*, **73**, 357–382.

Warner, A. (1975) "Pathways for ionic current flow in the early nervous system" in *Simple Nervous Systems* (eds. Usherwood, P. N. R., Newth, D. R.) Edward Arnold, London.

White, D. C. S. (1974) *Biological Physics* Chapman & Hall, London.

Whitear, M. (1971) Cell specialization and sensory function in fish epidermis *J. Zool. Lond.*, **163**, 237–264.

Wollacott, R. M. and Zimmer, R. L. (1978) "Metamorphosis of cellularioid bryozoans" in *Settlement and Metamorphosis of Marine Invertebrates* (eds. Chia, F-S., Rice, M. E.) Elsevier, New York and Oxford.

CHAPTER THREE

OPTICAL MECHANISMS IN THE HIGHER CRUSTACEA WITH A COMMENT ON THEIR EVOLUTIONARY ORIGINS

M. F. LAND

Introduction

Until about 20 years ago the standard textbook account of image formation in the malacostracan crustaceans was that provided by Exner's famous monograph of 1891 (see Waterman, 1961). Exner had proposed that arthropod eyes fall into two basic categories: apposition eyes in which each ommatidium has its own private optical system, and superposition eyes in which a large number of optical elements contribute to the image on a single rhabdom. The former mechanism is characteristic of diurnal eyes, and has an F-number that is typically around 2; the latter is found in nocturnal animals and gives a much brighter, though usually less well resolved image (F-number between 0.5 and 1) (Kirschfeld, 1974).

Exner showed that in superposition eyes the amount of ray bending that was required of the optical structures could not be accounted for by simple spherical refraction at the corneal surface, and he found it necessary to postulate a new kind of optical device—a lens cylinder—in which refraction occurs not at the outer and inner surfaces as in a conventional lens, but continuously along the length of the structure. This is achieved because the device has an inhomogeneous refractive index, high along the axis but decreasing roughly parabolically towards the walls of the cylinder. That this is the mechanism of refraction in superposition eyes of nocturnal insects is now universally accepted (Kunze, 1979). In the last few years such devices have actually been manufactured commercially (Iga and Yamamoto, 1977; see Land, 1980*a*).

In the Crustacea, Exner's lens-cylinder proposal began to run into difficulties in the early 1960's. Kuiper (1962) had found that the optical elements in crayfish eyes (which by other criteria ought to be of the superposition type) were of low refractive index, and, worse, homogeneous. These observations were confirmed by other workers, and led to a general disenchantment with both of Exner's important ideas: lens cylinders and the superposition mechanism itself (reviewed by Horridge, 1975). However, by the early 1970's interference microscope studies in particular had shown the essential accuracy of these two principles, at least in the case of nocturnal insects (Seitz, 1969; Horridge, Giddings and Stange, 1972; Hausen, 1973). What was still required was an explanation of Kuiper's result for the crayfish. How could superposition optics be a possibility without lens cylinders to bend the light? The answer was provided in 1975 by Vogt, working on the crayfish, and independently confirmed by myself (Land, 1976) for the eyes of a deep-sea shrimp. Vogt's postulate was beautifully simple: light paths that are almost identical to those produced by lens cylinders result when light is reflected from the surface of a plane mirror. The structures that make up the optical array in crayfish (and, it turns out, in all other long-bodied decapods) are not refracting elements at all, but square-sided plugs of jelly whose sides reflect light either because they have a multilayer mirror coating, or by total internal reflection as in a 90° prism (Vogt, 1975, 1977, 1980; Land, 1976, 1978, 1979*a*, 1980*a*).

The solution of this problem raised others. How common is this mechanism? Does it apply throughout the Decapoda? Throughout the Eucarida? Throughout the Malacostraca? Are there crustaceans that use the lens-cylinder mechanism instead? Has the mirror mechanism evolved once or many times? Does eye structure have anything useful to tell us about the evolution of the higher crustaceans that we did not know before? The results of studies on some of these questions are set out in outline in later sections of this paper, and they contain a number of surprises that suggest that the present classificatory system for the Malacostraca is not a very good one (and that it was better before 1880!). First, however, the optical structure of crustacean eyes is briefly reviewed.

A review of optical mechanisms

Three main types of optical system have been identified in the higher crustaceans, and with minor variations these seem to be the only three. These are (i) apposition eyes based on low refractive index lens cylinders (brachyuran crabs, all decapod larvae, some amphipods and stomatopods); (ii) superposition eyes with high refractive index crystalline cones (mysids and euphausiids); and (iii) superposition eyes with radially arranged mirror boxes (adult macruran or long-bodied decapods only). These types and some of their optical components are illustrated in Fig. 1. There is only one published review (Kunze, 1979) that deals with all three mechanisms, but not specifically with the versions of them found in

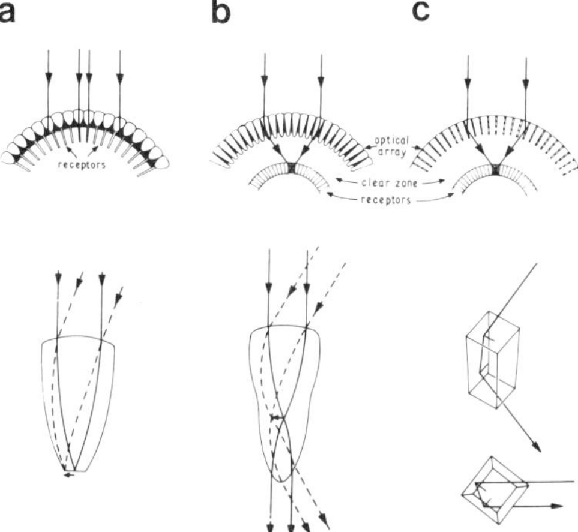

Figure 1 Three optical mechanisms in Crustacea. Upper row shows the overall layout and lower row details of the ray paths in individual optical elements.
(a) Apposition eye. Each rhabdom (typically 7–9 fused rhabdomeres) receives the image focused by a single refracting element. These are usually Exner lens cylinders (*below*) in which an image is formed by continuous internal refraction at the proximal tip of the crystalline cone.
(b) Refracting superposition eye. Light from a large region of the eye surface is focused onto a single rhabdom. The refracting devices are double length lens cylinders (*below*) that function as unity magnification inverting telescopes.
(c) Reflecting superposition eye. As (b) except that the optical elements are square-sided plugs of jelly with reflecting surfaces. The light paths for rays reflected from a single surface (*above*) are the same as in the refracting superposition eye. Oblique rays (*below*) are reflected from two surfaces, and if these are at right angles they behave as a single mirror perpendicular to the incident ray, just as in the case of single reflection.

crustaceans. Waterman (1961) gives a clear statement of the state of knowledge at that time, but there have been several important additions since then. In this section I will therefore try to outline the optics of the three types of eye, and indicate how each can be recognized by simple observations. A summary account is given in Land (1980*a*).

Apposition eyes (Fig. 1a) The most important optical feature of apposition eyes is that each receptor cluster contributing to a rhabdom has its own private optical system, the combination of lens system and receptors forming an ommatidium. In each ommatidium the lens, or equivalent structure, produces a small inverted image at the distal tip of the rhabdom, and the rhabdom itself receives a small portion of this image corresponding to a narrow angle (typically between 1 and 10 degrees) in outside space. The rhabdoms in adjacent ommatidia image adjacent solid angles with only a small amount of overlap.

In most diurnal insects the image-forming system is the cornea: a curved air-tissue interface which, like the human cornea, bends light by ordinary spherical refraction. In aquatic crustaceans a curved cornea is not a usable system because it has media with the same refractive index (effectively water; $n = 1.33$) on both sides, and so cannot refract light. Exner (1891) proposed an alternative that he called a lens cylinder. This is a structure between the cornea and the rhabdom that bends light rays continuously within it, not just at the interfaces. This is achieved by the structure having an inhomogeneous refractive index: high along the axis but falling in a roughly parabolic manner towards the surface of the cylinder. Exner demonstrated that this was undoubtedly the way images were formed in the eye of the xiphosuran *Limulus*, and this has been confirmed in detail recently (Land, 1979*b*). The optical properties of such structures were fully explored by Fletcher, Murphy and Young (1954). There is no direct proof that apposition eyes in the higher Crustacea work in this way, but by exclusion they must do (the problem is a technical one, the tissues involved are much softer than the *Limulus* cornea, and no-one has yet succeeded in measuring the refractive index profile). Intracellular recordings from crab receptors, however, show narrow fields of view, which means that there is an image at each rhabdom tip, and in the absence of an optically effective cornea that image can only be produced by lens-cylinder optics.

There are two main features that distinguish this type of eye from the others. First, the lens cylinders, which usually have the form of tapered cones, are contiguous with the rhabdoms, or very nearly so. That is, there is no "clear zone" of transparent homogeneous tissue separating the optical elements from the receptors (this is required in superposition eyes for the focusing of rays). Secondly, in fresh eyes there is nearly always a visible "pseudopupil", a small dark spot that appears to move around the eye as the observer views the eye from different directions (Figs. 4 and 5). The pseudopupil simply indicates the location of those ommatidia that share a common line of sight with the observer: the ommatidia that are looking in your direction must be absorbing light from you, and so must appear dark. Superposition eyes, whose effective pupils may be up to half the eye surface, do not show this phenomenon (a thorough discussion of the pseudopupil is given by Stavenga, 1979). In addition these eyes always have hexagonally faceted surfaces; this distinguishes them from reflecting superposition eyes (iii) but not refracting superposition types (ii).

Refracting superposition eyes (Fig. 1b) Superposition eyes of both types differ from apposition eyes in that each rhabdom receives light that entered the eye through a large number of facets, rather than just one. The individual contributions from each optical element are superimposed at the level of the retina, forming a single erect image. It was again Exner (1891) who showed how this was done. If one examines the paths of rays through the various lenses in Fig. 1b it becomes clear that each redirects light in such a way that the emergent beam lies on the same side of the lens axis as the entering beam, and that the angles the entering and emergent beam make with the lens axis are approximately the same (see Fig. 2c). It helps to think of the lenses as behaving rather like mirrors, since a mirror redirects light in just the manner described. A simple lens does not have these properties: the emergent beam focused by a single lens lies on the opposite side of the lens axis, for example. Ray paths like those in Fig. 1b could be produced if each optical element behaved as a two-lens telescope with unity magnification (an inverter) but, as Exner pointed out, the refractive indices of the actual lenses are too low for this mechanism to be the correct one (see Horridge, 1975). Instead he proposed that, as in *Limulus*, the optical elements (or crystalline cones) are lens cylinder devices, but instead of having a single focus at the proximal tip they have a focus somewhere near their centre. They are thus double-length lens cylinders, and just as a single-length lens cylinder behaves as a single lens, so these behave as two-lens devices; as unity magnification inverting telescopes in fact. Exner's work was mainly concerned with firefly eyes, and the correctness of his ideas has since been verified for fireflies by Seitz (1969). Chun (1896) believed the crystalline cones of euphausiids also behaved as Exner lens cylinders, and this has recently been confirmed (Land, Burton and Meyer-Rochow, 1979; Land and Burton, 1979).

The characteristic features of this kind of eye are, firstly, a peripherally arranged array of hard, highly refractile crystalline cones, which always have a bullet-shaped appearance (Fig. 2b). Secondly, there is a clear zone, free of optical obstructions, across which focusing takes place; and thirdly, the continuous retina of rhabdoms is situated well inside the eye, with a radius of curvature about half that of the eye itself. In some of the double-eyed euphausiids there are interesting departures from this geometry (Land, Burton and Meyer-Rochow, 1979) but they are still refracting superposition eyes. The crystalline cones are circular in cross section, and this is reflected in the hexagonal geometry of the corneal facet array.

Reflecting superposition eyes (Fig. 1c) The first correct description of the principle of image-formation in this kind of eye is very recent (Vogt, 1975); Exner believed these eyes employed the lens-cylinder mechanism outlined above, and in this he was mistaken. As pointed out in the last section, lens-cylinders behave rather like mirrors in the way they redirect light. The only important difference is that in reflecting superposition eyes the optical elements really are mirrors. The mirrors are the walls of flat-sided truncated pyramids with square cross sections that form an array just beneath the cornea. One of these mirror "boxes" was figured with exemplary accuracy by Grenacher (1879) in his description of the eye of *Palaemon*, but it was a century before the significance of his drawing became apparent (Land 1979*a*). If one considers only a two-dimensional cross-section of an eye of this kind (Fig. 1c) the principle of operation is obvious: light bouncing off each of the short radial mirrors is brought to a common focus at a point halfway out from the centre of the eye, and this is where the rhabdom layer is located. In three dimensions, however, the situation is a little more complicated, since most rays encounter the mirror plugs obliquely, and are reflected from two faces of each plug rather than one. This problem resolves itself rather neatly. Since the walls of the mirror-plugs are at right-angles to each other they behave as corner reflectors, and corner reflectors have the property (shown in Fig. 1c) that whatever the angle of incidence, the reflected ray always lies in a plane parallel to the incident ray. This means that a corner *behaves* as though it is a plane mirror that is always at right angles to the plane of the incident ray, and this in turn means that the simplified two-dimensional diagram in Fig. 1c is also valid for oblique rays that are reflected twice (Vogt, 1977, 1980; Land, 1979*a*).

The corners in corner reflectors must be at 90° for this to work. A 120° corner (which one would find in a hexagonally packed array) does not reflect like a single mirror. *This is why the eyes of all animals that use the reflecting superposition mechanism have square facets*, and this is the single most important diagnostic feature of these eyes (Fig. 4). The mirror boxes are unlike refracting crystalline cones not only in having a square cross-section, but also in being soft and not very refractile ($n \sim 1.41$ as opposed to a central n of about 1.52 in euphausiid cones). In some eyes the plugs are actually lined with multilayer mirrors (*Astacus*: Vogt, 1977, 1980), but in others (*Palaemonetes*) the mirror is simply the flat interface between the plug and surrounding tissue, and total internal reflection occurs, as between glass and air in a prism. In most other respects these eyes are similar to refracting superposition eyes; they have a clear zone, and a deep-lying retina.

The foregoing description applies strictly only to dark-adapted eyes. In the light many species show complicated pigment movements (reviewed by Kleinholz, 1961) which effectively convert the eyes into the apposition type, the mirror system becoming ineffective. In this state the eyes can show a pseudopupil and other characteristics of apposition eyes (Fig. 4a). The only reliable indicator of the reflecting mechanism is then the square corneal geometry, although the eye will certainly lose the pseudopupil in the dark, and probably also develop a large patch of glow, or eye-shine (Fig. 4b). This phenomenon, which is again diagnostic of superposition eyes of both types, is due to reflection from a tapetal layer behind the retina, and it is in principle exactly the same as the reflection from a cat's eye (see Stavenga, 1979; Kunze, 1979). It is unfortunately not an infallible criterion. Most mysids and macruran decapods have a reflecting tapetum, but the euphausiids do not.

A final but important point concerns the light-gathering power of the three different types of eye and the relation of this to habitat. The superposition eyes (ii) and (iii) give a much brighter image than the apposition type (i) and this, coupled with their larger receptors, means that under the same external lighting conditions the superposition eyes will provide a much higher photon capture rate per receptor. In insects, Kirschfeld (1974) has estimated that there is a 1000-fold difference in photon capture rate between a moth eye (superposition) and a bee eye (apposition). A similar figure would be expected in crustaceans as well, for the same reasons (Land, Burton and Meyer-Rochow, 1979). Superposition optics of both types are thus an adaptation to dim light conditions, which in Crustacea will usually mean the exploitation of deeper water habitats.

Distribution of optical types

Adult animals

Using the criteria set out in the preceding section, a survey of both the literature on the subject and of living and preserved material leads to a classification of eye types in higher Crustacea as set out in Table 1. The most important points are:

(a) The only two groups that definitely possess refracting superposition eyes (type ii) are the mysids and the euphausiids. This was already apparent from the anatomical studies of Grenacher (1879) and Chun (1896), and recent studies have confirmed the presence of a clear zone and highly refractile crystalline cones (Land, Burton and Meyer-Rochow, 1979). Kampa (1965) believed that there were light guides crossing the

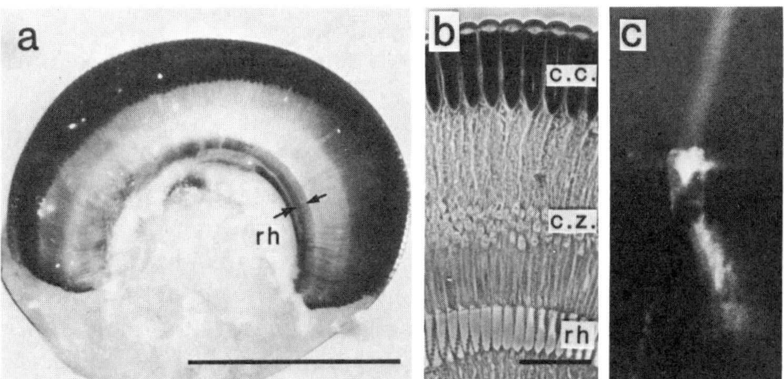

Figure 2 Eye of an adult euphausiid (*Meganyctiphanes norvegica*).
(a) Hemisection of whole eye. *rh* is the rhabdom layer situated around a sphere with half the radius of curvature of the whole eye. Note the geometrical identity to Fig. 1(b). Scale bar 1 mm.
(b) 1 μm section (phase contrast) showing crystalline cones (*c.c.*), clear zone (*c.z.*) containing receptor cell bodies, and the rhabdom layer (*rh*). Scale bar 100 μm.
(c) Ray path, made visible with fluorescein, through one or two crystalline cones. Light is refracted as in the lower part of Fig. 1(b). (From Land, Burton and Meyer-Rochow, 1979.)

Table 1 Eye structures and eye types in the higher Malacostraca

Taxonomic group[1] *Superorder* *Order* *Section* *Superfamily*	Facet geometry				
	Hexagonal	Square	Clear zone	Adult eye	Larval eye
Peracarida					
Isopoda	Yes	No	No	Apposition	—
Amphipoda	Yes	No	No[2]	Apposition	—
Mysidacea	Yes	No	Yes	Refracting superposition	
Eucarida					
Euphausiacea	Yes	No	Yes	Refracting superposition	Refracting superposition
Decapoda					
Penaeidea	No	Yes[3]	Yes	Reflecting superposition	Apposition
Caridea	No	Yes[3]	Yes	Reflecting superposition	Apposition
Stenopodidea	No	Yes[3]	Yes	Reflecting superposition	Apposition
Macrura	No	Yes[3]	Yes	Reflecting superposition	Apposition
Anomura					
Galatheidea	No	Yes[3]	Yes	Reflecting superposition	Apposition
Paguridea	Yes	No	No	Apposition	Apposition
Brachyura	Yes	No	No	Apposition	Apposition

Notes:

(1) Based on the classification used by Waterman and Chace (1961). No reliable information is available for the Peracaridan orders Thermosbaenacea, Spelaeogriphacea, Cumacea or Tanaidacea, which are omitted as are the presumably less related superorders Syncarida and Hoplocarida.

(2) There are apparent clear zones crossed by light-guides in some hyperiid amphipods (see text).

(3) Larvae all have hexagonal facets and no clear zone.

clear zone in euphausiids (which would have meant that these could have functioned as apposition eyes) but electron microscopy has shown that no such structures are present (Meyer-Rochow and Walsh, 1978), and it has also been established that the crystalline cones bend light in the correct way for superposition image production (Land, Burton and Meyer-Rochow, 1979, and Fig. 2c) and also that the cones have the appropriate refractive index gradient (Land and Burton, 1979). Mysid eyes have an almost identical structure to those of euphausiids, and although they have yet to be studied with the same degree of thoroughness, it seems inconceivable that their optical system is different in any important way.

(b) Reflecting superposition eyes (type iii) are found throughout the long-bodied decapods (the sections Penaeidea, Caridea, Stenopodidea and Macrura in the classification of Waterman and Chace, 1961). The

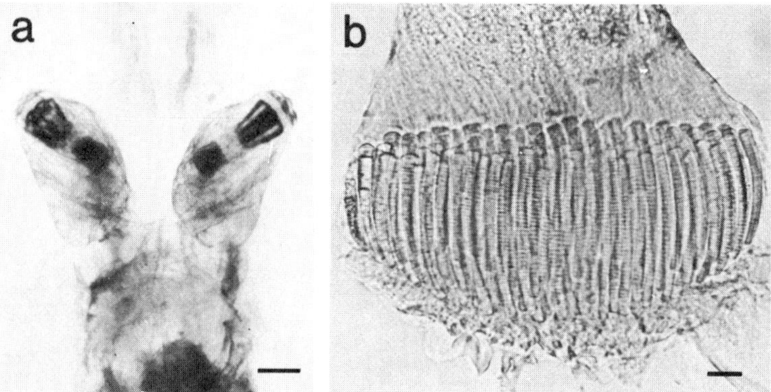

Figure 3 Eyes of furcilia larva of a euphausiid (*Thysanopoda tricuspidata*).
(a) Whole eyes showing cornea, crystalline cones, narrow clear zone and retina. Scale bar 100 μm.
(b) Detail of the retina. There are about 90 rhabdoms (compared with 7 crystalline cones) arranged in 3–4 rows. Scale bar 10 μm. See also Fig. 7.

only known exceptions to this rule are larval forms (see below) and a few benthic shrimps in which the optical structure of the eye appears to have been lost altogether. The other group of decapods with square-faceted eyes are the galatheids (squat lobsters) which are usually classified along with the pagurids (hermit-crabs) in the Anomura, a kind of dumping ground for unclassifiable decapods. In eye structure the galatheids resemble the macrurans (crayfish and lobsters) and not the crabs. This, however, is not true of the hermit crabs. They have hexagonally faceted apposition-type eyes like those of the true crabs (Brachyura).

(c) In many of the eyes with reflecting superposition optics there exist light adaptation mechanisms that can effectively convert them from the superposition to the apposition type between night and day. An example of this, in the shrimp *Palaemonetes varians*, is shown in Fig. 4. Black pigment moves out from beneath the receptors to fill the clear zone during the day; this zone is then traversed only by a series of narrow transparent tubes that join the mirror boxes to the rhabdoms, so that in the light-adapted condition each receptor is looking out through only one optical element. There are many variations on this theme (see Kleinholz, 1961) but their effects are the same. The light-adapted eye then exhibits a distinct black pseudopupil (Fig. 4a) as opposed to the large patch of eyeshine visible when the animal has been kept in the dark. The important point is that these are *basically* superposition eyes, because they have a superposition mechanism available to them. Ordinary apposition eyes (as in crabs) have neither the appropriate optics for the formation of superposition images nor a clear zone across which rays can be focused. In other words, whilst it is easy to convert a superposition eye into an

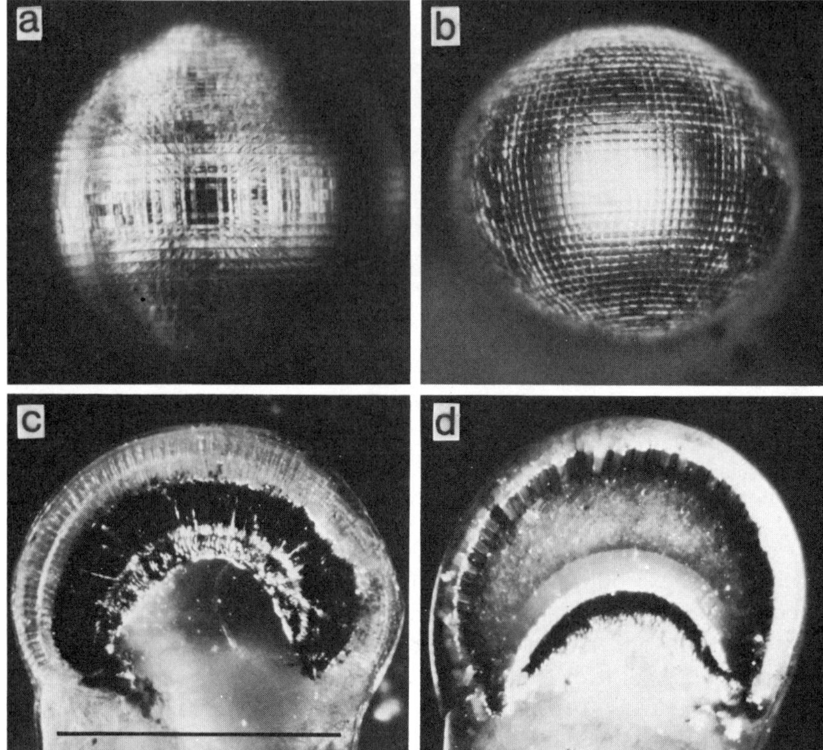

Figure 4 Appearance of the eyes of the decapod shrimp *Palaemonetes varians*.
(a) Light-adapted, showing pseudopupil.
(b) Dark-adapted showing patch of eye-shine corresponding to the superposition pupil. Note square geometry of the facet array (*cf.* Fig. 1(c)) and the tracery of reflecting pigment. Most reflection in this eye occurs by total internal reflection.
(c), (d) Hemisections corresponding to (a) and (b). In the light adapted state the "clear zone" is filled with black pigment, most of which resides beneath the basement membrane in the dark. The dark-adapted eye (d) has a transparent clear zone with receptor cell bodies; beneath this is the rhabdom layer backed by a white tapetum which is responsible for the eye-shine in (b). In (a) and (c) the eye behaves optically as an apposition eye (Fig. 1(a)). Scale bar on (c) is 1 mm and applies to all four figs.

apposition eye by rearrangement of pigment it is impossible to do the reverse.

(d) Apposition eyes appear to be the rule in all malacostracan groups other than those already mentioned. I know of no evidence for superposition image formation in the isopods, amphipods, stomatopods or the brachyuran decapods. In all these groups the optical elements lack the distinctive bullet-like appearance of the crystalline cones of euphausiids and mysids, there is no clear zone, and the ommatidia are always hexagonally packed. In some of the hyperiid amphipods that live in the deep ocean there may be a large transparent space between the eye surface and the retina which resembles a clear zone. The classic example of this is *Phronima* where there is a full 5 mm gap between the cones of the eye and the retina (Exner, 1891; Ball, 1977). This space, however, really *is* crossed by thick (10 μm) light guides continuous with the cones at one end and the rhabdoms at the other. There is an impressive black pseudopupil in the living animal (Land, 1980*b*), confirming that these are apposition eyes, and suggesting that the reason for the clear space is not optical, but perhaps concerned with camouflage in that it keeps the head relatively clear of dark pigment which would otherwise make the animal visible against the sea surface. The crystalline cone–light guide structures in the hyperiids appear simply to be rather elongated versions of the more typical cones of, say, the brachyuran crabs. Indeed, *Phronima* itself has a second pair of eyes in which the light guides are absent.

Larval animals

To establish possible phylogenetic relationships it is of great value to know whether there are similarities and differences between organs not only in the adults, but also in the larval stages. Larval euphausiid and larval decapod eyes only are briefly dealt with here.

The eye of a first instar larva of the decapod shrimp *Palaemon serratus* is shown in Fig. 5, and its appearance came as a real surprise to the author. The adult has an eye like that shown in Fig. 4, but the larval eye has hexagonal facets, a pseudopupil occupying about three facets, and a

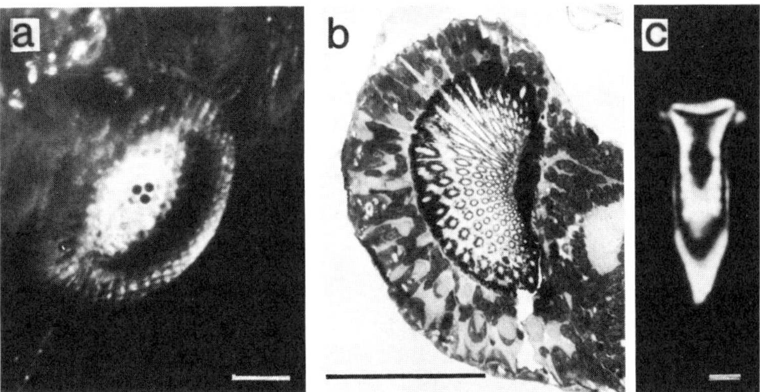

Figure 5 1st instar larval eye of *Palaemon serratus*.
(a) Gross appearance showing pseudopupil and hexagonal geometry. Scale bar 100 μm.
(b) 1 μm section showing outer rind of crystalline cones and cell bodies, pigment zone penetrated by small apertures (top left) and rhabdoms within. Scale bar 100 μm.
(c) Single crystalline cone (interference microscopy). The refractive index is about 1.43. Scale bar 10μm.

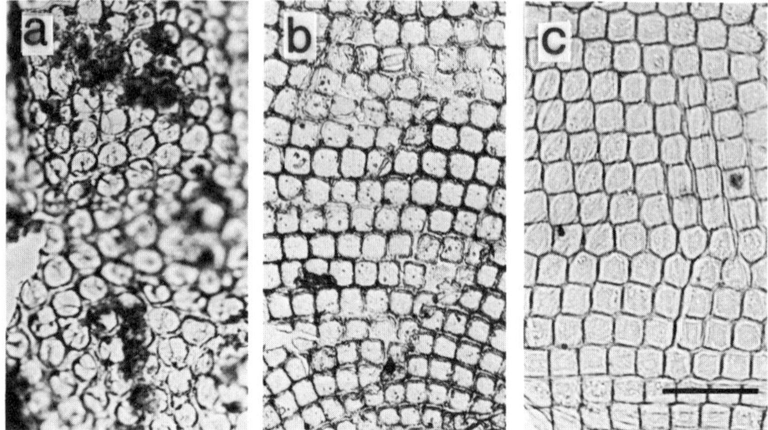

Figure 6 Cornea preparations of larvae of *Palaemonetes varians* at stages 11, 13 and 15 approximately, showing the progressive "squaring off" of the individual elements, and the array as a whole. Scale bar on (c) 100 μm.

general eye structure not unlike that of the light-adapted adult. This appearance is typical of the larval eyes of all the decapod larvae and stomatopod larvae so far seen.

As the shrimp develops, the optical facets gradually square off (Fig. 6). This does not occur at metamorphosis (moult 5) when the locomotor pattern of the animal changes, but rather late in development, between stages 11 and 15 when the animal has reached perhaps $\frac{2}{3}$ of its final size. Presumably by this stage the eye has begun to function (at least at night) as a reflecting superposition eye. Amongst the long-bodied decapods, then, there is a change during development from an apposition larval eye to a reflecting superposition adult eye, and it is a sound speculation that this change is functionally related to the fact that the larval forms all live near the surface in high light conditions, but that the adults in general live at deeper, dimmer levels in the water (Fincham, 1980).

Equally interesting is that larvae of crabs have eyes that are very similar to those of the shrimps, but that during development these do not undergo the "squaring-off" that one sees in shrimps. The eye of an adult crab is simply an enlarged, strengthened and somewhat more pigmented version of the larval eye, but retains the same basic design. Again this makes good ecological sense, since most crabs are semi-terrestrial as adults and would not need the extra light-gathering capacity of a superposition type of eye.

Larval euphausiids are completely different. Fig. 3 shows the eyes of the furcilia larva of *Thysanopoda tricuspidata*, a species in which the adult has a typical spherical refracting superposition eye. (The furcilia is not the first larval stage, but it is the earliest stage in which the eyes are clearly

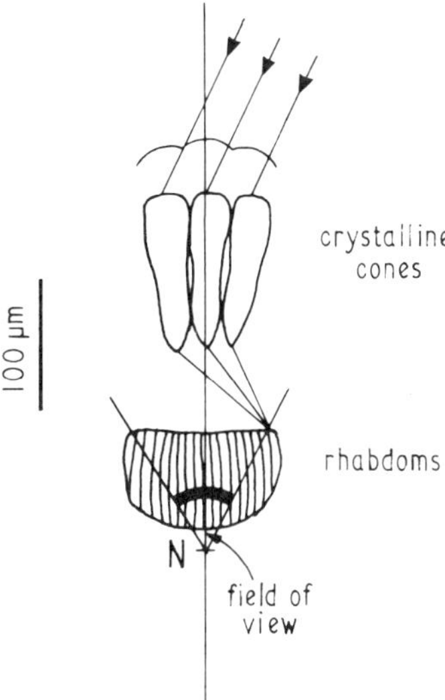

Figure 7 Optics of the furcilia eye of a euphausiid like that shown in Fig. 3. If the crystalline cones behave as in the adults (Fig. 2(c)) a superposition image will be formed on the distal tips of the receptors. *N* is the nodal point of the eye, which is the point of coincidence of the axes of the 7 cones. The field of view in the vertical plane is about 60°, but only about 20° horizontally. Individual receptors subtend about 4°.

functional and not hidden by the carapace). The eyes consist of 7 crystalline cones which look exactly like those of the adult. There is a relatively narrow clear zone (about 60 μm thick) and beneath that a retina containing about 90 rhabdoms. The mismatch between cone and rhabdom numbers immediately indicates that this is not an apposition eye, and if one draws optical ray paths through the crystalline cones, assuming that their optical properties are the same as those of the adult eye (Fig. 2c), it becomes clear that the larval eye will perform as a perfectly good image-forming superposition eye (Fig. 7).

Perhaps the strangest aspect of eye development in *T. tricuspidata* is the development of the larval eye in later stages. A new patch of eye develops just anterior to the furcilia eye, and grows steadily backwards, touching and finally surrounding the original 7 facets. This new eye becomes the adult eye, and at a relatively late adolescent stage the original 7 cones are actually ejected from it, leaving an easily visible hole in the mosaic, which is subsequently filled in with new cones. Thus, in this species of euphausiid at least, the larval eye is of the refracting superposition type, and so is the adult eye, but the latter replaces the former rather than being a modification of it as in the decapods. It is clear from these results therefore, that there is no point of contact between the design of eyes in the euphausiids and the decapods at any period of their respective ontogenies.

Evolutionary and taxonomic conclusions

Eyes as conservative characters

The best argument for believing that eye structure is at least as good an indicator of evolutionary origins as any other is that once an eye design that works well has evolved it is most unlikely that it will be abandoned for something different but equally complex that does essentially the same job. This argument would seem to apply particularly cogently to animals possessing reflecting and refracting superposition eyes (the long-bodied decapods and the euphausiids), since the mirror-lined box and lens cylinder mechanisms of achieving an image are both sophisticated and unusual, as well as being approximately similar in the quality and brightness of the images they produce. Not only is it hard to imagine how one might evolve into the other—without there being some near-blind intermediate—but there would be nothing to be gained either. This *a priori* argument seems to be strong enough to support the belief that the euphausiids and the decapods should not belong to the same superorder.

There is some direct evidence for the conservative nature of eye design from the consistency of eye type within each group. Thus *all* the euphausiids have refracting superposition eyes (as larvae and adults) and *all* the long-bodied decapods have reflecting superposition eyes as adults. There are no known exceptions (other than benthic or fossorial forms with clear evidence of degeneration) which might cause one to doubt whether eye design is a useful taxonomic criterion. This kind of evidence strengthens the belief that the long-bodied decapods (including the galatheids) represent a homogeneous group, a view that is not widely held by contemporary taxonomists.

Because superposition image formation is a relative rarity in the animal kingdom (it probably evolved several times in insects but only twice in Crustacea) one might reasonably argue that it is "difficult" to evolve. The same is not true for apposition image formation which is the standard mechanism throughout the insects and Crustacea and also occurs in the molluscs (*Arca*), annelids (*Branchiomma*), the myriapods and in the xiphosuran *Limulus*. In its most basic form, an apposition eye requires no special optics, just a series of receptors each at the bottom of a pigmented hole (see Milne and Milne, 1959; Land, 1980*b*). This distinction is of some value when deciding whether, on the basis of eye structure, two groups of animals are closely related, and taking into account the probability of convergent evolution. Thus it is more likely to be true that the mysids and euphausiids are related because both have refracting superposition eyes, than it is that the brachyuran crabs are closely related to either the amphipods or the stomatopods, just because they all have apposition eyes. The optical intricacy of superposition eyes, as well as their apparent rarity, argues for them as conservative characters, and by the same token it argues against using the same reasoning for apposition eyes.

A study of larval forms adds a little to these generalizations. The larvae of all decapods have similar eyes, which is comforting, but since these are of a rather basic apposition type it is not by itself a strong argument for grouping them together. The fact that larval euphausiids have refracting superposition eyes is, however, another strong argument for separating that group from the decapods. It is a pity that the mysids lack clear larval stages (they are born as miniature adults) and so there is only the structure of the adult eye to link them with the euphausiids.

A taxonomy based on eye design

On the basis of the evidence in this paper and on the arguments in the last section, and ignoring for the moment all other considerations, I propose the following statements as the three taxonomic conclusions one can draw from eye design that stand the greatest chance of being correct.*

(i) The Euphausiacea are only very distantly related to the Decapoda, because at no stage in their life cycle do they have an eye which is at all similar to either of the two decapod types. The super-order Eucarida (Calman, 1904) which currently contains both orders, is probably a false grouping.

(ii) The long-bodied decapods, including the anomuran galatheids, are derived from a common stock. This stock, early in its evolution, evolved a type of eye which is unique in the animal kingdom (there is a slight possibility that the reflecting superposition principle may also have evolved in some mayflies, see Horridge and McLean, 1978). The eyes of decapods probably arose by an elaboration of an ancestral apposition eye that resembled that of the present larvae. The short-bodied decapods (crabs and hermit crabs) either never made this transformation, or lost it through neoteny. These arguments imply that the Decapoda should be divided into two groups only, corresponding roughly to the Macrura and Brachyura division before the revision of the order by Boas (1880). The Anomura can possibly be abolished since eye structure splits the group down the middle. The current division of the decapods into Natantia and Reptantia (Borradaile, 1907), and the more recent Dendrobranchiata/Pleocyemata division based on gill structure proposed by Burkenroad (1963) and adopted by Glaessner (1969) find no support from considerations of eye design.

(iii) The Euphausiacea and Mysidacea should be grouped together because both have refracting superposition eyes, and are the only malacostracan groups that do. This, again, was the way they were

* Similar conclusions were reached by Fincham (1980) in an independent study.

Table 2 Comparison of eye types with different taxonomic schemes

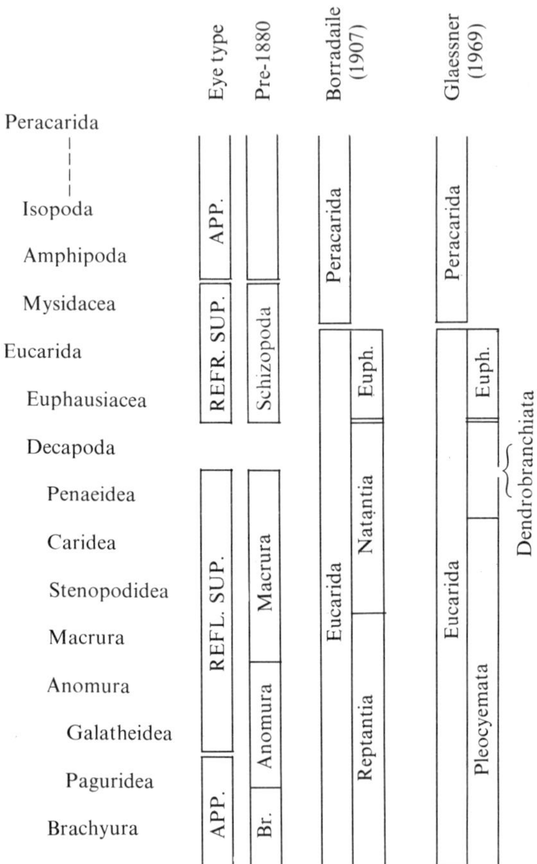

Abbreviations: APP., apposition; REFL. SUP., reflecting superposition; REFR. SUP., refracting superposition; Br., Brachyura; Euph., Euphausiacea.

grouped, as the order Schizopoda, before revision by Boas (1883). It is possible but unlikely that the same type of eye arose twice.

If a taxonomic system is intended to reflect the evolutionary history of a group, then one should expect a reasonable coincidence of those characters that can properly be regarded as conservative, and I have argued here that eye design is one such character. A taxonomy based on eye design alone supports closely the earliest classificatory schemes, prior to the revisions of Boas (1880, 1883), but contradicts, at least in part, all later schemes (Table 2). It is, of course, dangerous to depend on a single character like eye design as an indicator of evolutionary origins, and those that have been used in the past—exoskeleton, gill structure, larval development (see Gurney, 1942)—have equal claim to consideration as good taxonomic indicators. Unfortunately, we are dealing with a group whose major radiation occurred at least 250 million years ago and whose fossil record is poor—there are, for example, no fossil euphausiids. Such clues as comparative anatomy can provide must thus suffice in reconstructing their origins. I would like to think, therefore, that when the Malacostraca come up for their next revision the conclusions in this paper, and in particular the three statements listed above, will receive their due weight.

Acknowledgements

I am very grateful to Tony Fincham of the British Museum (Natural History) and to Arthur Baker of the Institute of Oceanographic Sciences, Wormley, U.K. both for access to their institutions' collections, and for valuable discussions about the implications of this study (they do not necessarily share my views!). Work at sea was supported by the NERC and at the University of Sussex by the SRC. This paper was written during a sabbatical term at the University of Oregon. Eugene, and it is a pleasure to thank Graham Hoyle for his hospitality, and Pam Hoyle for typing the manuscript.

REFERENCES

Ball, E. E. (1977) Fine structure of the compound eyes of the midwater amphipod *Phronima* in relation to behavior and habitat *Tissue Cell*, **9**, 521–536.

Boas, J. E. V. (1880) Studier over Decapodernes Slaegtskabsforhold *Dan. Selsk. Skr.* Ser. 6, **1**(2), 26–210.

Boas, J. E. V. (1883) Studien über die Verwandtschaftsbeziehungen der Malakostraken *Morph. Jb.*, **8**, 485–579.

Borradaile, L. A. (1907) On the classification of the Decapoda *Ann. Mag. nat. Hist.*, Ser. 7, **19**, 457–486.

Burkenroad, M. D. (1963) The evolution of the Eucarida (Crustacea, Eumalacostraca), in relation to the fossil record *Tulane Studies in Geology*, **2**(1), 3–16.

Calman, W. T. (1904) On the classification of the Crustacea Malacostraca *Ann. Mag. nat. Hist.*, Ser. 7, **13**, 144–158.

Chun, C. (1896) Atlantis. Biologische Studien über pelagische Organismen *Zoologica, Stuttgart*, **7**, 1–260.

Exner, S. (1891) *Die Physiologie der facettirten Augen von Krebsen und Insecten* Deuticke, Leipzig und Wien.

Fincham, A. A. (1980) Eyes and classification of malacostracan crustaceans *Nature*, **287**, 729–731.

Fletcher, A., Murphy, T. and Young, A. (1954) Solutions of two optical problems *Proc. R. Soc. Lond. A.*, **223**, 216–225.

Glaessner, M. F. (1969) "Decapoda" in *Treatise on Invertebrate Paleontology*, Part R (Arthropoda 4), Vol. 2 (ed. Moore, R. C.) Univ. of Kansas and Geol. Soc. Amer., 399–566.

Grenacher, G. H. (1879) *Untersuchungen über das Sehorgan der Arthropoden, insbesondere der Spinnen, Insekten und Crustaceen* Vanderhock und Ruprecht, Gottingen.

Gurney, R. (1942) *Larvae of the Decapod Crustacea* Ray Society, London.

Hausen, K. (1973) Die Brechungsindices im Kristallkegel der Mehlmotte *Ephestia kunniella* *J. comp. Physiol.*, **82**, 365–378.

Horridge, G. A. (1975) "Optical mechanisms in clear-zone eyes" in *The Compound Eye and Vision of Insects* (ed. Horridge, G. A.) Clarendon, Oxford, 255–298.

Horridge, G. A., Giddings, C. and Stange, G. (1972) The superposition eye of skipper butterflies *Proc. R. Soc. Lond. B.*, **182**, 457–495.

Horridge, G. A. and McLean, M. (1978) The dorsal eye of the mayfly *Atalophlebia* (Ephemeroptera) *Proc. R. Soc. Lond. B.*, **200**, 137–150.

Iga, K. and Yamamoto, N. (1977) Plastic focusing fiber for imaging applications *Appl. Opt.*, **16**, 1305–1310.

Kampa, E. H. (1965) The euphausiid eye; a re-evaluation *Vision Res.*, **5**, 475–481.

Kirschfeld, K. (1974) The absolute sensitivity of lens and compound eyes *Z. Naturforsch.*, **29c**, 592–596.

Kleinholz, L. (1961) "Pigmentary effectors" in *The Physiology of Crustacea*, Vol. 2 (ed. Waterman, T. H.) Academic Press, New York, 133–169.

Kuiper, J. W. (1962) The optics of the compound eye *Symp. Soc. exp. Biol.*, **16**, 58–71.

Kunze, P. (1979) "Apposition and superposition eyes" in *Handbook of Sensory Physiology*, VII, 6/A (ed. Autrum, H-J.) Springer-Verlag, Berlin, 441–502.

Land, M. F. (1976) Superposition images are formed by reflection in the eyes of some oceanic decapod crustacea *Nature*, **263**, 764–765.

Land, M. F. (1978) Animal eyes with mirror optics *Scient. Amer.*, **239**, 126–134.

Land, M. F. (1979*a*) Nature as an optical engineer *New Scientist*, **84**, 10–13.

Land, M. F. (1979*b*) The optical mechanism of the eye of *Limulus Nature*, **280**, 396–397.

Land, M. F. (1980*a*) Compound eyes: old and new optical mechanisms *Nature*, **287**, 681–686.

Land, M. F. (1980*b*) "Optics and vision in invertebrates" in *Handbook of Sensory Physiology*, VII, 6/B (ed. Autrum, H-J.) Springer-Verlag, Berlin.

Land, M. F. and Burton, F. A. (1979) The refractive index gradient in the crystalline cones of the eyes of a euphausiid crustacean *J. exp. Biol.*, **82**, 395–398.

Land, M. F., Burton, F. A. and Meyer-Rochow, V. B. (1979) The optical geometry of euphausiid eyes *J. comp. Physiol.*, **130**, 49–62.

Meyer-Rochow, V. B. and Walsh, S. (1978) The eyes of mesopelagic crustaceans: III. *Thysanopoda tricuspidata* (Euphausiacea) *Cell Tiss. Res.*, **195**, 57–79.

Milne, L. and Milne, M. (1959) "Photosensitivity in invertebrates" in *Handbook of Physiology*, Sect. 1, Vol. I (ed. Field, J.) Amer. Physiol. Soc., Washington D.C., 621–645.

Seitz, G. (1969) Untersuchungen am dioptrischen Apparat des Leuchtkaferauges *Z. vergl. Physiol.*, **62**, 61–74.

Stavenga, D. G. (1979) "Pseudopupils of compound eyes" in *Handbook of Sensory Physiology*, VII, 6/A (ed. Autrum, H-J.) Springer-Verlag, Berlin, 357–439.

Vogt, K. (1975) Zur Optik des Flußkrebsauges *Z. Naturforsch.*, **30c**, 691.

Vogt, K. (1977) Ray path and reflection mechanisms in crayfish eyes *Z. Naturforsch.*, **32c**, 466–468.

Vogt, K. (1980) Die Spiegeloptik des Flußkrebsauges (the optical system of the crayfish eye) *J. comp. Physiol.*, **135**, 1–19.

Waterman, T. H. (1961) "Light sensitivity and vision" in *The Physiology of Crustacea*, Vol. 2 (ed. Waterman, T. H.) Academic Press, New York, 1–64.

Waterman, T. H. and Chace, F. A. (1961) "General crustacean biology" in *The Physiology of Crustacea*, Vol. 1 (ed. Waterman, T. H.) Academic Press, New York, Chapter 1.

CHAPTER FOUR

BEHAVIOURAL CORRELATES OF PHOTORECEPTION IN *DAPHNIA*

STEPHEN YOUNG

Introduction

Two rival strategies for understanding sensory systems are represented in this book. One argues that an increasing knowledge of physics and engineering may help to unravel many sensory mysteries, while the other stresses that it is essential to remember the underlying biology of the organism to understand the function of a sense organ in the broader terms of its contribution to the animal's way of life. This paper, which presents data from a single crustacean species, the cladoceran *Daphnia magna*, describes my attempts to follow the first route, while being reluctantly forced towards the second.

Daphnia magna is traditionally used as a model for the smaller, planktonic Crustacea. It is a convenient laboratory animal, tough and easily reared, which feeds by filtering algae and bacteria, and reproduces largely parthenogenetically. Traditionally its visual system is implicated in maintaining an upright position and in locating patches of water coloured by food (Ringelberg, 1964; Baylor and Smith, 1957; Smith and Baylor, 1953). The straightforward appearance of the single large compound eye fits in with these undemanding roles. There are only 22 ommatidia in all, widely spaced around almost a complete sphere. Each ommatidium has a bulbous lens attached to a short squat fused rhabdom surrounded by black masking pigment (Fig. 1). The eye is highly mobile, "following" objects moved past the animal, and constantly exhibiting a fast tremor, which persists even in darkness. Behaviourally, the animal is most responsive to a blue stimulus seen through the top of its head, and to a yellow-green stimulus seen through the side of its head (Young, 1974).

This paper aims to show how these peculiar features are related to the visual world in which *Daphnia* lives.

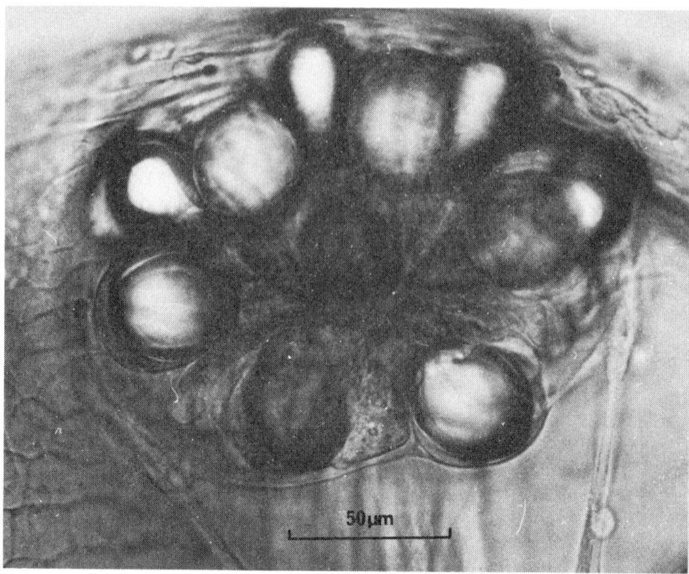

Figure 1 Eye of *Daphnia magna*. This is the eye of the clear-eye mutant, which lacks the black masking pigment, thus revealing the rhabdoms attached to the rear of the lenses.

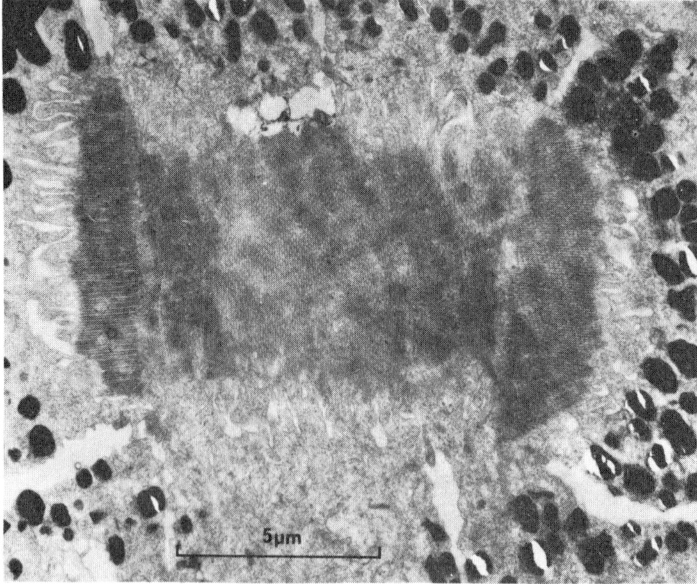

Figure 2 Cross section of *Daphnia* rhabdom, showing near-rectangular shape, and black pigment granules surrounding the rhabdom.

Receptive fields

The *Daphnia* eye is held together mainly by hydrostatic pressure (Downing, 1974), and the lenses are easy to separate from the rest of the eye. Their optical properties can be determined, and from these and measurements of rhabdom refractive indexes, it is possible to predict what sort of receptive field each receptor ought to have. The receptive field is a map of the relative decline in the response of the photoreceptor as a point source of light is moved progressively away from the straight ahead "on-axis" position. As *Daphnia* has rhabdoms with markedly rectangular cross section (Fig. 2) the contour map of a calculated receptive field (Fig. 3a) is asymmetrical, and, as the receptor is much closer to the lens than any focused image can get, there is a broad sensitivity to light over a wide field. This contradicts the common view that compound eye ommatidia have narrow fields. Heberdey and Kupka (1942) show a typical view of the *Daphnia* eye (Fig. 3b, top) with wide blind gaps between neighbouring receptors. Our calculations predict the state of affairs shown in Fig. 3b (bottom) with the 10% sensitivity regions of neighbours almost touching, despite a more realistic "worst-case" spacing between ommatidia. This makes for difficulties, because the existence of blind gaps between ommatidia provides an obvious rationale for the constant tremor of the eye: that it is scanning the gaps. Clearly anyone who wants to remove the gaps would be obliged to come up with a new explanation of the tremor. Faced with this daunting prospect we looked to our assumptions, which

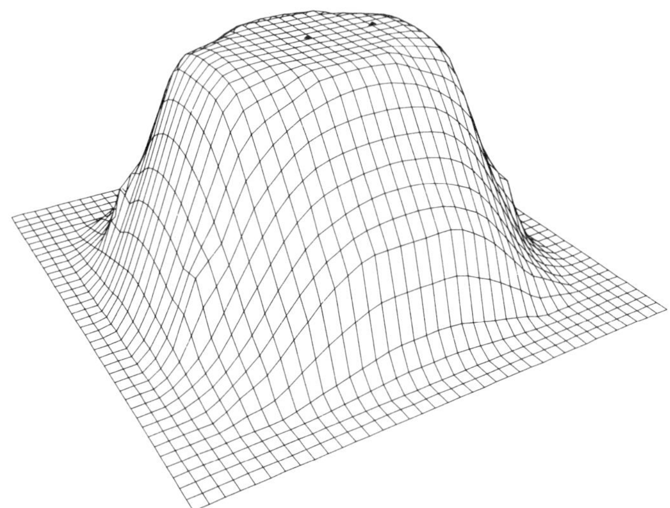

Figure 3a Perspective drawing of *Daphnia* receptive field, calculated from optical data. The z-axis is % response, and the x- and y-axes a polar plot of stimulus distance from the optical axis. The markers on the plateau are 5° apart.

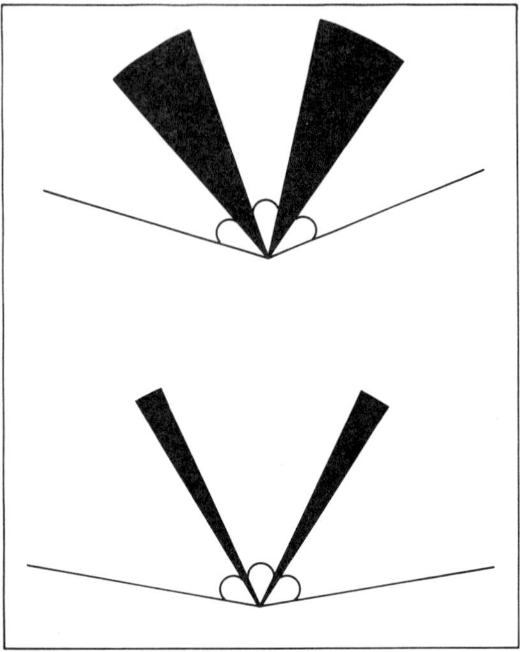

Figure 3b Blind gaps (blacked in) between neighbouring *Daphnia* ommatidia (top), as predicted by Heberdey and Kupka (1942), and (bottom) greatly reduced blind gaps, as predicted by receptive field shown in Fig. 3a.

were that the ommatidium could be regarded as a large, well-designed *f*/1.7 camera lens with a flat rectangular photocell mounted close to its rear surface. All diffraction and wave-guide effects were ignored, as was the considerable length of the photoreceptor. The first test of the reality of these assumptions was to use a real *Daphnia* lens suspended in an agar gel of appropriate refractive index, to replace the rhabdom with a microscope and a photomultiplier looking through a scale-sized rectangular aperture, and to rotate a point source of light around the lens. Fig. 4a shows the resulting array of x/y plotter outputs for fourteen lenses, each measured in the plane of both the long and the short axis of aperture. Fig. 4b shows that the median widths of these plots are, if anything, somewhat wider than the calculated receptor field (rf). The differences between the two plots for each lens are in the right direction, and are statistically reliable.

The next test was to see if it would be possible to use the behavioural response of a large eye movement evoked by a sudden light flash to make a direct check for the existence of blind zones. If these exist, it should be possible to find regions where the threshold for evoking a response with a small patch of light flashed briefly is much elevated. This experiment proved extremely difficult in practice, but we finally did find one animal prepared to return its eye reliably to the same starting position over the period of many hours required to measure thresholds at 5° intervals all

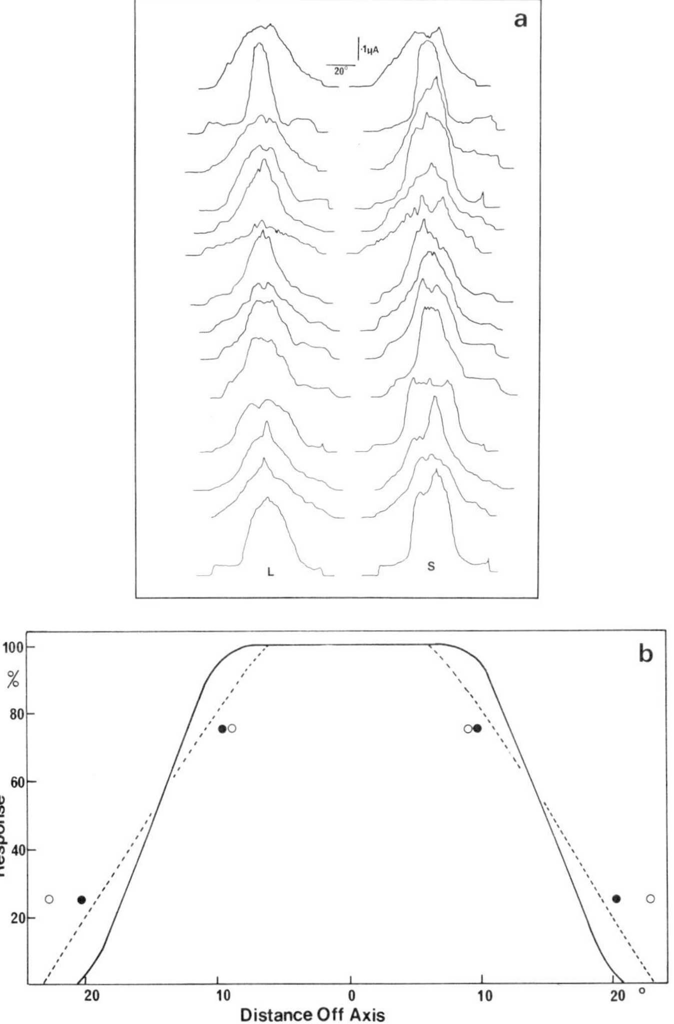

Figure 4 (a) Photomultiplier receptive fields. For each trace, the x-axis is the angular position of the stimulus light, and the y-axis the multiplier anode current. Each pair of traces comes from a single lens, tracking along long (L) and short (S) sides of the rectangular rhabdom mask.

(b) Median widths of multiplier receptive fields at 25% and 75% of maximum height.

● ● S condition
○ ○ L condition
——— S prediction } from model shown in Fig. 3a.
– – – L prediction

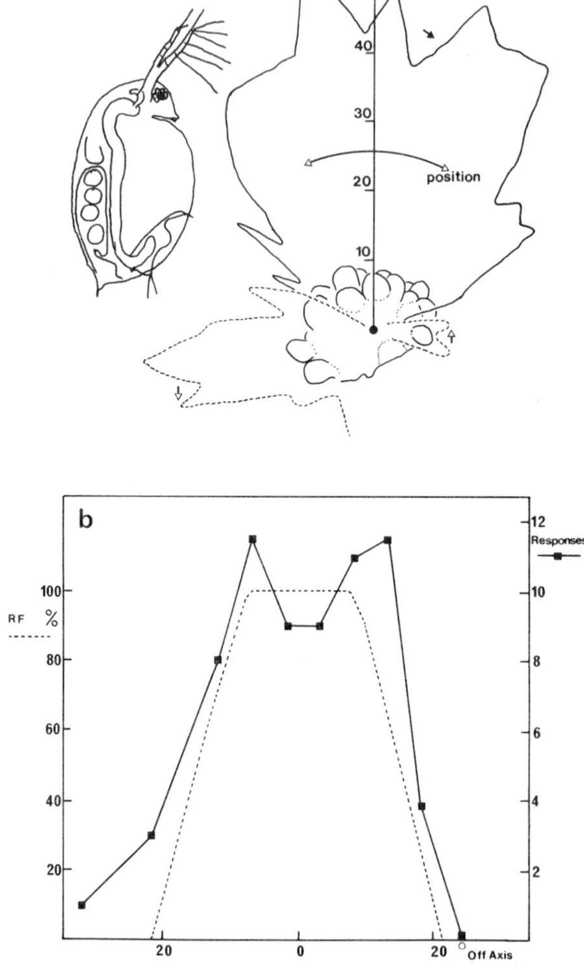

Figure 5 (a) Polar plot of sensitivity measured at 5° intervals around a *Daphnia* eye. θ axis gives stimulus position relative to eye. (Orientation of whole animal shown by sketch.) R-axis is total number of eye movement responses elicited by a series of 50 test flashes of graded intensity. Arrows show eye movement direction.

(b) Extreme ventral portion of Fig. 5a (——■——), compared to average calculated receptive field profile (— — — —).

around the circumference of the eye. The results show that the response is complex, because some regions of the eye evoke a dorsal, and some a ventral movement of the eye. In between, there are regions which give a dorsal movement for a bright flash, and a ventral one for a dim flash, with no response to intermediate intensities (Fig. 5a). However, at the extreme ventral edge of the eye there is a narrow band in which a dorsal movement

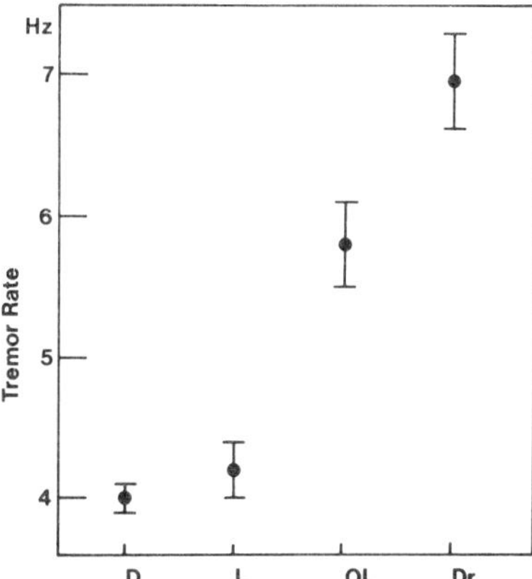

Figure 6 *Daphnia* eye tremor frequency. Bars show standard errors (on means of 12, 12, 8, and 7 animals) from left to right. D = dark, L = light, OL = open loop, Dr = driven.

response seems likely to be mediated by a single pair of ommatidia. Fig. 5b shows that the threshold distribution in this region is a reasonably good fit to the calculated receptive field. Four more animals showed the same pattern of dorsal and ventral eye movement response, and in no case could a convincing blind gap be found.

Eye tremor

In *Daphnia magna* the tremor rate is comparatively unaffected by light intensity, though colour has a strong effect. The tremor can be entrained by a flashing stimulus, and the eye will follow the stimulus as its flash rate

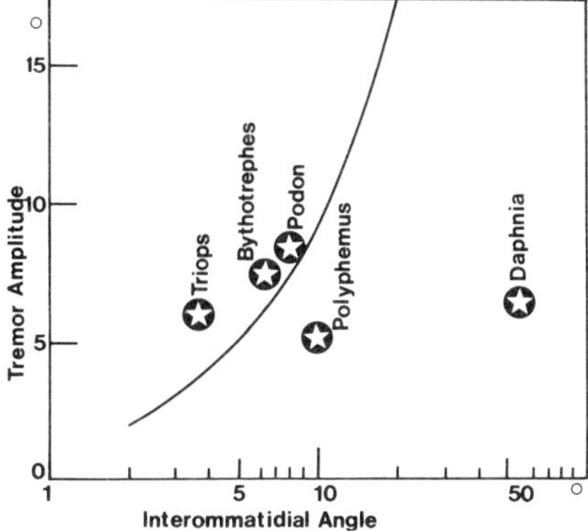

Figure 7 Average eye movement amplitudes for 5 crustaceans. All from single frame cine film analysis. Solid line gives tremor amplitude directly proportional to interommatidial angle. (*Podon* and *Daphnia* data from records in Downing (1971).)

is increased, up to about 7 Hz. Similarly, an increase in tremor frequency can be achieved by engineering an "open loop" in which the eye movement detector automatically switches off the light source thus triggering a new movement (Fig. 6). The tremor amplitude is typically around 5° to 10°, much less than the inter-ommatidial angle. This sort of eye tremor is shared by many related small crustaceans, and, despite considerable differences in the complexity of the eyes involved, invariably seems to involve a rocking movement of amplitude around 7° (Fig. 7). This observation seems to make it very unlikely that an explanation of tremor will be found in the structure, optics, or neural connections in the eyes concerned. Any straightforward theory on these lines will predict a clear relationship between tremor amplitude and interommatidial angle. Moreover, there are two close relatives of these animals, with similar-looking eyes, which operate completely without tremor in the case of *Chirocephalus*, and with extremely infrequent movements, in the case of *Artemia*. I think it is significant that both these dissenters swim constantly

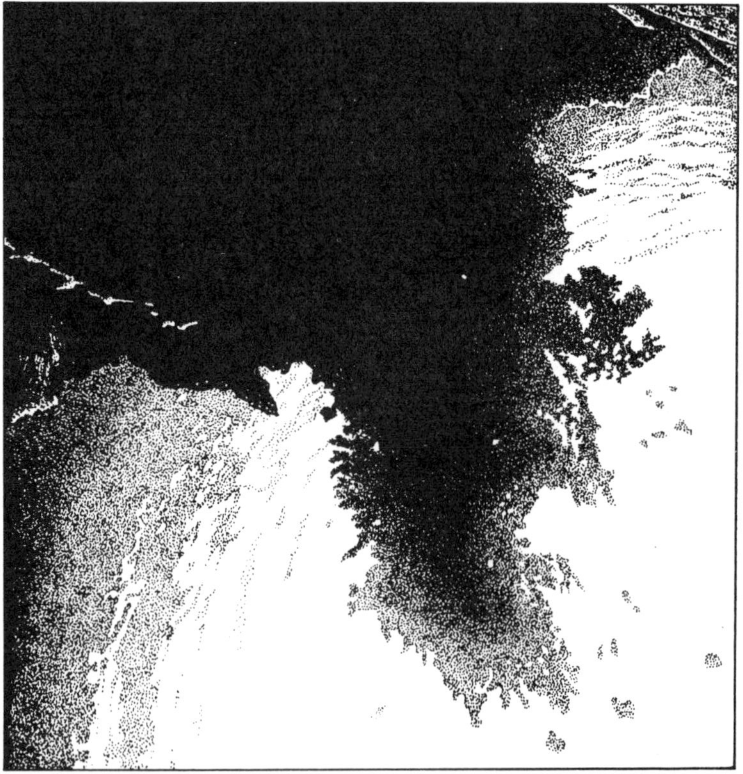

Figure 8 Water surface viewed from underneath, showing about $\frac{1}{4}$ of Snell's window, with mangrove root in the foreground. (Drawn by W. D. G. Cox from photograph by J. Lythgoe.)

on their backs with a head down orientation, unlike the animals with tremor, which watch the undersurface of the water. Several authors have suggested that daphnids use the constant angular position of Snell's window (Fig. 8) to maintain their body axis at some preferred angle to the vertical. My conclusion about the role of tremor is that it must relate to the visual environment rather than the eye structure, and that the curiously static Snell's window is a good candidate for the environmental feature the tremor helps detect. It may be that stimuli of constant angular size tend to adapt readily, or it may not be a coincidence that the ripple zone at the edge of the disc of light on the photograph is around 8° wide.

Food searching

Dingle (1962) has shown that *Daphnia* will collect underneath shallow transparent trays containing algae, floating on the water surface, thus confirming the involvement of vision in food location. Baylor and Smith (1957) report that *Daphnia* swim vigorously, with a large horizontal vector, in blue light, while tending to smaller vertical movements in red light.

These two observations are often used to support a model in which the animals become trapped in food-rich regions by curtailment of their

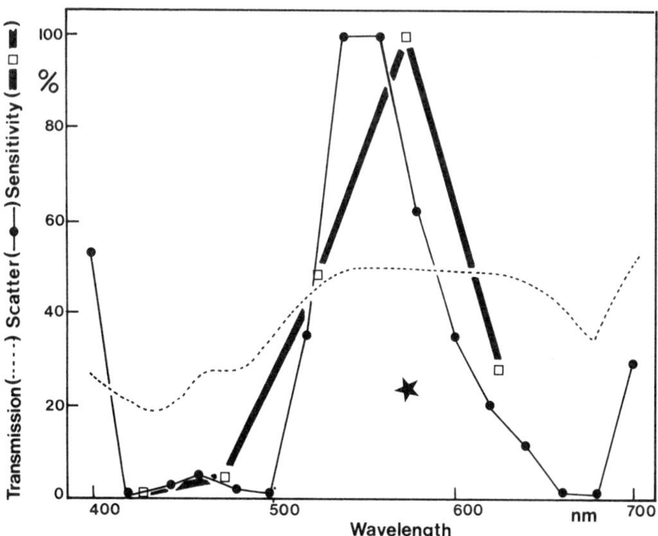

Figure 9 ------ Light transmitted by sonicated and centrifuged *Chlorella*
—●— Light scattered by suspension of intact *Chlorella*
■□■ *Daphnia* visual sensitivity—derived from thresholds for eye tremor following response, with illumination through the side of the animal's head (all as a function of light wavelength).

swimming movements by the red light to be found there. I have always raised the naïve objection that algae are green, not red, only to be told that light transmitted by green plants has a large red component.

What actually happens if a tube of algal suspension is put in a spectrophotometer is that it "looks" to the spectrophotometer to be very dark grey. If you sonicate and centrifuge the suspension, it now appears yellowish green (Fig. 9), but if a collimated beam from an intense source is directed through a large rectangular cell containing a suspension of intact algal cells, the spectral composition of the light scattered at right angles to the illuminating beam (Fig. 9) is predominantly bright green. Sideways scattered light from algal cells must be the main stimulus for any *Daphnia* food-locating mechanism, and hence it seems unlikely that any mechanism involving inhibition of locomotion by red light will function in practice. We have attempted to quantify Baylor's red and blue dances by observing three-dimensional tracks of individual *Daphnia* swimming in a rectangular tank containing filtered pond water. Narrow band interference filters were used to provide monochromatic illumination, adjusted to constant energy (48 mW/m^2) with a vacuum thermopile. The tracks were produced by two observers simultaneously watching the animal through a small aperture, one through the front and one through the side of the tank. Every five seconds each observer marked the apparent position of the animal on a piece of acetate sheet attached to the tank wall, and sequentially numbered each mark. Allowing for refraction at the air/water interface, the intersection of the two "eyelines" gave the position of the

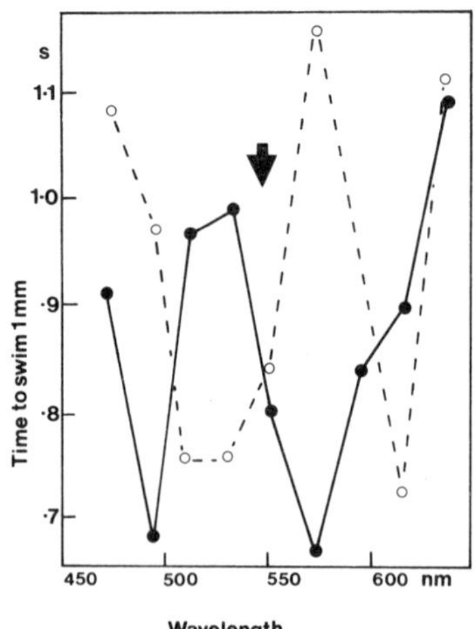

Figure 10 *Daphnia* "loitering index" as a function of light wavelength.
——●—— Black-eyes
— — ○ — — Clear-eyes
Arrow shows peak of light scattered by *Chlorella*.

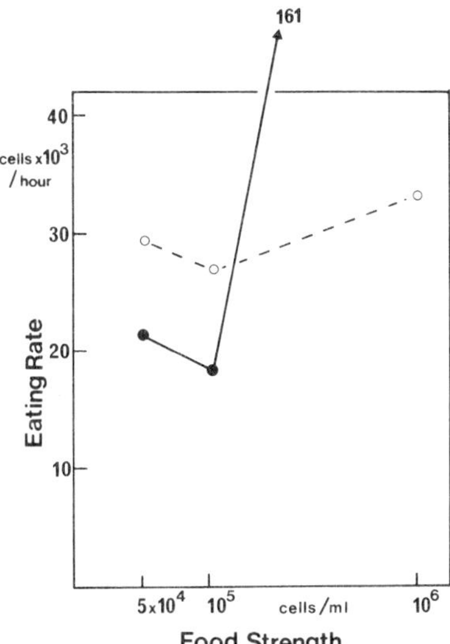

Figure 11 *Daphnia* eating rate as a function of food strength.
——●—— Black-eyes
— — — ○ — Clear-eyes

Daphnia. We computed total distance from start to finish of a two-minute test period, total horizontal vector, total vertical vector (both round the track), total angle turned through (cumulative angles between track segments in the plane of adjacent segments), and total distance around the track. Only the last was statistically significantly affected by light colour. Fig. 10 shows the results plotted as a loitering index, in terms of the time required to cover 1 mm. Loitering does show a peak in the green, as well as in the red. The dashed line gives the data from a group of clear-eye mutant *Daphnia*, which lack the black melanin masking pigment in their compound eyes. These have anomalous light reception, being hypersensitive especially to light through the side of the head, and clearly lack the necessary swimming behaviour to "find" dense algal clumps. Interestingly, their actual food intake, measured by comparing the reductions in algal concentration brought about by groups of twenty *Daphnia* browsing in 100 ml batches of algal suspension, show that clear-eyes can gain more food from weak suspensions than normal animals, but are much poorer at feeding from rich suspensions (Fig. 11) (Watts and Young, 1980).

Feeding

Daphnia first filters algae from a pumped water stream onto a grating made of interlocking hairs, then scrapes them off the grating towards its mandibles to form boluses, which are finally swallowed. We have measured the rates of the filter limb beats, movement of the mandibles, and the swallowing of boluses over a range of food concentrations, temperatures, and light regimes. The bolus swallowing is unaffected by food concentration, and the clear-eyes have the same rate as the normals. However, they show a reduced filtering rate overall, as compared to normal, and a compensating increase in mandible rate. We found these differences between the two morphs disappeared if the lighting was altered so that the animals were illuminated through the top of their head, rather than through the side of the head (Fig. 12). This came as a surprise, because McMahon (1965) had shown that light intensity had no effect on feeding rate over a range from complete darkness to 12 W/m^2. Our own measures of filter limb beat rate did show reliable differences between light (1 W/m^2) and dark, though a brief period in the reverse state had little

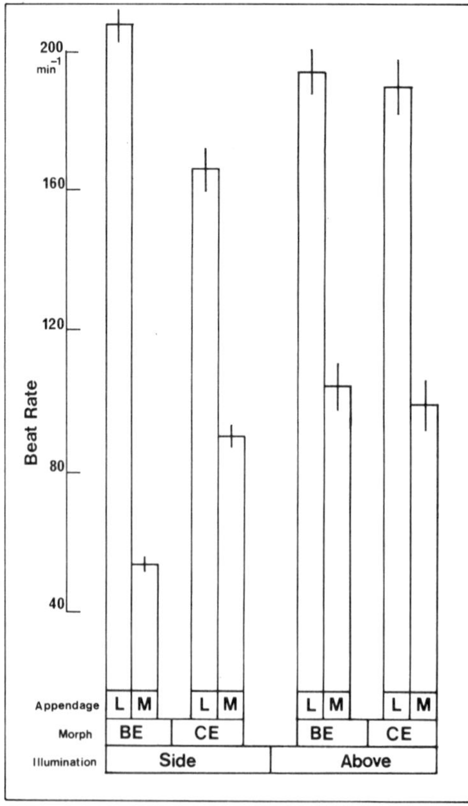

Figure 12 There is a difference between black-eyes (BE) and clear-eyes (CE) for both filter limb (L) and mandible (M) beat rates, but only when illumination comes from the side. All data with food concentration of 10^5 algae/ml, at 20°C. Bars give standard errors from analysis of variance residuals.

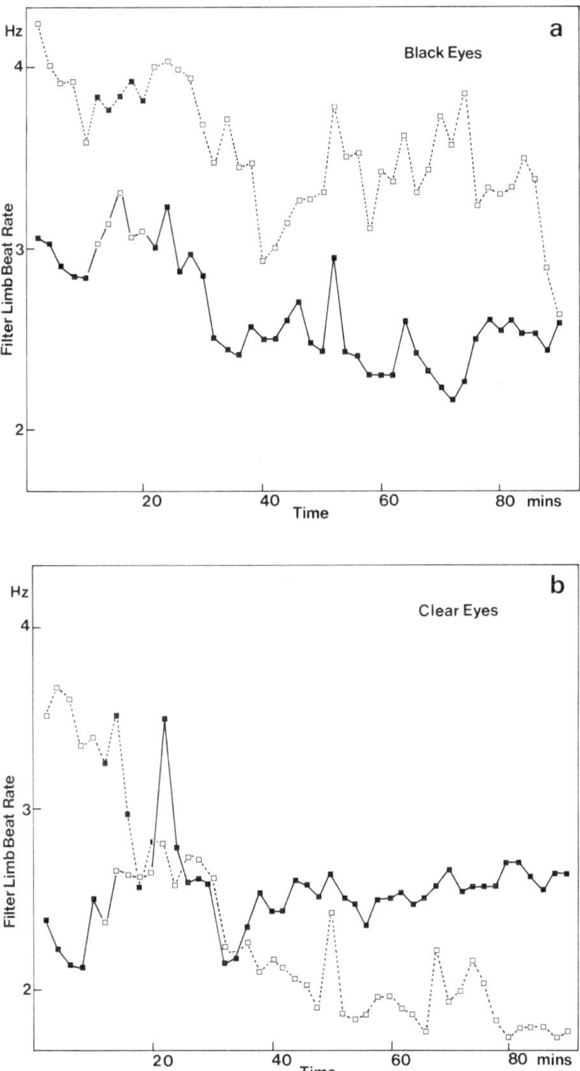

Figure 13 (a) Filter limb beat rates over a 90 m period for dark- (——■——) and light- (— — □ — —) adapted *Daphnia*. The second 10 m of the period is spent with the light regime reversed. Illumination, 1 W/m^2, temperature 20°C, food concentration 5×10^4 algae/ml.

(b) Similar data for clear-eyes. In both cases points are medians for two minute test periods. Ten animals are available for the first thirty minutes of the trial, subsequently there are five replicates.

effect. Paradoxically, as usual, the clear-eyes have their long term "setting" reversed by the brief period of light regime reverse (Fig. 13). These are long term adaptation effects, and do not provide an explanation of the differences in filtering rate with light coming from different directions noted in the previous experiment.

If the total light reaching the animal is held constant at 1 W/m^2, and the ratio of top to side light varied, normal *Daphnia* show a significant change in feeding rate as the sidelight proportion increases from 6 % to 20 %, after which there is no further change. This effect does not occur with clear-eyes, and is independent of the actual concentration of food available.

Conclusion

Our current working hypothesis for the mechanism controlling *Daphnia* filtering rate is that the ratio of side to toplight provides the animal with an estimator of food concentration, because the richer the food, the higher the proportion of sideways scattered light. Fig. 9 compares the relative sensitivity of the eye in a sideways direction with the light scattered by an algal suspension. The star indicates the much reduced sensitivity of the upward looking photoreceptors, which peak in the blue, at maximum for the sideways looking ones. Thus the upward looking receptors are most responsive to blue sky, while the sideways looking ones respond to suspended algal material.

The *Daphnia* eye seems well fitted to optimize food-seeking and efficient feeding, though the complexity of the spectral response curve for swimming behaviour warns against any straightforward deduction about the relationship between receptor sensitivity and the final behaviour. The black masking pigment in the eye is necessary to keep the upwards and sidewards systems optically separated. Without it, the clear-eyes are incapable either of finding rich food supplies, or of coping effectively with them by initiating an efficient rate of filtering.

REFERENCES

Baylor, E. R. and Smith, F. E. (1957) "Diurnal migration of plankton crustaceans" in *Recent Advances in Invertebrate Physiology* (ed. Scheer, B. T.) University of Oregon Publications, Eugene, 21–35.

Downing, A. C. (1974) The hydraulic suspension of the *Daphnia* eye—a new kind of universal joint? *Vision Res.*, **14**, 647–652.

Downing, A. C. (1971) *Form perception in* Daphnia. Thesis, University of Cambridge.

Dingle, H. (1962) Occurrence and ecological significance of colour responses to some crustacea *Am. Nat.*, **96**, 151–160.

Heberdey, R. F. and Kupka, E. (1942) Helligkeitsunterscheidensvermögen von *Daphnia pulex Z. vergleich. Physiol.*, **31**, 89–111.

McMahon, J. W. (1965) Some physical factors influencing the feeding behaviour of *Daphnia magna* Strauss *Can. J. Zool.*, **43**, 603–611.

Ringelberg, J. (1964) The positively phototactic reaction of *Daphnia magna* Strauss: a contribution to the understanding of diurnal vertical migration *Neth. J. Sea Res.*, **2**, 319–406.

Smith, F. E. and Baylor, E. R. (1953) Color responses in Cladocera and their ecological significance *Am. Nat.*, **87**, 49–55.

Watts, E. and Young, S. (1980) Components of *Daphnia* feeding behaviour *Journal of Plankton Research*, **2**, 203–212.

Young, S. (1974) Directional differences in the colour sensitivity of *Daphnia magna J. exp. Biol.*, **61**, 261–267.

CHAPTER FIVE

PROPERTIES OF HAIR CELLS IN THE MAMMALIAN COCHLEA

IAN RUSSELL

Introduction

The transducer elements in the sensory epithelia of acoustico lateralis receptors are the hair cells, and they reach their pinnacle of sensitivity and frequency response in the mammalian cochlea. In the past, the properties of the cochlear hair cells have been inferred from comparisons between their sensory input (vibrations of the basilar membrane) and their output represented in their contribution to the extracellular receptor potentials and in the discharges of the auditory nerve fibres. Quite recently it has been possible to measure the responses of cochlear hair cells by making intracellular recordings from them. This chapter reviews what we know about these responses and compares the properties of hair cells in the cochlea with those of other acoustico lateralis receptors.

Functional morphology of cochlear hair cells

The sensory epithelium of the cochlea, the organ of Corti, consists of a strip of cells attached to the basilar membrane. This forms a helical ribbon, wide at the apex of the cochlea and narrow at its base, which separates the endolymph of the scala media from the perilymph of the scala tympani. Distributed along the length of the organ of Corti are the sensory cells: a single row of inner hair cells and three rows of outer hair cells (Fig. 1).

The inner and outer hair cells differ from each other not only in their shape, number and location in the organ of Corti, but in their innervation, the organization of their stereocilia, and the relation of these to the tectorial membrane. The latter characteristics may be important in the

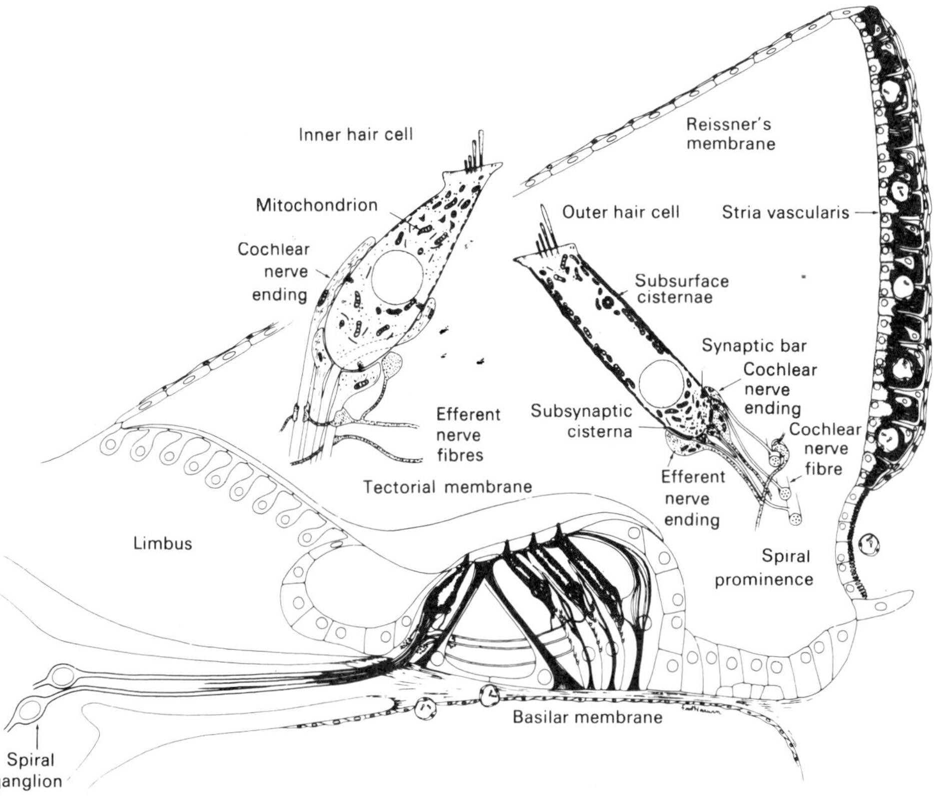

Figure 1 Drawing of the cochlear duct, second turn, guinea pig (reprinted from Smith, 1975).

different roles the inner and outer hair cells apparently play in sensory transduction in the cochlea.

The ovoid inner hair cells are less numerous than the cylindrical outer hair cells, but receive the greatest proportion of the afferent innervation. Approximately 95% of the afferent fibres in the auditory nerve form synapses with the inner hair cells, each hair cell receiving an average of 20 afferent fibres (Spoendlin, 1970). The outer hair cells receive the remaining afferent fibres; one fibre innervating many hair cells. The afferent innervation differs in other important respects. Fibres destined for the inner hair cells emerge from a series of small canals, the habenula perforata in the spiral lamina, and radiate to hair cells immediately adjacent to the pore. The fibres are well myelinated up to the point where they emerge from the habenulae, and the synapses are characterized by an electron dense presynaptic body in the hair cell, which is surrounded by a halo of vesicles. Fibres destined for the outer hair cells travel along the length of the basilar membrane in spiral fashion for distances up to 1.5 mm before making synaptic contact. They are poorly myelinated, and morphological signs of functional synaptic contact are rare (Spoendlin, 1970). Interestingly, their central destination is in question. Poorly myelinated fibres are virtually absent in the root of the eighth nerve and it has been proposed by Spoendlin (1978) that these fibres may not form central connections. Support for this conjecture stems from his observations that sectioning the cochlear nerve causes massive degeneration of the radial fibres, but leaves the spiral fibres undamaged. Thus we are left with implications from the morphology that little if any sensory information is relayed from the outer hair cells to the central nervous system.

In contrast to this, the outer hair cells receive a massive efferent innervation which, in relation to the afferent innervation, terminates presynaptically on the hair cell membranes (Fig. 1). The efferent synapses are morphologically characterized by sub-synaptic cysternae, double or multiple membrane bounded lamellae which lie parallel to the plasma membrane. They extend beneath the basal-lateral walls of the outer hair cells, and stop close to the apical surface. Inner hair cells also receive an efferent innervation, but this largely terminates post-synaptically on the afferent nerve terminals (Fig. 1). Thus, in relation to their innervation inner hair cells appear to provide the sensory input to the auditory system, while the outer hair cells are the end organs of the efferent system.

It is generally accepted that hair cells in the acoustico-lateralis system are excited by shear displacement of their stereocilia towards the kinocilium (Flock, 1971). Kinocilia are present early in the development of cochlear hair cells but these disappear at birth and only their basal bodies remain (Bredburg, Ades and Engström, 1972). Kinocilia are believed to damp the frequency characteristics of hair cells and the absence of kinocilia in cochlear hair cells has been associated with their high frequency responses (Hudspeth and Corey, 1977).

It has been established, by direct experimental observation in the frog sacculus, that hair cells are excited by shear displacement of their stereocilia, and the kinocilium is not involved in the transduction process (Hudspeth and Jacobs, 1979). In the mammalian cochlea, shear displacement of the hair cell stereocilia is believed to be caused by relative movements between the basilar and tectorial membranes. The stereocilia are orientated on the proximal side of the basal body in relation to the limbus (Fig. 1) and, on the basis of their morphological polarization, it has been proposed that hair cells are depolarized by movements of the basilar membrane towards the scala media (Davis, 1965).

The stereocilia are not true cilia but bear close similarity to the microvilli of cells in the intestinal mucosa (Mooseker and Tilney, 1975).

The stereocilia are club-shaped and the fibrillar core continues as a root into the electron dense matrix of the cuticular plate (Fig. 1). Here the fibrils fan out from the root and form helical structures in the matrix of the cuticular plate adjacent to the roots.

In view of the nature of hair cell excitation, the mechanical properties of the stereocilia are important in determining the characteristics of the stimulus hair cells receive. Flock and Cheung (1977), and Flock, Flock and Murray (1977) investigated the structural composition and mechanical properties of hair cells in the crista ampullaris of frogs and discovered that the fibrillar core of the stereocilia are composed of the contractile protein actin, and more recently myosin filaments have been detected in the cuticular plate (Macartney, Comis and Pickles, 1980). This has led to the interesting speculation that transduction in hair cells may involve active, motile processes. For example, in the cells of the intestinal mucosa, where the microvilli are also composed of actin rooted into a fibrillar matrix (the terminal web), which also contains myosin, the microvilli are motile and their mechanical properties are sensitive to metabolic changes in their environment (Mooseker, 1975; Mooseker and Tilney, 1975). In relation to these findings the presence of the subsynaptic cysternae of the efferent system takes on fresh significance. Electron probe studies indicate that Ca^{2+} is associated with these structures (Thornhill, personal communication). Thus there is considerable stimulus to investigate the role of the efferent system and its postsynaptic action on hair cells. Are the subsynaptic cysternae equivalent to the T system of muscle fibres and does stimulation of the efferent system influence the mechanoelectric properties of hair cells?

The efficiency of the mechanical coupling of the hair cells to the overlying tectorial membrane is, in part, determined by the stiffness of the stereocilia bundle (Harris, 1968). This stiffness will depend upon the stiffness of individual stereocilia, their mechanical coupling to each other and their spatial arrangement. The stiffness of individual stereocilia has been qualitatively determined in hair cells of the amphibian crista ampullaris by Flock *et al.* (1977). They moved the stereocilia around with microprobes and observed that they behaved like stiff rods and were readily snapped. The stiffness is a property of the actin core and not the membrane, which was selectively dissolved by the detergent Triton X-100. Stereocilia are coupled to each other by a web of triplet or doublet filamentous bridges between the stereocilia. Hudspeth and Jacobs (1979) and Flock *et al.* (1977) have observed that stereocilia move as a bundle in response to mechanical displacement, even after selective removal of the plasma membrane. The implications of this are that the filamentous bridges mechanically connect the stereocilia to each other, and the filaments penetrate the plasma membrane.

The spatial distribution of stereocilia on the apical surfaces of hair cells is very regular, and characteristic of different hair cells. Early in development the patterns of distribution of stereocilia in inner and outer hair cells appear to be similar (Pujol and Abonnene, 1977), but these later differentiate into palisades of stereocilia on the apical surfaces of inner hair cells, and more numerous stereocilia in W-shaped rows on the outer hair cells. In inner and outer hair cells the stereocilia in the row closest to the basal body are tallest, and successive rows decrease in height in stepwise fashion. The arrangement of stereocilia on the inner hair cells is fairly constant in the different turns of the cochlea. However between the basal and apical turns of the cochlea the angle between the two arms of the W arrangement of stereocilia of outer hair cells becomes progressively more acute. The functional significance of this characteristic and ordered distribution of stereocilia on the surfaces of hair cells is unknown but apparently important for hair cell transduction.

Flock *et al.* (1977) have proposed that the regular spacing between the stereocilia is maintained by electrostatic repulsion between the negative charges on the surfaces of the stereocilia. If hair cells are exposed to aminoglycosides, such as streptomycin, which have strong affinity for these negative charges, the spacing between the stereocilia is reduced and they may eventually fuse (Wersäll, Bjökroth, Flock and Lindquist, 1973). Recent electrophysiological measurements on lateral line organs give an indirect indication that low concentrations of amino glycosides may cause a change in stiffness in the coupling between the cupula and hair cells. That this is due to a change in the spatial relationships between stereocilia is still a matter for speculation (Kroese and van der Berken, 1980).

The different properties of the sensory epithelia of the acoustico lateralis system depend to a large extent on the properties of the accessory structures and the way the hair cells are coupled to them. In the cochlea, the way inner and outer hair cells are mechanically coupled to the tectorial membrane has been a central issue in the study of its functional morphology for a number of years. Electronmicroscopical observations by Kimura (1966) and Lim (1972) reveal that the tips of the stereocilia of outer hair cells are firmly embedded in the underside of the tectorial membrane, while those of inner hair cells barely make contact with it. The implications of these morphological observations are that the stereocilia of outer hair cells will be moved directly by the displacements of the tectorial membrane in relation to the organ of Corti, but the stereocilia of inner hair cells will be moved by viscous drag of fluid streaming around them. Thus the displacement of the free-standing stereocilia of inner hair cells will be proportional to basilar membrane velocity. The interpretation of these ultra-structural studies is plagued by the uncertainty that the relationships between inner and outer hair cells and the tectorial membrane may be a product of the histology (Engström and Engström, 1978).

These uncertainties have, to some measure, been resolved by electrophysiology.

The nature of inner and outer hair cell receptor potentials

The cochlea behaves as a frequency analyser capable of resolving the components of a complex sound. Mechanical measurements of basilar membrane vibration to pure tones show that the amplitude of vibration varies along the length of the basilar membrane, with the maximum depending in a graded way upon the frequency of the tone (von Bekesy, 1960; Johnstone and Boyle, 1967; Rhode, 1971). The basal turns respond maximally to high frequencies and the apex to low frequencies.

Extracellular receptor potentials have been recorded from various regions of the cochlea, including the round window, in association with the vibrations of the basilar membrane. The potential evoked by a tone burst consists of an alternating waveform that resembles the acoustic waveform, and hence the waveform of vibration of the basilar membrane. The potential has been called the *cochlear microphonic* (CM). The cochlear microphonic is usually offset either above or below the recording baseline, depending on where it is recorded, and this has been called the summating potential. It is of considerable interest to discover what relative contribution the inner and outer hair cell populations make to these potentials, since extracellular potentials have formed the basis for comparison with neural responses and measurements of basilar membrane motion for many years. It is also evident from these extracellular measurements that cochlear hair cells respond to high frequencies of auditory stimulation. However afferent fibres in the acoustico lateralis system are excited by the presynaptic release of chemical transmitter (Furukawa and Ishii, 1967; Flock and Russell, 1973, 1976; Sand, Ozawa and Hagiwara, 1975), and since transmitter release is a voltage dependent phenomenon (Katz, 1969), it seems reasonable to expect that the high frequency potential changes associated with acoustic transduction would be filtered out by the capacitative impedance of the hair cell membranes. So what are the special adaptations of the receptor potential which permit the responses of hair cells to high frequency auditory stimulation to be transmitted to the afferent nerve terminals?

Intracellular recordings have been made from inner hair cells in the basal turn of the guinea pig cochlea (Russell and Sellick, 1977, 1978, 1980; Sellick and Russell, 1980). The cells were identified by iontophoretic injection of Procion and Lucifer yellow, and the resting membrane potentials were found to be between −20 and −45 mV. The hair cells were recorded from a region of the organ of Corti where their characteristic frequencies were between 15–22 kHz; however, it was possible to elicit receptor potentials from them in response to low frequency auditory

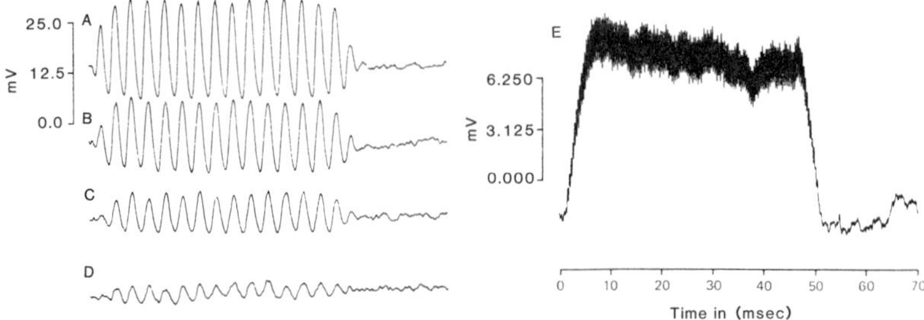

Figure 2 Intracellular receptor potentials from a hair cell with a resting potential of -35 mV recorded in the 16 kHz region of the basilar membrane. A–D, responses to 300 Hz tone 90–50dB in 10dB steps; E, response to 3 kHz at 80 kHz at 80 dB. Sound pressure levels in dB re 2×10^{-5} Nm^{-2}.

stimulation (300 Hz) providing the stimulus intensity was high (c. 100dB SPL).

In response to symmetrical, sinusoidal pressure changes measured at the tympanic membrane, the depolarizing phase of the receptor potential is about three times greater than the hyperpolarizing phase (Fig. 2). This rectification of the receptor potential in the direction of depolarization is a property common among hair cells of the acoustico-lateralis system (Flock and Russell, 1973, 1976; Hudspeth and Corey, 1977; Fettiplace and Crawfurd, 1978), and is clearly seen in the transfer function illustrated for an inner hair cell in Fig. 3.

The hair cells are depolarized during the phase of rarefaction of the sound stimulus. During this phase, the basilar membrane moves towards the scala media, and according to a model proposed by Davis (1965), this causes a shearing motion of the hair cell stereocilia towards the basal body. Thus cochlear hair cells share a common functional and morphological polarization with other hair cells in the acoustico-lateralis system (Flock, 1971; Hudspeth and Corey, 1977).

When the frequency of auditory stimulation is progressively increased, the phasic (AC) component of the receptor potential becomes attenuated about a DC level whose magnitude is determined by the stimulus intensity and the rectifying properties of the transduction process. Above 1 kHz the DC component of the receptor potential dominates the voltage responses of the inner hair cells (Fig. 2) and the AC component virtually disappears.

It has been proposed that the attenuation of the AC component of the receptor potential is due to the capacitative impedance of the hair cell membrane (Russell and Sellick, 1978). In order to test this hypothesis the membrane time constants and low pass cut-off frequencies (-3dB points) of the ratio of AC and DC components of the receptor potential of several hair cells were determined (Sellick and Russell, 1980). In each case there

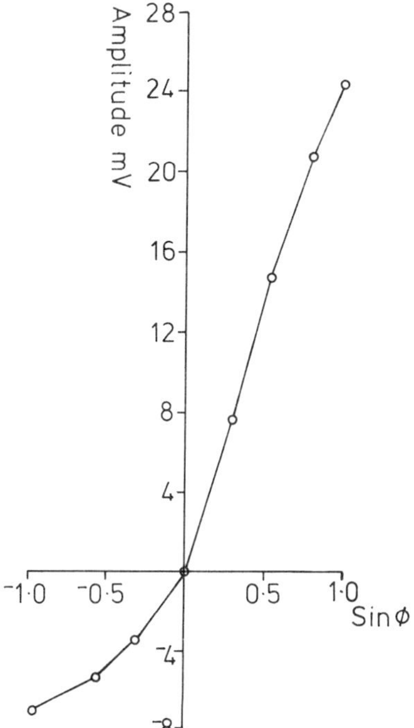

Figure 3 Transfer characteristics of a cochlear hair cell measured in response to a 200 Hz tone at 100dB SPL. The ordinate represents the amplitude of the receptor potential in millivolts, and the abscissa is the sinusoidal displacement of the basilar membrane (reprinted from Russell, 1980).

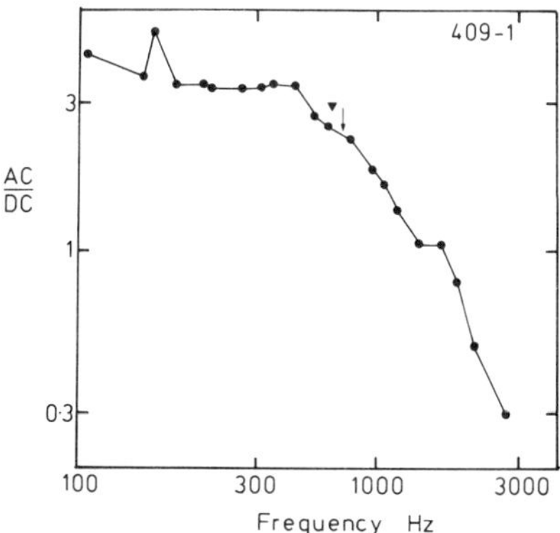

Figure 4 The relationship between the ratio of AC and DC components of the receptor potential versus frequency of a single hair cell. The arrow indicates the 3dB point and ▼ indicates the cut-off frequency determined from the electrical time constant (reprinted from Sellick and Russell, 1980).

was close agreement between the two measurements (Fig. 4). Below the cut-off frequency, the ratio between the AC and DC components is 3, and above this frequency the ratio decreases by about 6dB/octave, which is to be expected from a passive R–C network with time constants similar to those measured in the hair cells (0.89–0.19 ms, mean 0.43 ms in 15 cells).

These measurements support the earlier hypothesis that the AC component is reduced by the capacitative impedance of the hair cell, so that at high frequencies of auditory stimulation, the DC component predominates.

The frequency-dependent form of the inner hair cell receptor potentials is closely related to the patterns of discharge activity which have been recorded from auditory nerve fibres, and presumably account for them. Below 1 kHz, fibres in the auditory nerve are phase locked to the stimulus with a high degree of synchronization, above this, synchronization decreases with frequency and disappears above 4 kHz (Rose, Brugge, Anderson and Hind, 1968).

Thus the asymmetrical operating characteristics of the inner hair cells appear to be an adaptation for producing voltage responses from hair cells at high frequencies of auditory stimulation. It is significant that the point of maximum inflexion of this curve coincides with its operating point at the resting potential. Thus, a DC component will be generated at high frequencies of auditory stimulation even when the stimulus levels are small.

In contrast to the inner hair cell receptor potential, intracellular receptor potentials from outer hair cells are symmetrical and almost an order of magnitude smaller than those from inner hair cells (Fig. 5). Furthermore large DC potentials have never been recorded from them in response to high frequency tones, an observation which has been confirmed by Tanaka *et al.* (1980) and Dallos (personal communication).

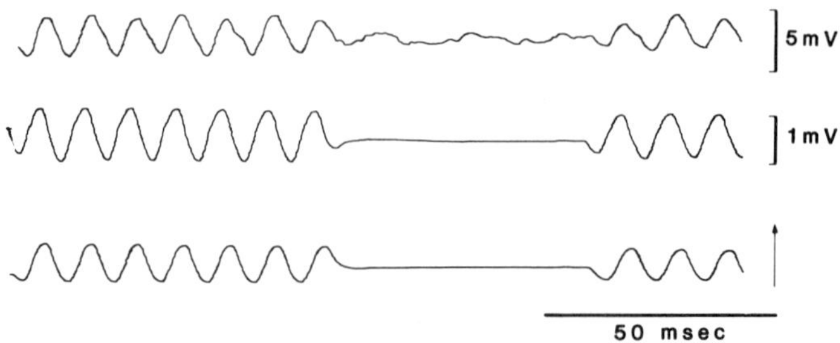

Figure 5 Intracellular recording of receptor potential from an outer hair cell in the basal turn of the guinea pig cochlea in response to a 125 Hz tone at 100dB re 2×10^{-5} Nm^2. *Middle trace:* organ of Corti microphonic potential. *Lower trace:* sound pressure recorded from auditory meatus. Arrows indicate direction of rarefaction (reprinted from Russell and Sellick, 1980).

Their small amplitude may reflect only a small receptor current flowing through them during excitation. Alternatively, they may be electrically transparent in relation to the inner hair cells. Support for the possibility that outer hair cells have low impedance is drawn from the observation that the tissues of the organ of Corti are dominated by extracellular potentials originating in the outer hair cells (the organ of Corti CM) (Fig. 5). The flow of current from the outer hair cells into the supporting cells may be facilitated by electrotonic coupling between adjacent supporting cells, based on the observation that fluorescent dyes flow readily between them. It remains to be seen if outer hair cells are electrotonically coupled to neighbouring cells.

The symmetrical receptor potentials of outer hair cells have an interesting implication for their functional limitations. At high frequencies of auditory stimulation they generate little or no DC component, and, therefore, will not excite afferent fibres at these frequencies, if it is assumed that neural transmission between hair cells and their afferent innervation is a voltage dependent process. In view of their ultrastructural peculiarities it is of considerable interest to discover if the afferent innervation of outer hair cells is functional at any frequency of auditory stimulation.

In conclusion it seems that the outer hair cells are predominantly responsible for generating the extracellular CM, and inner hair cells generate the extracellular summating potential. Thus we are in agreement with Dallos and Cheatham (1976) who first put forward this proposition based on extracellular receptor potential recordings from normal cochleae and in cochleae where the outer hair cells had been selectively destroyed by ototoxic poisoning.

Inner hair cells respond to basilar membrane velocity

The electronmicroscopical observations by Kimura (1966) and Lim (1972) which indicate that the stereocilia of outer hair cells are attached to the tectorial membrane, while the stereocilia of inner hair cells are not, has received support from electrophysiological studies in the cochlea of normal guinea pigs, and in guinea pigs whose outer hair cells were destroyed by treatment with kanamycin, an ototoxic agent. Dallos, Billone, Durrant, Wang and Raynor (1972) recorded CM differentially across the basilar membrane in different turns of the cochlea while producing trapezoidal movements of the basilar membrane by displacing the stapes with a low frequency triangular oscillation (since it has been established that basilar membrane motion in the guinea pig is proportional to stapes velocity—Dallos, 1970; Wilson and Johnstone, 1975). In those regions of the cochlea in which the outer hair cells remained undamaged by the kanamycin treatment, the CM reflected the basilar membrane displacement, and the potential waveforms were trapezoidal, while in other regions, usually the basal, high frequency regions, where only inner hair cells remained, the CM was reduced and its waveform reflected the differential or velocity of basilar membrane motion. The response of the inner hair cells to basilar membrane velocity was determined by comparing the amplitude and phase of CM recorded from regions of the basilar membrane devoid of outer hair cells and in normal cochleae in response to sinusoidal stimulation (Dallos, 1973). It was found that in kanamycin-poisoned animals, the sensitivity of the CM increased at a rate which was 6dB/octave faster than in normal animals over the range 100–500 Hz, and at 100 Hz, the phase led normal CM by 90°. This phase lead was not sustained however, and fell to about 45° for the frequency range 300–2000 Hz. On the basis of these observations Dallos *et al.* proposed that inner hair cells responded to basilar membrane velocity while outer hair cells responded to basilar membrane displacement.

One objection to these experiments is that the responses of the inner

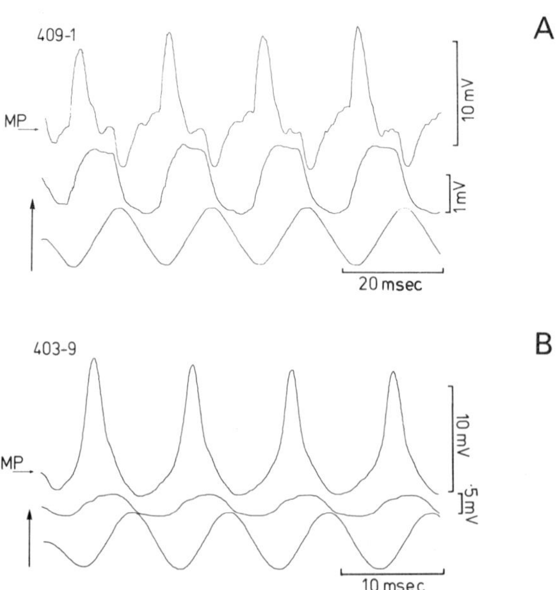

Figure 6 Receptor potentials recorded intracellularly from inner hair cells in the basal turn of the guinea pig cochlea in response to a 52 Hz triangular acoustic stimulus at 100dB SPL (A) and (B) a 102 Hz sinusoidal tone at 80dB SPL. In both records, upper trace: receptor potential; middle trace: CM recorded adjacent to the recording site; lower trace: sound pressure recorded at tympanic membrane. MP indicates membrane potential, −40 mV, −30 mV. Arrows in bottom trace indicate direction of rarefaction. Sound intensities in dB are 2×10^{-5} Nm^{-2}.

hair cells to basilar membrane velocity, in those regions denuded of outer hair cells by kanamycin, is a product of experimental manipulation and not the normal response. An attempt was made to avoid this criticism by making intracellular recordings from inner hair cells and comparing their receptor potentials with the extracellularly recorded CM during sinusoidal and trapezoidal stimulation of the basilar membrane (Sellick and Russell, 1980; Russell and Sellick, 1980).

The receptor potential recorded intracellularly from an inner hair cell, and the CM recorded from a gross electrode in the scala tympani, in response to triangular sound pressure variations are illustrated in Fig. 6 (top). The trapezoidal shape of the CM indicates a response to the first derivative of the sound pressure variation, i.e. to the basilar membrane displacement, whereas the inner hair cell receptor potential is clearly the second differential of the sound pressure, indicating that it is proportional to basilar membrane velocity. The inner hair cell potentials are characteristically rectified and they also apparently respond to basilar membrane velocity during sinusoidal stimulation (Fig. 6, bottom).

The phase and amplitude of the inner hair cell receptor potentials were measured to discover if the inner hair cells responded to basilar membrane velocity over the frequency range 20–4000 Hz. It was anticipated that the intracellular potentials would be delayed and attenuated by the electrical time constants of the hair cell membranes and these were measured and taken into account in the calculation of the phase and amplitude relations of the receptor potentials.

The amplitude characteristics of the receptor potential for a cell with a measured time constant of 0.22 ms (3dB point 723 Hz) are illustrated in Fig. 7. Over the frequency range 28–300 Hz, the receptor potential amplitude increases at 12dB/octave, while the CM increases at 6dB/octave. This is to be expected if the receptor potential is proportional to basilar membrane velocity, and the CM is proportional to displacement. Above 300 Hz, the amplitude of the receptor potential reaches a plateau and then declines at 12dB/octave. These relationships become more apparent if the ratio of the receptor potential amplitude and CM is plotted with respect to frequency, since the results are then standardized for constant stapes velocity.

This is illustrated in Fig. 8 where the relationship between the ratio of AC : CM versus frequency may be approximated as a plateau between 300–700 Hz with rising and falling slopes of 6dB/octave. If the receptor potential/CM ratio is corrected for the decrement of the receptor potential produced by the hair cell time constant, the resulting curve has the characteristics of a high pass filter with a 3dB point close to 200 Hz. One interpretation of these results is that the rising slope of the curve represents the velocity response of the hair cell, at 200 Hz the hair cell begins to respond to basilar membrane displacement, and at 700 Hz and

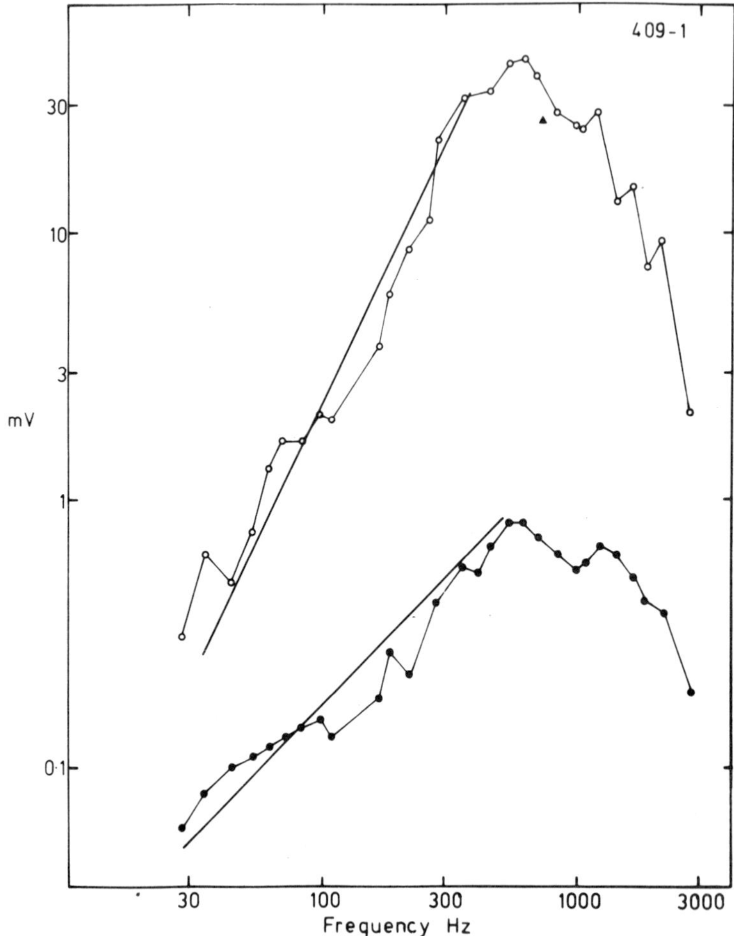

Figure 7 The relationships between the amplitude of the IHC intracellular receptor potential and CM versus frequency for constant SPL at 80dB SPL. ○ and ● indicate the amplitude of the receptor potential and CM respectively. The lines on the upper and lower curves indicate 12 and 6dB/octave slopes respectively. ▲ indicates the cut-off frequency, determined from the electrical time constant, of the hair cell (reprinted from Sellick and Russell, 1980).

above the phasic component of the receptor potential is attenuated by the capacitative impedance of the hair cell membrane. This interpretation is also supported by analysis of the phase differences between the receptor potential and sound pressure measured at the tympanic membrane and the CM (Sellick and Russell, 1980; Russell and Sellick, 1980).

Analysis of the phase and amplitude characteristics of the IHC receptor potential indicate that for the hair cell illustrated, the receptor potential is

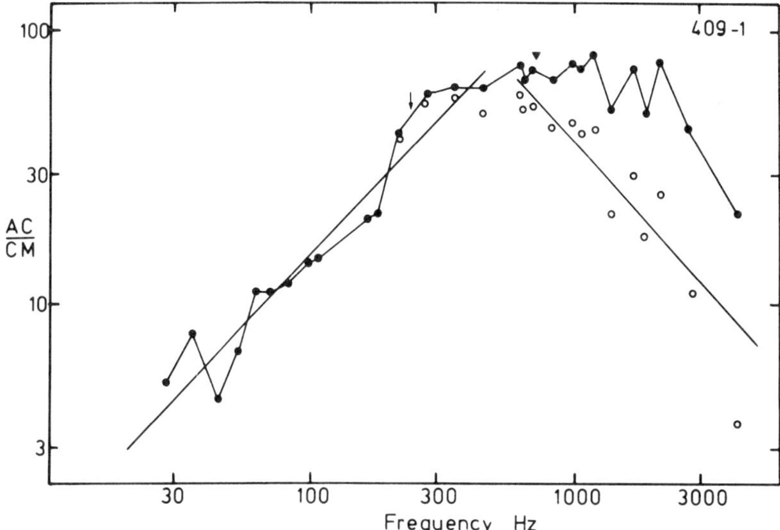

Figure 8 The relationship between the ratio of IHC receptor potential and CM versus frequency for the hair cell illustrated in Fig. 7. The arrow indicates the 3dB point of the mechanical high pass filter and ▼ indicates the cut-off frequency of the hair cell determined from the electrical time constant. ○: raw data; ●: data corrected for membrane time constant. Rising and falling lines represent slopes of 6dB/octave (reprinted from Sellick and Russell, 1980).

proportional to basilar membrane velocity below 200 Hz, and above this, it behaves as a displacement detector. This process has the characteristics of a high pass filter, and in each cochlea the points at which the hair cells change their response from basilar membrane velocity to displacement are remarkably similar, although the measurements of membrane time constant may vary considerably in different cells.

These intracellularly recorded responses are in agreement with Dallos *et al.*'s (1972) notion that IHCs respond to basilar membrane velocity but only below about 200 Hz. Above this frequency the IHC cilia become entrained to basilar membrane displacement.

Thus, evidence from our experiments would suggest that outer hair cells are excited by the shear displacement between the basilar and tectorial membranes, while the inner hair cells respond to fluid movements in the subtectorial space. In other words, inner and outer hair cells respond to different products of basilar membrane vibration.

The fluid coupling of the inner hair cell stereocilia may have a protective role, preventing them from being biased by sustained, large amplitude displacements of the basilar membrane. Protection against biasing is important for the function of the IHCs at high frequencies when the AC component of the receptor potential is very small and transmitter release, from the afferent synapse, is governed by the DC component. This is a product of the asymmetrical transfer function of the hair cell and it is important that the operating point of the hair cell remains at a point of inflection on the transfer function so that a rectified receptor potential and, consequently, a DC component is produced.

The special environment of hair cells and speculations about its role

The hair cells of acoustico-lateralis receptors are located in epithelia which separate fluids of different ionic composition. The apical surfaces of the hair cells face endolymph which is rich in K^+, while the innervated basal and lateral membranes face perilymph which is similar in ionic composition to other extracellular fluids (Smith, Lowry and Wu, 1954; Russell and Sellick, 1976; Peterson, Frischkopf, Lechene, Oman and Weiss, 1978). The high potassium concentrations are maintained by metabolically labile electrogenic pumps which are believed to be located in supporting cells of the sensory epithelium or in specialized cells adjacent to it, e.g. the stria vascularis of the cochlea. In the cochlea (see Sellick and Johnstone, 1975 for a review) and lateral line organs of *Xenopus* (Russell and Sellick, 1976) the electrogenic pumps cause a positive potential adjacent to the apical surface of the hair cell of +80 mV and +50 mV in the scala media and cupulae respectively. However, in other acoustico-lateralis receptors, notably the vestibular and auditory systems of lower vertebrates (Corey and Hudspeth, 1979; Peterson *et al.*, 1978) this potential is absent or very small.

What is the functional significance of this special ionic and electrical environment, and how might it influence the properties of the hair cells?

The presence of high K^+ concentrations adjacent to the sensory epithelium of the hair cell and a positive driving force for this ion across the apical membranes of these cells has led to the proposal that K^+ carries the receptor current in hair cells of the cochlea and the vestibular and lateral line systems (Sellick and Johnstone, 1975; Russell and Sellick, 1976). The use of K^+ to carry the receptor current in hair cells has considerable functional significance principally because it places no special energy demands on the hair cells. The energy necessary for creating the electrochemical gradient for K^+ across the apical membranes of the hair cells is provided by the supporting cells. Moreover, no energy is expended in removing the K^+, which might be expected to accumulate in the cytoplasm of the hair cells during transduction. K^+ will flow down the naturally occurring concentration gradient at the basilateral surfaces of the hair cell which are exposed to Na^+-rich perilymph or extracellular fluid.

Thus hair cells are not subject to the type of sensory adaptation found in other receptors, e.g. crustacean stretch receptors (Nakajima and Onodera, 1969) in which the receptor current is carried by cations which are not normally accumulated in the cytoplasm. The switching on of electrogenic pumps to rid the cell of excess cations causes a hyperpolarization of the membrane potential and sensory adaptation.

The conductance change associated with the transduction process is not selective for K^+ and receptor potentials have been recorded from the sensory epithelia of the sacculus in goldfish (Matsuura, Ikeda and Furukawa, 1971), and the sacculus in the frog (Hudspeth and Corey, 1977) when the hair cells were exposed to sodium rich perilymph instead of their normal potassium rich micro-environments. These observations have been confirmed in voltage clamp and ion substitution studies on the nature of the conductance change associated with transduction in hair cells of the frog sacculus by Corey and Hudspeth (1979). They find that the conductance change is non-selective, and the conductance channel is at least as large as, and resembles, the non-specific acetylcholine-activated channel of the motor end plate which has an internal diameter of 0.65 nM (Dwyer, Adams and Hille, 1979).

It has been proposed that the role of the endocochlear potential and the endocupular potential of lateral line receptors is to provide a positive driving force for K^+ across the apical surface of the hair cell (Sellick and Johnstone, 1975; Russell and Sellick, 1976) and that the size of the larger driving force for the receptor current in the cochlea may, in part, account for the remarkable sensitivity of the hair cells. However, the endocupular potential may have an important role in regulating the electrical excitability of the hair cells, and consequently their sensitivity.

In a recent paper, Corey and Hudspeth (1979) have observed that the resistances of hair cells in the frog sacculus (normally 200–300 MΩ) drop to 6–7 MΩ when the hair cells are depolarized from −60 mV to −50 mV. They attribute this delayed rectification to a voltage-dependent K^+ conductance since it is largely abolished by the presence of 3,4-diaminopyridine (Meves and Pichon, 1977). Because of this delayed rectification, a receptor current which generates a receptor potential of 20 mV in a hair cell of the frog sacculus at a resting potential of −60 mV, produces a receptor potential of only 0.5 mV at a resting potential of −40 mV. It may be that latent voltage-dependent conductances exist in the sensory membranes of cochlear hair cells. If so, then one role of the endocochlear potential may be to hyperpolarize the sensory membrane to levels where their slope conductances are very steep. Thus small changes in receptor current would result in the relatively large receptor potentials which have been seen in cochlear hair cells.

The positive, potassium rich microenvironment which tends to hyperpolarize the sensory membrane, will also tend to depolarize the basal presynaptic membrane of the hair cell. Moreover, it is probably this depolarization which is responsible for the steady release of afferent transmitter which is manifested as the spontaneous, excitatory, postsynaptic potentials and afferent impulses that have been recorded from afferent nerve terminals in the cochlea (Russell and Sellick, unpublished), and elsewhere in the acoustico-lateralis system (Flock and Russell, 1973; Sand *et al.*, 1975; Furukawa and Ishii, 1967). The spontaneous release of transmitter also increases the sensitivity of the afferent fibres to mechanical stimulation. For example the relationship between the presynaptic and postsynaptic potentials at the classical squid giant synapse is sigmoidal (Katz and Miledi, 1971), so that for small levels of presynaptic depolarization, the resulting postsynaptic depolarization is disproportionately small. The release of transmitter at the hair cell synapse in the absence of sensory input represents a shift of the operating point of the synapse along the presynaptic voltage axis so that it is operating in a steeper part of the input–output function. Unlike the afferent synapses of

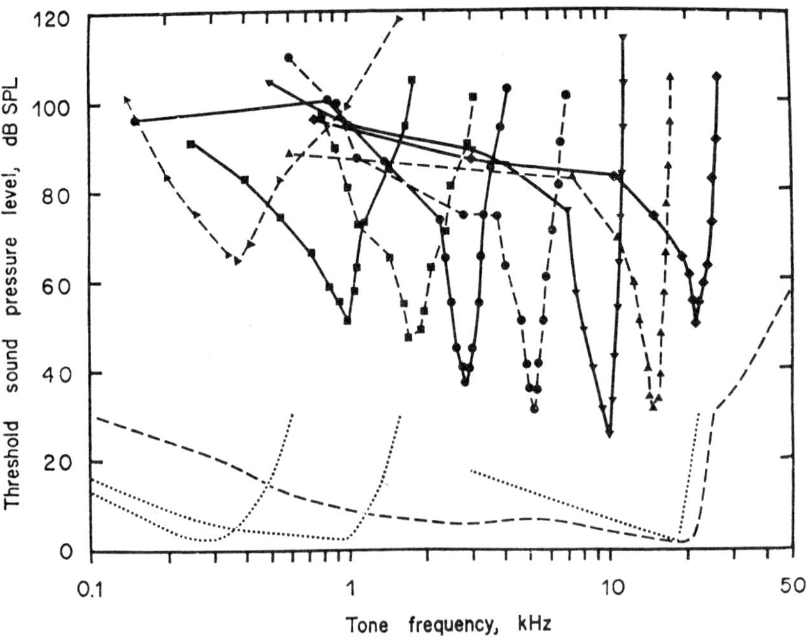

Figure 9 The curves through the data points are frequency threshold curves obtained from the auditory nerve of the guinea pig. These fibres have very sharply defined characteristic frequencies as compared with the isoresponse curves for the basilar membrane shown below. Lower dotted curves: analogous curves derived from the measurements of the vibration amplitude of the guinea pig basilar membrane by von Bekesy (1944) (curves with radius at 0.3 and 0.95 kHz); by Johnstone, Taylor and Boyle (1970) (dotted line with radius at 20 kHz); and by Wilson and Johnstone (dashed curve with radius at 20 kHz) (reprinted from Evans, 1975).

some electroreceptors (Bennett, 1976) the slope of the presynaptic–postsynaptic voltage relationship may not be very steep. In cochlear hair cells the threshold for neural excitation in the afferent fibres seems to be associated with a hair cell depolarization of about 2 mV (Russell and Sellick, 1978).

The frequency responses of inner hair cells

Perhaps the most interesting problem in auditory physiology is the discrepancy between the frequency selectivity of the basilar membrane motion and that of the auditory nerve fibres. This is illustrated in Fig. 9, based on a paper by Evans (1975). It depicts isoresponse curves for basilar membrane motion measured in different turns of the cochlea, and for different afferent fibres. The curves represent the stimulus intensity required to obtain a particular amplitude of basilar membrane vibration or neural discharge rate whose values are arbitrarily determined. There are clear differences between the frequency selectivity of the basilar

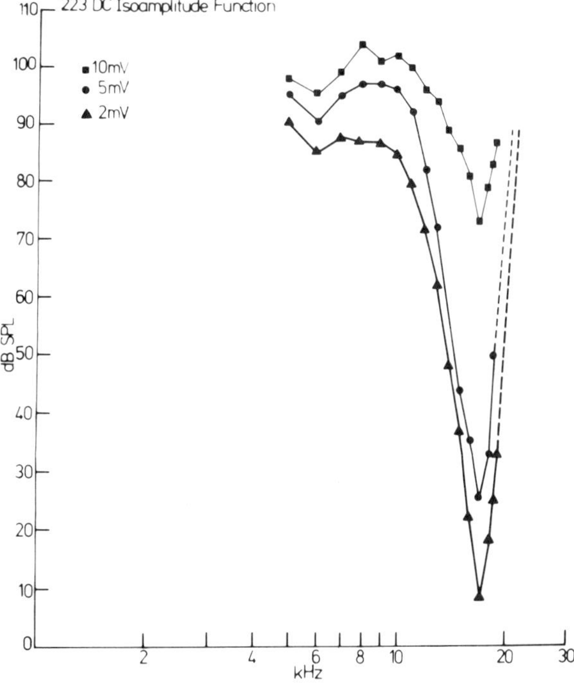

Figure 10 Isoamplitude curve for the DC component of an inner hair cell in the basal turn of the guinea pig cochlea (reprinted from Russell and Sellick, 1978).

membrane motion and responses of the auditory nerve fibres, differences which have led to considerable speculation. The location of the sharpening process has been somewhat obscured by the fact that the extracellular CM, which represents the responses of the hair cells, is broadly tuned and resembles the frequency selectivity of the basilar membrane motion (Yates and Johnstone, 1976). However, it was proposed by Dallos and Cheatham (1976) that CM is dominated by the responses of the outer hair cells, a view now supported by intracellular recordings from cochlear hair cells (Russell and Sellick, 1980). The vast majority of afferent fibres in the mammalian cochlea innervate inner hair cells. In view of this, the frequency selectivity of inner hair cells was determined as a first step towards investigating the basis for the sharply defined characteristic frequencies of the auditory fibres (Russell and Sellick, 1977, 1978). An example of the frequency tuning curve for a single inner hair cell is illustrated in Fig. 9, and shows that the threshold response curves of primary auditory fibres, and iso response curves of hair cells are remarkably similar. This discovery indicated that the sharply defined frequency characteristics are due to mechanisms present in the inner hair cells or between the basilar membrane vibration and the process of transduction in the inner hair cells, namely in the micromechanics of the subtectorial space.

The role of outer hair cells in the frequency selective mechanism of the cochlea remains obscure. Their apparently broad frequency characteristics (Dallos, 1973; Russell and Sellick, in preparation) may be due to their different mechanical coupling to basilar membrane vibration. Namely that they respond to the relative shear displacement between the basilar and tectorial membranes while inner hair cells respond to fluid movements in the subtectorial space. However, the role of outer hair cells in the frequency selective process is important in controlling the mechanical input to the inner hair cells. Destruction of outer hair cells by ototoxic poisoning causes loss of threshold and frequency selectivity in auditory nerve fibres (Dallos, Ryan, Harris, McGee and Ozademar, 1977; Evans and Harrison, 1976).

An electrical tuning mechanism, based on the individual properties of hair cells, has been proposed for hair cells in the turtle cochlea (Fettiplace and Crawfurd, 1978, 1980). However, voltage dependent conductances have yet to be sought in hair cells of the mammalian cochlea. Moreover, any tuning mechanism which is based on individual differences between inner hair cells has to cope with the enormous frequency range in the mammalian cochlea.

Acknowledgements

Work reviewed in this paper was done jointly with Peter Sellick, to whom I am indebted, and experiments illustrated in Figs. 2 and 3 were done in collaboration with Dr. Mike Merzenich. This research was supported by a grant from the MRC.

REFERENCES

Bekesy, G. von (1960) in *Experiments in hearing* (ed. Wever, E. G.) McGraw-Hill, New York.

Bennett, M. V. L. (1976) "Transmission at receptor synapses" in *Mechanisms in transmission of signals for conscious behaviour* (ed. Desiraju, T.) Elsevier, Amsterdam, 345–366.

Bredberg, G., Ades, H. W. and Engström, H. (1972) Scanning electromicroscopy of the normal and pathologically altered organ of Corti *Acta Otolaryngol.* Suppl., **301**, 3.

Corey, D. P. and Hudspeth, A. J. (1979) Ionic basis of the receptor potential in a vertebrate hair cell *Nature*, **281**, 675–677.

Dallos, P. (1970) Low frequency auditory characteristics: species dependence *J. Acoust. Soc. Am.*, **48**, 489–499.

Dallos, P. (1973) "Cochlear potentials and cochlear mechanics" in *Basic mechanisms in hearing* (ed. Møller, A.) Academic Press, New York, London, 335–376.

Dallos, P., Billone, M. C., Durrant, J. D., Wang, C-y. and Raynor, S. (1972) Cochlear inner and outer hair cells: functional differences *Science*, **177**, 356–358.

Dallos, P. and Cheatham, M. A. (1976) Production of cochlear potentials by inner and outer hair cells *J. Acoust. Soc. Am.*, **60**, 510–512.

Dallos, P., Ryan, A., Harris, D., McGee, T. and Ozademar, O. (1977) "Cochlear frequency selectivity in the presence of hair cell damage" in *Psychophysics & Physiology of Hearing* (ed. Evans, E. F., Wilson, J. P.) Academic Press, New York, London, 249–261.

Davis, H. (1965) A model for transducer action in the cochlea *Cold Spring Harbor Symp. Quant. Biol.*, **30**, 181–190.

Dwyer, T. M., Adams, D. J. and Hille, B. (1979) Ionic selectivity of end-plate channels *Biophys. J.*, **25**, 67a.

Engström, H. and Engström, B. (1978) Structures of the hairs on cochlear sensory cells *Hearing Res.*, **1**, 49–66.

Evans, E. F. (1975) The sharpening of cochlear frequency selectivity in the normal and abnormal cochlea *Audiology*, **14**, 419–442.

Evans, E. F. and Harrison, R. V. (1976) Correlation between cochlear outer hair cell damage and deterioration of cochlear nerve tuning properties in the guinea pig *J. Physiol.*, **256**, 43–44.

Fettiplace, R. and Crawfurd, A. C. (1978) The coding of sound pressure and frequency in cochlear hair cells of the terrapin *Proc. R. Soc. Lond. B*, **203**, 209–218.

Fettiplace, R. and Crawfurd, A. C. (1980) The origin of tuning in turtle cochlear hair cells *Hearing Res.* (in press).

Flock, A. (1971) "Sensory transduction in hair cells" in *Handbook of Sensory Physiology*, Vol. 1 (ed. Loewenstein, W.) Springer, Berlin, 396–441.

Flock, A. and Cheung, H. C. (1977) Actin filaments in sensory hairs of inner ear receptor cells *J. Cell. Biol.*, **75**, 339–343.

Flock, A., Flock, B. and Murray, E. (1977) Studies on the sensory hairs of receptor cells in the inner ear *Acta Otolaryngol.*, **83**, 85–91.

Flock, A. and Russell, I. J. (1973) Efferent nerve fibres: postsynaptic action on hair cells *Nature*, **243**, 89–91.

Flock, A. and Russell, I. J. (1976) Inhibition by efferent nerve fibres: action on hair cells and afferent synaptic transmission in the lateral line canal organ of the Burbot, *Lota lota J. Physiol.*, **257**, 45–62.

Furukawa, T. and Ishii, Y. (1967) Neurophysiological studies on hearing in goldfish *J. Neurophys.*, **30**, 1377–1403.

Harris, G. (1968) Brownian motion in the cochlear partition *J. Acoust. Soc. Am.*, **44**, 176–186.

Hudspeth, A. J. and Corey, D. P. (1977) Sensitivity, polarity and conductance changes in the response of vertebrate hair cells to controlled mechanical stimuli *Proc. Nat. Acad. Sci.*, **74**, 2407–2411.

Hudspeth, A. J. and Jacobs, R. (1979) Stereocilia mediate transduction in vertebrate hair cells *Proc. Nat. Acad. Sci.*, **76**, 1506–1509.

Johnstone, B. M. and Boyle, A. J. F. (1967) Basilar membrane vibration examined with the Mössbauer technique *Science*, **158**, 389–390.

Katz, B. (1969) *The release of neural transmitter substances* Liverpool University Press, Liverpool.

Katz, B. and Miledi, R. (1971) The effect of prolonged depolarization on synaptic transfer in the stellate ganglion of the squid *J. Physiol.*, **216**, 503–512.

Kimura, R. S. (1966) Hairs of the cochlear sensory cells and their attachment to the tectorial membrane *Acta Otolaryngol.*, **61**, 55–72.

Kroese, A. B. A. and van der Berken, J. (1980) Dual action of ototoxic antibiotics on sensory hair cells *Nature*, **283**, 395–397.

Lim, D. J. (1972) Fine morphology of the tectorial membrane *Arch. Otolaryngol.*, **96**, 199–215.

Macartney, J. C., Comis, S. D. and Pickles, J. O. (1980) Myosin in the cochlea—a basis for active motility *Nature* (in press).

Matsuura, S., Ikeda, K. and Furukawa, T. (1971) Effects of Na^+, K^+ and ouabain on microphonic potentials of the goldfish inner ear *Jap. J. Physiol.*, **21**, 563.

Meves, H. and Pichon, Y. (1977) The effect of internal and external 4-aminopyridine on the potassium currents in intracellularly perfused squid giant axons *J. Physiol.*, **268**, 511–532.

Mooseker, M. S. (1975) Brush border motility *J. Cell. Biol.*, **71**, 417–433.

Mooseker, M. S. and Tilney, L. G. (1975) Organization of an actin filament membrane complex *J. Cell. Biol.*, **67**, 725–743.

Nakajima, S. and Onodera, K. (1969) Adaptation of the generator potential in crayfish stretch receptors under constant length and constant tension *J. Physiol.*, **200**, 187–204.

Peterson, S. K., Frischkopf, L. S., Lechene, C., Oman, C. M. and Weiss, T. F. (1978) Element composition of inner ear lymphs in cats, lizards and skates by electron probe micro-analysis of liquid samples *J. comp. Physiol.*, **126**, 1–14.

Pujol, R. and Abonnene, M. (1977) Receptor maturation and synaptogenesis in the golden hamster cochlea *Arch. Oto-Rhino-Laryng.*, **217**, 1–12.

Rhode, W. S. (1971) Observations of the vibration of the basilar membrane in squirrel monkeys using the Mössbauer technique *J. acoust. Soc. Amer.*, **49**, 1218–1231.

Rose, J. E., Brugge, J. F., Anderson, D. J. and Hind, J. E. (1968) "Patterns of activity in single auditory nerve fibres of the squirrel monkey" in *Hearing mechanisms in vertebrates* (ed. de Reuck, A. V. S., Night, J.) Churchill, London, 144–156.

Russell, I. J. (1980) "The responses of vertebrate hair cells to mechanical stimulation" in *Neurones without Impulses* (ed. Bush, B., Roberts, A.) Cambridge University Press (in press).

Russell, I. J. and Sellick, P. M. (1976) Measurement of potassium and chloride ion concentrations in the cupulae of the lateral lines of *Xenopus laevis J. Physiol.*, **257**, 245–255.

Russell, I. J. and Sellick, P. M. (1977) Tuning properties of cochlear hair cells *Nature*, **267**, 858–860.

Russell, I. J. and Sellick, P. M. (1978) Intracellular studies of hair cells in the mammalian cochlea *J. Physiol.*, **284**, 261–290.

Russell, I. J. and Sellick, P. M. (1980) The responses of inner hair cells to low frequency auditory stimulation in the guinea pig cochlea (in preparation).

Sand, P., Ozawa, S. and Hagiwara, S. (1975) Electrical and mechanical stimulation of hair cells in the mudpuppy *J. Comp. Physiol. A*, **102**, 13–26.

Sellick, P. M. and Johnstone, B. M. (1975) Productions and role of inner ear fluid *Prog. Neurobiology*, **5**, Part 1.

Sellick, P. M. and Russell, I. J. (1980) The responses of inner hair cells to basilar membrane velocity during low frequency auditory stimulation in the guinea pig cochlea *J. Hearing Res.* (in press).

Smith, C. A. (1975) "The inner ear: its embryological development and microstructure" in *The Nervous System*, Vol. **3**: *Human communication and its disorders* (ed. Tower, D. B.) Raven Press, New York, 1–18.

Smith, C. A., Lowry, O. H. and Wu, M. L. (1954) The electrolytes of the labyrinthine fluids *The Laryngoscope*, **64**, 141–153.

Spoendlin, H. (1970) "Auditory, vestibular, olfactory and gustatory organs" in *Ultrastructure of the peripheral nervous system and sense organs* (ed. Bischoff, A.) G. Thieme, Stuttgart, 173–263.

Spoendlin, H. (1978) "The afferent innervation of the cochlea" in *Evoked electrical activity in the auditory nervous system* (ed. Naunton, R. F., Fernandez, C.) Academic Press, NewYork, San Francisco, London, 21–42.

Tanaka, Y., Asanurna, A. and Yanagisawa, T. (1980) Potentials of outer hair cells and their membrane properties in cationic environments *Hearing Research* (in press).

Wersäll, J., Björkroth, B., Flock, A. and Lundquist, P. G. (1973) Experiments on ototoxic effects of antibiotics *Adv. Otorhinolaryngol.*, **20**, 14.

Wilson, J. P. and Johnstone, J. R. (1975) Basilar membrane and middle ear vibration in guinea pig measured by capacitative probes *J. Acoust. Soc. Am.*, **57**, 705–723.

Yates, G. K. and Johnstone, B. M. (1976) Localized cochlear microphonics recorded from the spiral lamina *J. Acoust. Soc. Am.*, **59**, 476–479.

CHAPTER SIX

CHEMORECEPTORS: THEIR STRUCTURE AND FUNCTION

J. BOECKH

Introduction

Basic functional characteristics of chemoreceptors are already found at the level of unicellular organisms such as bacteria and protozoa. It is well known for instance that *Escherichia coli* can detect and discriminate amongst a variety of chemical stimuli with high sensitivity and accuracy. Attractive stimuli (amino acids or carbohydrates) that indicate valuable nutrients are distinguished from repellents, which enables *E. coli* to avoid a source of noxious material by moving away from it (Adler, 1974). Apparently, devices for transmembrane transport serve as receptors for such substances, which can be regarded as chemical stimuli. Via an intracellular chain of reactions the receptors influence the movements of the flagella which drive the organism forward or backward. *E. coli* bacteria detect amino acids at concentrations of 10^{-8} M, and they respond to differences in concentration as low as 1 in 10^4 over a distance of 2 μm, which is the length of the bacterium (Koshland, 1974).

In higher organisms, especially in the eumetazoa, specialized organs are found which serve as detectors for chemical stimuli in the outside world. Their structure and function will be the topic of this review. They are involved in many vitally important functions such as detection and investigation of food, investigation of the environment and especially the habitat, finding partners for reproduction and detection of their readiness to reproduce, and communication by means of chemical signals (pheromones) between sexual and social partners. Other chemo-detective devices like hormone receptors, postsynaptic receptors, or the internal chemoreceptors monitoring CO_2 content or pH of the body fluid, will not be considered.

Morphology of chemosensory organs and their receptor cells

Among soft-bodied invertebrates, the chemoreceptive organs of molluscs have been closely investigated. A variety of organs have been described, consisting of groups or scattered individual receptor cells on tentacles, rhinophores and in the osphradium of gastropods whilst certain cells in the suckers and the olfactory pit of cephalopods are also believed to serve as chemoreceptors (Graziadei, 1964; Kohn, 1961; Wells *et al.*, 1965; Bailey and Laverack, 1966; Jahan-Parwar, 1972, 1977). At present the data obtained for this group of animals are only of moderate significance in establishing general concepts of chemoreceptor processes.

The situation is different in arthropods, especially insects, where abundant data exist on the structure and function of chemoreceptors. Chemical sense organs of arthropods have been investigated for more than 100 years. Most of these organs occur as *sensilla*, which are cuticular hairs, pegs or plates on the surface or in pits on the antennae, mouthparts and other body appendages. An extensive review on the subject is given by Altner and Prillinger (1980). Each sensillum is supplied with one, a few, or even several hundreds of sensory cells which are located underneath the cuticle. Their dendrites run towards the hair lumen within a cuticular sheath, and they are subdivided into an inner and an outer segment by a neck which contains a ciliary structure of nine peripheral pairs of tubules. The outer segments sometimes divide up into many fine branches. In contact chemoreceptive sensilla the terminal tip of the sensillum is perforated by a pore through which the dendrites are exposed to the exterior. Olfactory hairs and plates of insects have numerous pores or slits in the sensillum wall which provide channels for molecules to penetrate towards the dendrites. The number of chemoreceptor cells in the whole animal can reach hundreds of thousands. A honeybee antenna or a maxillary palp of a cockroach is densely covered with sensilla, and the receptor cells do not fit side by side into a hypodermical layer underneath, but instead form sac-like protrusions in the inner haemolymph space. In certain moths, the antennae, together with their side branches, are covered with long trichoid sensilla which form a net with a mesh width of about 10–20 μm (Steinbrecht, 1971). An odour molecule in an air current flowing through this lattice is nearly 100% likely to hit the cuticular surface of the antenna where it can be adsorbed and rapidly transported towards the pores in the hair walls by means of a two-dimensional diffusion along the cuticle (Adam and Delbrück, 1968). In this way a male silk moth filters literally all the molecules of female sexual attractant from an air stream passing through the cross section of his antennae (Kaissling and Priesner, 1970). Whether the properties of the cuticle or the substances filling the pores in the hair walls influence the approach of molecules to the receptor dendrites is still a matter of speculation.

In vertebrates an olfactory epithelium is found in the nasal cavity which is ventilated by respiratory movements. The distal portions of the receptor cells are generally equipped with cilia or microvilli. A vomeronasal organ with an opening to the oral cavity is densely packed with receptor cells which again show numerous microvilli. In mammals this organ is "ventilated" by means of a pump which sucks fluid and dissolved odour molecules into the lumen of the organ. Snakes are believed to "catch" odour molecules by darting the tongue out of the mouth and drawing them into the cavity of the organ. The receptor cells of the olfactory and the vomeronasal epithelium send their axons into the glomeruli of the olfactory bulb and the accessory bulb respectively. For more extensive reviews of this subject see Graziadei (1973, 1975), and Altner and Kolnberger (1975). Chemoreceptor cells without axons, the taste cells, are found in taste buds which are distributed over the tongue and the oral cavity of vertebrates. In certain fish they are found in abundance on the body surface, especially on the barbels of catfish (Atema, 1971). A taste bud consists of supporting cells and up to 50 sensory cells. The distal portions of the sensory cells carry microvilli, and they are exposed to the surface of the tongue via a small common pore. The receptor cells are innervated by afferent axons of the facial and the glossopharyngeal nerves which run into the brain stem. This subject is reviewed by Bradley (1971), Murray (1971, 1973), Graziadei (1975), and Sato (1980).

Both olfactory as well as taste cells of vertebrates undergo continual replacement. Receptor cells in mammalian taste buds have a lifetime of only a few days (Beidler and Smallman, 1965; Graziadei and Metcalf, 1975; Graziadei and Monti-Graziadei, 1978). The epithelial formations of olfactory and taste cells permit access by stimulus molecules probably only at the distal portions of the receptor cells (Kerjaschki, 1977). Here the surface of the receptor cells is greatly enlarged by microvilli and cilia. However, it is not yet clear whether these structures are required for the sensory process, as there are reports that olfactory cells without cilia still function as receptors (Tucker, 1967). The epithelia are covered with mucous fluids which certainly play a role as solvents for the stimuli which (as in olfaction) reach the receptors in aqueous solution. It has even been hypothesized that the mucous layer serves as a chromatographic layer, in which compounds are transported at different speeds, according to their physicochemical properties, along the surface of the olfactory epithelium (Mozell, 1970). It should also not be forgotten that free nerve endings of the trigeminal and vagal nerves very probably function as chemoreceptors in the nasal and the pharyngeal cavities (Tucker, 1971).

Reactions and reaction ranges of chemoreceptor cells

The first detectable event after the impact of a stimulus at the receptor cell is a conductance change in the dendritic membrane, which can be recorded as a receptor potential. In some insect sensilla a supporting battery is provided for the receptor current by a transepithelial potential between the peridendritic space and the haemolymph space on the other side of the basal lamina. This potential results from ionic transport out of supporting cells into the peridendritic space. The supporting cells are the trichogen and the tormogen cells which produce the hair shaft and the socket of the hair during ontogenesis (Thurm, 1974). At a generator region near the receptor cell soma the receptor current gives rise to nerve impulses which are conducted to the central nervous system. Impulses in afferent fibres of taste nerves are elicited by synaptic transmission between receptor cells in the taste buds and the fibres.

The time course of the response is in many cases phasic-tonic. Often, the plateau rate is decreased continuously during the reaction, so that the activity may cease while the stimulus is still present. Frequently strong adaptation is observed; a second, superimposed or subsequent stimulus evokes a lower amplitude. In the frog olfactory epithelium, inhibition is often observed as well as a superposition of excitatory and inhibitory events, which results in complicated time courses of response (Gesteland *et al.*, 1965; Duchamp *et al.*, 1974). The initial peak excitation is of significance for the perception of stimulus transients. During sniffing or antennal movements sharp on- and offsets of stimuli are produced which in turn result in high changes of excitation. Such rapid changes will also occur when odours are transported by air currents over long distances and arrive not as continuous streams but rather in discontinuous clouds. With steeply rising stimuli insect olfactory (and also taste) cells produce impulse rates of more than 400 for a short time. Vertebrate and mollusc chemoreceptor cells respond at much lower rates.

Dose response characteristics of many chemoreceptor cells are sigmoidal in a semilogarithmic plot. Often the curves rise monophasically, but there are instances where maxima appear at medium intensities while at higher intensities the responses are of lower amplitude. This might be due to overloading of the receptors and fast adaptation or to the way the data are evaluated and plotted. The shape of the curve seems to depend on counting intervals of impulses and the weighing of peak rates etc. (Revial *et al.*, 1978; Seelinger, 1977). Since one does not know the measure which is applied by central neurones to determine afferent excitatory levels, there is no way to decide which plot is more relevant in terms of signal transfer.

Individual cells may cover concentration ranges of up to 4 decadic steps between threshold and saturation. However, summated responses of whole nerves or whole epithelia are reported to follow an increase of the stimulus over 7 or more decadic steps (Tucker, 1963; Caprio, 1975). In these cases the reaction range of the whole organ might be subdivided into smaller domains of intensities each of which is covered by an individual cell population with steep and individually characteristic slopes. Thus a reasonable sensitivity for small differences in intensities is maintained in the single group as well as a broad band of total range in the organ.

Reaction thresholds of individual receptor cells have been demonstrated as low as is physically possible. As long as 20 years ago it was clearly shown in behavioural experiments that dogs and eels can detect odorants at concentrations of 10^3 molecules per cm^3 of medium (Neuhaus, 1956*a*, *b*; Teichmann, 1959). In man very low thresholds are also reported; for instance, for certain mercaptans it is highly probable that individual receptor cells in the human nose respond to the impact of single molecules (Stuiver, 1958). Kaissling was able to demonstrate that male silkmoths react to concentrations of only several hundreds of molecules of female sex attractant per cm^3 of air. At this concentration it is highly improbable that one cell out of the 25 000 total pheromone receptors receives more than one molecule. Thus it can be concluded that a single molecule can trigger a nervous impulse in such a cell (Kaissling and Priesner, 1970). In electrophysiological experiments it has been shown that at threshold concentration 320 odour-induced impulses are superimposed on 3600 spontaneously fired impulses in the whole receptor cell population. This value is just above the theoretically critical value for a detectable signal-to-noise distance ($3 \cdot \sqrt{n}$). Near threshold, the receptors seem to function as molecule counters. One molecule elicits one impulse, two molecules lead to two impulses, etc. With higher concentrations the sigmoid characteristic appears which means that the receptors work on a proportional basis. In the course of the steep part of the curve each tenfold increase in intensity results in a given and constant increase of reaction. From these data it can be concluded that it is the capture of molecules by supporting structures, and the number and density of receptor cells, rather than receptor sensitivity, which determines whether low reaction thresholds of the whole organ can be achieved.

The central machinery of the olfactory system seems in keeping with this performance. The high grade of convergence of receptor cell axons at central neurones in the olfactory bulb of vertebrates and the antennal lobes of insects permits a precise detection of the arrival of odour molecules at the receptor cell level, even if only a small fraction of the receptors was hit. Such a spatial summation of receptor inputs can be shown physiologically in insects, where central neurones respond to stimulation of receptors at different parts of the antenna. In the saturniid moth *Antheraea* about 200 000 receptor cells for female sexual attractant terminate in a certain "macroglomerular complex" of the antennal lobe of the male, where widely branching deutocerebral neurones take up these inputs. At a stimulus concentration where only every hundredth receptor receives a molecule, the central neurone fires reproducibly and safely with considerable numbers of impulses (Boeckh and Boeckh, 1979). A macro-glomerulus with a similar convergence of receptors onto central neurones is also found in the male cockroach (Ernst *et al.*, 1977). Such a performance of the olfactory system of course permits orientation over long distances or detection of minute amounts of molecules during tracking. Receptor cells on the vertebrate tongue and contact chemoreceptors of insects in general need more molecules of "their" stimuli. In aquatic animals such as catfish or lobster, very low "taste" thresholds are reported (for review see Bardach, 1975) which can be as low as 10^{-13} M in the case of littoral crustaceans (Fuzessery and Childress, 1975).

The neural basis of coding of taste and odour quality

There are several theoretical possibilities for a neural code for odour and taste quality. The first works on the principle of labelled lines—for each stimulus type a separate receptor type exists. The second possibility would be a co-operation of receptors or receptor types, in which each stimulus is coded by a characteristic pattern composed of the responses of several receptors. A third way would be to change the time course of the response of a receptor (the temporal pattern). Examples of the third case are found in vertebrates and insects. Frog olfactory receptor cells are known to change the time course of their impulse pattern when stimulated with different compounds (Gesteland *et al.*, 1965; Duchamp *et al.*, 1974). Pheromone receptor cells of the silk moth display characteristically different time courses of receptor potentials and impulse rates when stimulated with the pheromone or certain other substances (Kaissling, 1974). Similar results are reported from chemoreceptors on the antennae of terrestrial isopods (Seelinger, 1977).

Before examples of the first and second possibilities are described, a general remark should be made about the problem of the chemical specificity of chemoreceptor cells. With the exception of CO_2 receptors on the honeybee antenna, no chemoreceptor cell is known which is excited by a single compound only. In all other cases, several substances are effective stimuli, and it is extremely difficult to predict which compounds of the multitude of organic substances might also be effective. When physiologists started to use compounds which are, or might be, constituents of natural chemical stimuli, considerable progress was made in determining adequate stimuli. One prominent example is the work which was done on pheromones and pheromone receptors in insects (for reviews see Kaissling, 1971; Priesner, 1973, 1979). Meanwhile, such highly effective compounds have been found in a number of cases, and it is reasonable to assume that each of these constitutes at least part of the core of the spectrum for the corresponding receptor cell type. In addition to these powerful stimulants, the spectrum for any cell also contains other compounds which are less effective. Whether such a wide band of substances is effective because of a broad tuning of the receptor sites or whether different types of receptor molecules are present in a given cell, is an open question for most cases. Wieczorek (1976) was for instance able to show that more than one receptor site exists on a special type of contact chemoreceptor cell in the larvae of a noctuid moth.

A classical example for chemoreceptor cells working on the basis of labelled lines are the contact chemoreceptors of insects which have been intensively studied especially in blowflies and caterpillars (for reviews see Schoonhoven and Dethier, 1966; Dethier, 1976). In each sensillum of a given morphological type a constant number of receptor cells exists, each cell having its separate and characteristic spectrum. In the blowfly, one cell responds to carbohydrates with certain molecular configurations, such as sucrose (sugar receptor), another cell responds to water, a third and fourth type to anions and cations present in salts such as sodium chloride (salt receptors) (for review see Hansen, 1974). In behavioural experiments it was shown that stimulation of the sugar receptor cell alone elicits a feeding response in a blowfly while stimulation of the salt cell evokes rejection. Amino acid receptor cells in crustaceans seem to belong to a similar type of exclusively tuned receptor cells (Bauer and Hatt, 1980). Most of the pheromone-sensitive receptor cells in insects are also very narrowly tuned and without overlap of spectra. The corresponding stimuli are effective only on this group of receptors, thus being perceived by separate input lines which are not shared by other odorants. Often such cells occur in great numbers (up to 200 000 in certain moths), and all respond uniformly throughout the population. Because of these properties they have been named as "odour specialists" (Schneider *et al.*, 1964). They are very useful for investigations where large numbers of reproducible results are required.

In the honeybee, a prominent species in research on olfaction, the receptor cells are also reported to be grouped in populations with separate spectra. These spectra seem to comprise many compounds, thus the receptors are broadly tuned. Receptor cells within a group might perhaps react differently regarding their preferential sensitivity for certain compounds within the group's spectrum. Also, the slopes of the dose-response curves might vary from one cell to the other. In this way a neural basis would exist not only for a fine discrimination between odours from different group spectra, but also for discrimination between odours within a given group spectrum (Vareschi, 1971).

A well-known case of coding according to the principle of the "across-fibre" pattern is found in the vertebrate taste system. The first recordings from single fibres in the chorda tympani of the rat revealed that nearly every fibre responds to representatives of all four basic taste qualities which have long been known to exist in man: sucrose (for sweet), hydrochloric acid (for sour), sodium chloride (for salty) and quinine hydrochloride (for bitter) (Pfaffmann, 1941, 1955). A similar situation was found with individual receptor cells in taste buds (Kimura and Beidler, 1961). From behavioural and neurophysiological investigations it was concluded that four basic taste qualities exist for many mammals (Nowliss and Frank, 1977). Taste fibres in the chorda tympani and the glosso-pharyngeal nerves respond to representatives of more than one taste quality, so the spectra overlap. However, there is a gross subdivision of the fibres according to their preferential sensitivity to the four basic groups of stimuli. There are "salt best, sugar best, quinine best, and acid best" groups of fibres, the rank order of efficiency for the four groups of stimuli being constant in each fibre type. Thus, each taste stimulus will be effective in more than one fibre type, but according to the relative specificity will be more effective for one type than for others. In this way a characteristic pattern of response across the four types is the code for taste quality, for each stimulus a characteristic profile of responses arises, the height of the profile signalling the stimulus intensity. There are exceptions to this scheme, as for instance in Old World monkeys, where special sugar fibres were detected which respond exclusively to a series of carbohydrates.

Woolston and Erickson (1979) having evaluated a considerable amount of data on gustatory brain stem neurones come to the conclusion that labelled lines do not exist in the gustatory pathway, and that there is no grouping into a limited number of fibre types. They assume that patterns across a great variety of fibres of different preferential sensitivity code for stimulus quality.

In several insects, large populations of sensory cells are subdivided into clearly established types. There is hardly any variation in the preferential sensitivity between individual receptor cells within such a type, and the spectra of the types overlap. Many food odour receptor cells belong to this category, and it might be speculated that even all olfactory cells on an antenna are grouped into a limited number of types which include pheromone sensitive cells as well (Mustaparta, 1975; Kaib, 1974; Sass, 1976, 1979).

In principle, this system of coding seems a reasonable compromise between maximum sensitivity and maximum number of codewords. Many different characteristic patterns of response can be produced from a small number of receptor types if their spectra overlap, and there remains a large enough number of individuals of each type to maintain a high probability for a given molecule to hit an appropriate receptor.

An extreme case of this system seems to be used in the frog olfactory receptor cells (Revial *et al.*, 1978), and in some populations of cells in insect antennae (Schneider *et al.*, 1964; Mustaparta, 1975). There, each receptor cell has its individual and unique odour spectrum which is different from the spectra of all other cells, but which overlaps these other spectra. In such a case the number of codewords is practically unlimited.

In insects, such cells were believed to serve as olfactory receptors in a broader and more general sense than do the highly specialized and narrowly tuned specialists for special stimuli, such as pheromones. Therefore, these have been given the name "odour generalists" (Schneider *et al.*, 1964).

The biological stimulus situation

There is hardly any biologically important chemical stimulus which arrives at the sense organ as a single compound. A caterpillar feeding on a leaf, a carnivore biting a piece of flesh from its prey or a male moth smelling the air around a female are all exposed to at least a few, or even a great many, compounds which in combination make up the complete stimulus (the leaf taste, the flesh taste, the female sexual odour). In some moths, and the American cockroach, the female sex attractant consists of relatively few compounds, each of which is an adequate stimulus for a separate receptor cell type. The complete odour excites all these cell types in a given male (Kochansky *et al.*, 1975; Priesner, 1979). But it is not only the presence of certain compounds which is important. In several genus of saturniid, tortricid, and noctuid moths, the same compounds are used by different species. In these cases, the species-specific mixtures of the compounds are the specific signal (Kochansky *et al.*, 1975; Roelofs, 1979). For species which live together in the same habitat and which do not possess other isolation mechanisms to use against one another, it is of vital interest not only to detect the various components but also their relative amounts. Basically the same holds for the taste receptors of a blowfly or of a caterpillar. In most situations, more than one receptor cell type will be stimulated, because there will be more taste substances in a leaf than simply sucrose. The nervous system decides the overall taste on the basis of activity from many different inputs, which arise in characteristic manner according to the mixture of stimuli present (Dethier, 1973, 1976; Schoonhoven and Dethier, 1966).

In the American cockroach it has been shown that complex odours consisting of many compounds such as those found in different types of fruit or other foodstuffs, again are effective stimuli for a whole collection of receptor types on the antenna. Since many of these compounds occur in more than one type of foodstuff, the pattern of compounds present in different concentration is analysed by the receptors in the following way; each receptor type is excited to a certain degree according to its differential sensitivity to these compounds and according to the relative amount of the different substances. There is no specialized banana- or orange-receptor type; each type of stimulus will evoke a pattern where certain types are more affected than others, thus eliciting a highly characteristic pattern for this odour over a considerable part of the whole receptor population (Sass, 1979). In this way, the odour is analysed for its components and their relative amounts by the receptors.

The central nervous system, which has to interpret these complicated profiles of excitation at the receptor level, does so by comparing the inputs of different receptor types at central neurones. Their output is a result of this process which allows for a specific response not only to the constituents of a complex odour but to the whole odour. This has been shown in the pheromone pathway in two insect species (Boeckh *et al.*, 1977; Boeckh and Boeckh, 1979) and also for some food odour sensitive neurones in the olfactory pathway of *Periplaneta americana* (Boeckh *et al.*, 1976).

Is there evidence for a topographical representation of chemosensory quality?

A gross subdivision of chemosensory input into taste (or contact chemoreception) and olfaction is easily demonstrated in terrestrial vertebrates by the anatomical separation and classification of the sense organs and the corresponding central pathways. Even in fish and tadpoles the taste buds are more concerned with perception of food substances, while the nasal receptors are responsible for long-distance orientation, e.g. in the homing salmon, or in the perception of alarm substances in cyprinid fish (Atema, 1971; Bardach, 1975). In insects, antennae carry not only olfactory sensilla but also contact chemoreceptive organs and on the maxillary palps of cockroaches, olfactory sensilla are found. Here, only the sensillum type is an indication as to whether olfactory or gustatory stimuli are perceived. This subdivision does collapse, however, if one considers the data of Rüth (1975) and Seelinger (1977) who were able to show that receptor cells in sensilla which clearly belong to the contact chemoreceptor type (terminal pore) respond to vapours of "classical" odorous compounds such as fatty acids and alcohols.

A topographical localization of different olfactory quality can be seen in several cases. In the frog nasal epithelium there are regions of preferential sensitivity for certain compounds (Mustaparta, 1971). Spatial distribution of this type was also found in mammals (Costanzo and Mozell, 1976; Thommesen and Døving, 1977). Apparently, receptors with similar response characteristics are assembled in certain regions (Kauer and Moulton, 1974). In the glomerular layer of the olfactory bulb there are also regions where certain odours are especially effective (Pinching and Døving, 1974; Stewart *et al.*, 1979). The axons of receptor cells for female sexual attractants of some moths and cockroaches terminate in special "macroglomerular" regions in the antennal centres. Special groups of neurones take up the information from there and transmit it via separate bundles into higher olfactory centres (see above).

From the evidence described, it therefore appears that chemosensory specificity is reflected by a corresponding anatomical specificity. This conclusion might sound trivial. However, as the result of combined physiological and anatomical investigations, it is of considerable value for a closer approach to the network which is responsible for the evaluation of the chemosensory input data.

REFERENCES

Adam, G. and Delbrück, M. (1968) "Reduction of dimensionality in biological diffusion processes" in *Structural Chemistry and Molecular Biology* (eds. Rich, A., Davidson, N.) Freeman, San Francisco, 198–215.

Adler, J. (1974) "Chemotaxis in Bacteria" in *Biochemistry of Sensory Functions* (ed. Jaenicke, L.) Springer Verlag, Berlin-Heidelberg-New York, 107–131.

Altner, H. and Kolnberger, I. (1975) "The application of transmission electron microscopy on the study of the olfactory epithelium of vertebrates" in *Methods in Olfactory Research* (eds. Moulton, D. G., Turk, A., Johnston, J. W. Jr.) Academic Press, London-New York-San Francisco, 163–190.

Altner, H. and Prillinger, L. (1980) Ultrastructure of invertebrate chemo-, thermo-, and hygroreceptors and its functional significance *Int. Rev. Cytol.*, **67**, 69–139.

Atema, J. (1971) Structures and functions of the sense of taste in the catfish (*Ictalurus nataliis*) *Brain Beh. Evol.*, **4**, 273–294.

Bailey, D. F. and Laverack, M. S. (1966) Aspects of the neurophysiology of *Buccinum undatum* (Gastropoda) *J. exp. Biol.*, **44**, 131–148.

Bardach, J. (1975) "Chemoreception of aquatic animals" in *Olfaction and Taste V* (eds. Denton, D. A., Coghlan, J. P.) Academic Press, New York-San Francisco-London, 121–132.

Bauer, U. and Hatt, H. (1980) Demonstration of three different types of chemosensitive units in the crayfish claw using a computerized evaluation *Neuroscience Letters*, **17**, 209–214.

Beidler, L. M. and Smallman, R. L. (1965) Renewal of cells within taste buds *J. Cell. Biol.*, **27**, 263–273.

Boeckh, J., Boeckh, V. and Kühn, A. (1977) "Further data on the topography and physiology of central olfactory neurons in insects" in *Olfaction and Taste VI* (eds. le Magnen, J., MacLeod, P.) IRL, London-Washington, 315–321.

Boeckh, J. and Boeckh, V. (1979) Threshold and odor specificity of pheromone-sensitive neurons in the deutocerebrum of *Antheraea pernyi* and *A. polyphemus* (Saturnidae) *J. comp. Physiol.*, **132**, 235–242.

Boeckh, J., Ernst, K. D., Sass, H. and Waldow, U. (1976) Zur nervösen Organisation antennaler Sinneseingänge bei Insekten unter besonderer Berücksichtigung der Riechbahn *Verh. Dtsch. Zool. Ges.*, 1976, 123–139.

Bradley, R. M. (1971) "Tongue Topography" in *Handbook of Sensory Physiology IV*, Chemical Senses 2. Taste (ed. Beidler, L. M.) Springer Verlag, Berlin-Heidelberg-New York, 1–30.

Caprio, J. (1975) "Extreme sensitivity and specificity of catfish gustatory receptors to amino acids and derivatives" in *Olfaction and Taste V* (eds. Denton, D. A., Coghlan, J. P.) Academic Press, New York-San Francisco-London, 157–161.

Costanzo, R. M. and Mozell, M. M. (1976) Electrophysiological evidence for a topographical projection of the nasal mucosa onto the olfactory bulb of the frog *J. gen. Physiol.*, **68**, 297–312.

Dethier, V. G. (1973) Electrophysiological studies of gustation in Lepidopterous larvae. II—Taste spectra in relation to food plant discrimination *J. comp. Physiol.*, **82**, 103–134.

Dethier, V. G. (1976) *The hungry fly* Harvard University Press, Cambridge-London.

Duchamp, A., Revial, M. F., Holley, A. and MacLeod, P. (1974) Odour discrimination by frog olfactory receptors *Chemical Senses and Flavour*, **1**, 213–233.

Ernst, K. D., Boeckh, J. and Boeckh, V. (1977) A neuroanatomical study on the organization of the central antennal pathway in insects *Cell Tiss. Res.*, **176**, 285–308.

Fuzessery, Z. M., Childress, J. J. (1975) Comparative chemosensitivity to amino acids and their role in the feeding activity of bathypelagic and littoral crustaceans *Biol. Bull.*, **149**, 522–538.

Gesteland, R. C., Lettvin, J. Y. and Pitts, W. H. (1965) Chemical transmission in the nose of the frog *J. Physiol. Lond.*, **181**, 525–559.

Graziadei, P. (1964) Electron microscopy of some primary receptors in the sucker of *Octopus vulgaris Z. Zellforsch.*, **64**, 510–522.

Graziadei, P. (1973) "The ultrastructure of vertebrate olfactory mucosa" in *The Ultrastructure of Sense Organs* (ed. Friedman, I.) New Holland Publishing Company, Amsterdam-London, 267–305.

Graziadei, P. (1975) "Application of scanning electron microscopy and autoradiography in the study of olfactory mucosa" in *Methods in Olfactory Research* (eds. Moulton, D. G., Turk, A., Johnson, W.) Academic Press, London-New York-San Francisco, 191–240.

Graziadei, P. P. C. and Monti-Graziadei (1978) "Continuous nerve cell renewal in the olfactory system" in *Handbook of Sensory Physiol. IX* (ed. Jacobson, M.) Springer Verlag, Berlin-Heidelberg-New York, 55–83.

Graziadei, P. and Metcalf, J. F. (1975) Autoradiographic study of frog's olfactory mucosa *Amer. Zool.*, **10**, 559.

Hansen, K. (1974) "α-glucosidases as sugar receptor proteins in flies" in *Biochemistry of Sensory Functions* (ed. Jaenicke, L.) Springer Verlag, Berlin-Heidelberg-New York, 207–233.

Jahan-Parwar, B. (1972) Behavioral and electrophysiological studies on chemoreception in *Aplysia Amer. Zoologist*, **12**, 525–537.

Jahan-Parwar, B. (1977) "Structure and function of the chemoreceptor sheet in *Aplysia*" in *Olfaction and Taste VI* (eds. le Magnen, J., MacLeod, P.), IRL, London-Washington, 353.

Kaib, M. (1974) "Die Fleisch- und Blumenduftrezeptoren auf der Antenne der Schmeißfliege Calliphora vicina *J. comp. Physiol.*, **95**, 105–121.

Kaissling, K. E. (1971) "Insect olfaction" in *Handbook of Sensory Physiology*, Vol. IV, Chemical Senses I. Olfaction (ed. Beidler, L. M.) Springer Verlag, Berlin-Heidelberg-New York, 243–273.

Kaissling, K. E. (1974) "Sensory transduction in insect olfactory receptors" in *Biochemistry of Sensory Functions* (ed. Jaenicke, L.) Springer Verlag, Berlin-Heidelberg-New York, 243–273.

Kaissling, K. E. und Priesner, E. (1970) Die Riechschwelle des Seidenspinners *Naturwiss.*, **57**, 23–28.

Kauer, J. S. and Moulton, D. G. (1974) Response of olfactory bulb neurones to odour stimulation of small nasal areas in the salamander *J. Physiol.*, **243**, 717–737.

Kerjaschki, D. (1977) "Some freeze-etching data on the olfactory epithelium" in *Olfaction and Taste VI* (eds. le Magnen, J., MacLeod, P.) IRL, London, 75–85.

Kimura, K. and Beidler, L. M. (1961) Microelectrode study of taste receptors of rat and hamster *J. cell. comp. Physiol.*, **58**, 131–140.

Kochansky, J. J., Tette, J., Taschenberg, F. F., Cardé, R. T., Kaissling, K. E. and Roelofs, W. L. (1975) Sex pheromone of the moth *Antheraea pernyi J. Insect Physiol.*, **21**, 1977–1983.

Kohn, A. J. (1961) Chemoreception in gastropod molluscs *Amer. Zoologist*, **1**, 291–308.

Koshland, D. E. (1974) "The chemotactic response in bacteria" in *Biochemistry of Sensory Functions* (ed. Jaenicke, L.) Springer Verlag, Berlin-Heidelberg-New York, 133–160.

Mozell, M. M. (1970) Evidence for a chromatographic model of olfaction *J. gen. Physiol.*, **56**, 46–63.

Murray, R. G. (1971) "Ultrastructure of taste receptors" in *Handbook of Sensory Physiology*, Vol. IV, Chemical Senses II. Taste (ed. Beidler, L. M.), Springer Verlag, Berlin-Heidelberg-New York, 31–50.

Murray, R. G. (1973) "The ultrastructure of taste buds" in *The Ultrastructure of Sense Organs* (ed. Friedmann, I.) North Holland Publishing Company, Amsterdam-London, 1–81.

Mustaparta, H. (1971) Spatial distribution on receptor responses to stimulation with different odours *Acta physiol. Scand.*, **82**, 154–166.

Mustaparta, H. (1975) Responses of single olfactory cells in the pine weevil *Hylobius abietis* L. (Col. Curculionidae) *J. comp. Physiol.*, **97**, 271–290.

Neuhaus, W. (1956*a*) Die Riechschwelle von Duftgemische beim Hund und ihr Verhältnis zu den Schwellen unvermischter Duftstoffe *Z. vergl. Physiol.*, **38**, 238–258.

Neuhaus, W. (1956*b*) Die Unterscheidungsfähigkeit des Hundes für Duftgemische *Z. vergl. Physiol.*, **39**, 25–43.

Nowliss, G. H. and Frank, M. (1977) "Qualities in hamster taste: behavioral and neural evidence" in *Olfaction and Taste VI* (eds. le Magnen, J., MacLeod, P.) IRL, London, 241–248.

Pfaffmann, C. (1941) Gustatory afferent impulses *J. cell. comp. Physiol.*, **17**, 243–258.

Pfaffmann, C. (1955) Gustatory nerve impulses in rat, cat and rabbit *J. Neurophysiol.*, **18**, 429–440.

Pinching, A. J. and Døving, K. B. (1974) Selective degeneration in the rat olfactory bulb—following exposure to different odours *Brain Res.*, **82**, 1095–204.

Priesner, E. (1973) Artspezifität und Funktion einiger Insektenpheromone *Fortschr. Zool.*, **22**, 49–135.

Priesner, E. (1979) "Sensory encoding of pheromone signals and related stimuli in male moths" in *Insect Neurobiology and Pesticide Action* Society of Chemical Industry, London, 359–366.

Revial, M. F., Duchamp, A. and Holley, A. (1978) Odour discrimination by frog olfactory receptors: a second study *Chemical Senses and Flavour*, **3**, 7–21.

Roelofs, W. (1979) "Production and perception of lepidopterous pheromone blends" in *Chemical Ecology* (ed. Ritter, F. J.) Elsevier/North Holland, Amsterdam-New York-Oxford, 159–167.

Rüth, E. (1975) Elektrophysiologie der Sensilla chaetica auf den Antennen von *Periplaneta americana J. comp. Physiol.*, **105**, 55–64.

Sass, H. (1976) Zur nervösen Codierung von Geruchsreizen bei *Periplaneta americana J. comp. Physiol.*, **107**, 49–65.

Sass, H. (1979) Olfactory receptors on the antenna of *Periplaneta*: Response constellations that encode food odours *J. comp. Physiol.*, **128**, 227–233.

Sato, T. (1980) Recent advances in the physiology of taste cells *Progr. in Neurobiol.*, **14**, 25–67.

Schneider, D., Lacher, V. and Kaissling, K. E. (1964) Die Reaktionsweite und das Reaktionsspektrum von Riechzellen bei *Antheraea pernyi* (Lepidoptera, Saturniidae) *Z. vergl. Physiol.*, **48**, 632–662.

Schoonhoven, L. M. and Dethier, V. G. (1966) Sensory aspects of host-plant discrimination by Lepidopterous larvae *Arch. Neerland. Zool.*, **16**, 497–530.

Seelinger, G. (1977) Der Antennenendzapfen der tunesischen Wüstenassel *Hemilepistus reaumuri*, ein komplexes Sinnesorgan (Crustacea, Isopoda) *J. comp. Physiol.*, **113**, 95–103.

Seelinger, G. (1977) Morphologische und elektrophysiologische Untersuchungen am Antennen-Endzapfen der sozialen tunesischen Wüstenassel *Hemilepistus reaumuri* (Audovin und Savigny). Doctoral dissertation, University of Regensburg.

Steinbrecht, R. A. (1971) Zur Morphometrie der Antenne des Seidenspinners *Bombyx mori* L.: Zahl und Verteilung der Riechsensillen (Insecta, Lepidoptera) *Z. Morph. Tiere*, **68**, 93–126.

Stewart, W. B., Kauer, J. S. and Shepherd, G. M. (1979) Functional organisation of rat olfactory bulb analysed by the 2-deoxy-glucose method *J. comp. Neurol.*, **185**, 715–734.

Stuiver, M. (1958) The biophysics of the sense of smell. Doctoral thesis, Rijksuniversiteit, Groningen.

Teichmann, H. (1959) Über die Wirkung des Geruchssinnes beim Aal (*Anguilla anguilla*, L.) *Z. vergl. Physiol.*, **42**, 206–254.

Thommesen, E. and Døving, K. B. (1977) Spatial distribution of the EOG in the rat, a variation with odour quality *Acta physiol. Scand.*, **99**, 270–280.

Thurm, U. (1974) "Mechanisms of electrical membrane responses in sensory receptors, illustrated by mechanoreceptors" in *Biochemistry of Sensory Functions* (ed. Jaenicke, L.) Springer Verlag, Berlin-Heidelberg-New York, 367–390.

Tucker, D. (1963) "Olfactory, vomeronasal and trigeminal receptor responses to odorants" in *Olfaction and Taste I* (ed. Zotterman, Y.) Pergamon Press, New York, 49–69.

Tucker, D. (1967) Olfactory cilia are not required for olfaction *Fed. Proc.*, **26**, 544.

Tucker, D. (1971) "Non-olfactory responses from the nasal cavity: Jacobson's organ and the trigeminal system" in *Handbook of Sensory Physiology*, Vol. IV, Chemical Senses I. Olfaction Springer Verlag, Berlin-Heidelberg-New York, 151–181.

Vareschi, E. (1971) Duftunterscheidung bei der Honigbiene: Einzelzellableitungen und Verhaltensreaktionen *Z. vergl. Physiol.*, **75**, 143–175.

Wells, M. J., Freeman, N. H. and Ashburner, M. (1965) Some experiments on the chemotactile sense of octopuses *J. exp. Biol.*, **43**, 533–563.

Wieczorek, H. (1976) The glucoside receptor of the larvae of *Mamestra brassicae* L. (Lepidoptera, Noctuidae) *J. comp. Physiol.*, **106**, 159–176.

Woolston, D. C. and Erickson, R. P. (1979) Concept of neuron types in gustatoria in the rat *J. Neurophysiol.*, **42**, 1390–1409.

CHAPTER SEVEN

THE TRANSDUCER MECHANISMS OF SENSE ORGANS

C. J. DUNCAN

Introduction

We have, as yet, no precise description of the sequence of biochemical events that underlie the process by which the energy of the stimulus is converted by a sense organ into a pattern of nervous impulses. Are there common processes in the transducer mechanisms of different sense organs? Are there any simple model systems that will help us to understand transducer mechanisms and which may illustrate how sense organs have evolved? The transformation of energy in biological systems is central to our understanding of cellular physiology, and in this paper some partial answers to these questions are provided.

The response of a sense organ, in terms of impulse frequency generated, is usually regarded as being proportional to the logarithm of the intensity of stimulation, at least over a limited range (Granit, 1955), although it seems probable that the true relationship is that of a rectangular hyperbola (Duncan, 1963, 1967). The initial response of a sense organ that is detectable electrophysiologically is the *receptor potential.* Both its amplitude and rate of rise are graded and are dependent on stimulus intensity (Katz, 1950; Gray and Sato, 1953; Diamond, Gray and Inman, 1958; Kimura and Beidler, 1961; Loewenstein, 1961) and, again, the relationship between the stimulus energy and the response appears to be that of a rectangular hyperbola in a variety of sense organs (Duncan, 1963, 1967), (but see the qualifications below.) Thus, there is a simple linear relationship between the amplitude of the receptor potential and the frequency of impulses (Katz, 1950). Since receptor (or generator) potentials are apparently a common step in sense organ physiology, being their basic output mechanism, an understanding of their genesis is an advance towards a description of the transducer mechanism of sensory receptors.

Molecular mechanisms controlling cation-permeability in excitable cells

It is accepted that the receptor potential is a localized, non-propagated event that is caused by a change in cation-permeability at the plasmalemma; this is usually and predominantly (although not necessarily exclusively—Ottoson, 1964) an increase in permeability to Na^+. In the retinal rods, however, this change is a decrease in P_{Na} (Hagins, Penn and Yoshikami, 1970). Thus, Diamond *et al.* (1958) showed that perfusion of the capillary system of the Pacinian corpuscle with Na^+-free saline produced a rapid abolition of nerve impulses and the receptor potential fell to some 10% of its original value; the persistence of a residual potential is not surprising and has been discussed elsewhere (Wareham, Duncan and Bowler, 1974). The common feature therefore in this form of energy transduction is a change in P_{Na} (either an increase or a decrease), but we would expect that the way that this is achieved would differ in different sense organs.

In 1963, it was suggested that cation-permeability in excitable cells was controlled by a mechanoenzyme system in the plasma membrane formed from an ATPase which was dependent on divalent cations for activation and which had actomyosin-like properties (Duncan, 1963, 1967). Since then, a great deal of work has been done, using ATPase preparations as ionophores when inserted into black lipid membranes. The familiar Na^+-K^+-ATPase can act in this way, but the Ca^{2+}-ATPase of the sarcoplasmic reticulum (S.R.) is of particular interest. It can be split by carefully controlled tryptic digestion into three components, each of which can be purified by SDS column chromatography or by SDS-preparative gel electrophoresis and then re-inserted into black lipid membranes (Shamoo and Goldstein, 1977). These constituent components are:

(a) A 20 000 dalton fragment with Ca^{2+}-dependent and Ca^{2+}-selective ionophoric activity (Shamoo, 1978) which is termed the *gate*. However, the Ca^{2+}-dependency or -selectivity of this fragment was not as pronounced as that of the intact enzyme or when combined with fragment (b). Ruthenium red specifically inhibits Ca^{2+}-Mg^{2+}-ATPase activity and also the ionophoric activity of the intact enzyme and of this 20 000 dalton fragment.

(b) A 30 000 dalton fragment which represents the site of ATP hydrolysis; it contains the site of phosphorylation and of *N*-[^{3}H]-ethylmaleimide binding. ATP hydrolysis at the hydrolytic site requires the presence of two Ca^{2+} which are then transported after ATP hydrolysis.

(c) A 45 000 dalton fragment which possesses non-specific ionophoric activity and which forms a *non-selective channel* across the plasma membrane.

Fig. 1 shows the different ways in which these elements could be combined to produce a non-selective channel, a selective channel, a non-selective pump or a selective pump (see Abramson and Shamoo,

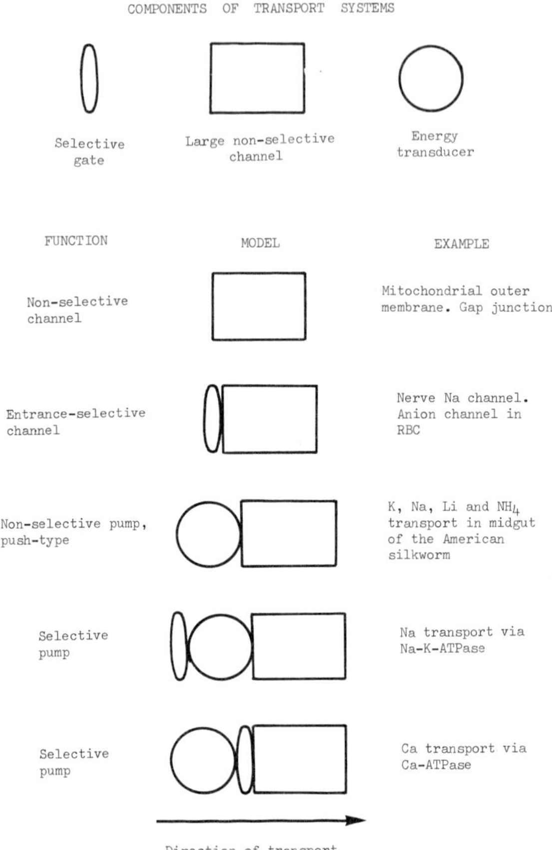

Figure 1 The components of the Ca^{2+}-ATPase of the S.R. produced by selective tryptic digestion, and the ways in which they could theoretically be assembled so as to form different molecular systems for the movement of ions across cellular membranes. The selective gate is formed from the 20 000 dalton component; the non-selective channel from the 45 000 dalton component and the energy transducer from the 30 000 dalton component. After Shamoo and Goldstein (1977).

1978, for further details). The ways in which such molecular systems could have evolved can be clearly seen in this figure which is adapted from Shamoo and Goldstein (1977).

It is known that the Na^{+}-K^{+}-ATPase (Post, Taniguchi and Toda, 1974), the Ca^{2+}-ATPase (Knowles and Racker, 1975) and the Ca^{2+}-pump of the erythrocyte membrane (Rossi, Garrahan and Rega, 1978) can all be made to operate in the reverse direction by suitable manipulations of ionic concentrations or gradients, so synthesizing ATP by the phosphorylation of ADP. Since such a transfer of phosphate to ADP by the Ca^{2+}-ATPase of the S.R. is also markedly dependent on pH and on the H^+ concentration gradient, it can be seen that these systems are related to the mechanism of mitochondrial oxidative phosphorylation and that the ATPases are central to all cellular energy transformations.

It has been suggested (Duncan, 1967) that the cation-permeability channels are formed from the ionophoric properties of ATPase molecules. In sense organs (and perhaps in other excitable cells), it seems probable that such channels are formed from all three elements, gate, non-specific channel *and* the hydrolytic site, rather than from the gate and channel alone, as suggested by Shamoo and Goldstein (1977; see Fig. 1), and that the hydrolytic site may be implicated in the changes in cation-permeability of the receptor potential.

Ca^{2+}-ATPases and the regulation of cation-permeability at sense organs

The detailed results concerning the response of the Pacinian corpuscle show that, although the relationship between the rate of rise of the receptor potential and the stimulus intensity is apparently that of a rectangular hyperbola over much of the working range (see above), a marked deviation is found at low stimulus energies, where the plot is sigmoidal (Gray and Sato, 1953). It is interesting that such a graph corresponds with the activation of Ca^{2+}-ATPases of brain or myofibrils by Ca^{2+} (Portzehl, Zaoralek and Gaudin, 1969; Duncan, 1976) and also that Ca^{2+}-Mg^{2+}-ATPase activity has now been detected in single Pacinian corpuscles (Kukushkina and Cherepnov, 1976).

It is therefore reaffirmed that the common component of the transducer mechanism of sense organs is a divalent cation ATPase with actomyosin-like properties, capable of configurational changes, that controls monovalent cation permeability in a graded fashion and hence regulates the receptor potential (Duncan, 1967). The view that the Ca^{2+}-Mg^{2+}-ATPase is implicated in the regulation of the passive permeability properties of the membrane (as well as in active ion transport) has now been summarized by Jilka and Martonosi (1977). Furthermore, Tada, Yamamoto and Tonomura (1978) have now summarized the evidence concerning the similarity in Ca^{2+}-ATPase, in Na^+-K^+-ATPase and in myosin ATPase in the molecular mode of coupling between the chemical reactions (a rapid equilibrium between the key intermediates) and the molecular motion of the enzyme (rotatory movement), which indicates that the mechanisms of energy-transducing processes in cation transport and muscle contraction are essentially similar (see Duncan, 1967).

Transducer mechanisms in different sense organs

The permeability control system of the axon is directly sensitive to the potential across the membrane. Sense organs, on the other hand, have obviously specialized in the different ways in which the stimulus energy is coupled to the common ATPase system regulating permeability. In brief, the following general principles and possibilities can be seen. The action can be either direct or indirect. Examples of direct modulation of the ATPase are probably mechanoreceptors (Pacinian corpuscle) and thermoreceptors. On the other hand, in some chemoreceptors the molecular deformation associated with the combination of the chemical stimulus with its receptor on the free border of the cell has to be signalled to the lateral plasma membrane; equally the photoisomerization of the rhodopsin on the discs of the vertebrate retinal rod is structurally and electrophysiologically disconnected from the plasma membrane and some form of communication is necessary.

Thus, any one of the following systems could be utilized to alter, modulate or tune the permeability control system:

(a) Direct membrane deformation (possibly involving changes in enzyme-substrate or enzyme-activator relationships).

(b) Ca^{2+} acting as an internal messenger, leading to Ca^{2+}-activation of the ATPase. The possible involvement of Ca^{2+} in the transducer mechanism of vertebrate retinal rods is discussed below, but Ca^{2+} has also been implicated in the response of *Limulus* photoreceptors (Brown and Blinks, 1974; Fein and Lisman, 1975); in the phototransduction in *Aplysia* neurones following Ca^{2+}-release from the pigment granules (Brown, Baur and Tuley, 1975; Henkart, 1975); and in the transducer mechanism of the crayfish stretch receptor (Chaplain, 1975).

(c) Phosphorylation of the Ca^{2+}-ATPase, regulated by cyclic nucleotides and Ca^{2+}. The possible importance of cAMP in acting as a second messenger and in regulating cation-permeability in excitable cells is well documented (Nathanson, 1977), and MacLennan and Holland (1975) have suggested that phosphorylation of the Ca^{2+}-ATPase is a factor controlling ion flow through such ionophores. Menevse, Dodd and Poynder (1977) have now shown that phosphodiesterase inhibitors and dibutyryl-cAMP cause a reversible reduction in the amplitude of the frog electro-olfactograms (cGMP derivatives were ineffective). They conclude that cAMP is specifically involved in the transducer step in primary olfactory neurones and that odorants binding to different types of receptor have a common transduction mechanism.

(d) Involvement of the Ca^{2+}-dependent regulator (CDR = modulator protein = calmodulin). A protein modulator that exhibits multiple Ca^{2+}-dependent, regulatory functions has been identified; it activates phosphodiesterase (Wang and Desai, 1977) and adenylate cyclase (Brostrom *et al.*, 1975) and so regulates cyclic nucleotide levels; it activates Ca^{2+}-Mg^{2+}-ATPase and Ca^{2+} transport (Larsen *et al.*, 1978; Jarrett and Penniston, 1978); it can suppress the troponin I inhibition of actomyosin ATPase (Amphlett, Vanaman and Perry, 1976; Dedman, Potter and Means,

1977); it is the activator protein of myosin light chain kinase (Yagi *et al.*, 1978). Ca^{2+} confers a more helical structure to CDR, thereby permitting it to interact with the apoenzyme to form an active holoenzyme. The Ca^{2+}-Mg^{2+}-ATPase of the erythrocyte exists therefore in two states. When free of CDR it has a low apparent Ca^{2+}-affinity and low V_{max}; when associated with CDR it has a high Ca^{2+} affinity and high V_{max} (Scharff, 1978). Thus there are once again close affinities between the Ca^{2+}-Mg^{2+}-ATPase, actomyosin, Ca^{2+} and the cyclic nucleotides.

(e) Ca^{2+}-Mg^{2+}-ATPase of the erythrocyte membrane has been shown to be activated by tropomyosin, the regulatory protein of muscle (Ohnishi, 1977) which also modifies the ouabain sensitivity of the Na^+-K^+-ATPase (Charlemagne *et al.*, 1980).

From this brief summary we can see the variety of ways in which the reception of the stimulus energy can be transferred to the ionophore. Second messengers (Ca^{2+}, cAMP, cGMP) will be involved in many instances, as in the indirect transducer mechanisms.

Model systems for sense organs

The way in which the sensory responses of *Amoeba* can be used as a model for the transducer mechanism of the Pacinian corpuscle has been detailed elsewhere (Duncan, 1967). It has been emphasized previously how many sensory transducers are based structurally on cilia (Duncan, 1967, 1977), for example retinal rods, olfactory cells, the grasshopper chordotonal organ (Moran *et al.*, 1977) and the stereocilia of vertebrate hair cells (Hudspeth and Jacobs, 1979). The vertebrate retinal rod is of particular interest in this respect; the modification of its outer segment (ROS) from a cilium has been traced during morphogenesis and the remnants of the microtubular structure and the centriole persist in the mature cell. The retinal discs of the ROS form by infolding of the plasma membrane of the cilium (De Robertis, 1960). It has been suggested that a molecular reorientation of the visual pigment causes a change in the Ca^{2+}-permeability of the discs, so allowing the release of Ca^{2+} stored therein which acts as an intracellular messenger, amplifying and coupling the photochemical signal from the disc to the plasma membrane (Yoshikami and Hagins, 1971; Zuckerman, 1973). One variant of this hypothesis (which introduces the possibility of an amplifier cascade and also overcomes difficulties concerning the amount of Ca^{2+} released) is that the Ca^{2+} released activates a phosphodiesterase that catalyses the destruction of cGMP which otherwise, indirectly, promotes the opening of Na^+ channels in the surface membrane (Miller and Nichol, 1979). This hypothesis has received support from the following experiments:

(a) Ca^{2+} is concentrated in dark-adapted discs (Bownds *et al.*, 1971);

(b) Ca^{2+} release has been demonstrated on bleaching (Poo and Cone,

1973; Hendriks, Daemen and Bonting, 1974; Liebman, 1974; Mason, Fager and Abrahamson, 1974; Kaupp and Junge, 1977; Smith, Fager and Litman, 1977; Kaupp, Schnetkamp and Junge, 1979);

(c) a Ca^{2+}-ATPase is localized in ROS (Sack and Harris, 1977);

(d) measurements with aequorin show that $[Ca^{2+}]_i$ rises in *Limulus* photoreceptors during illumination (Brown and Blinks, 1974);

(e) treatment of ROS with Ca^{2+} causes their hyperpolarization (Hagins and Yoshikami, 1974);

(f) injection of Ca^{2+}, causing an increase in $[Ca^{2+}]_i$, hyperpolarizes the rod membrane, mimicking the receptor potential (Brown, Coles and Pinto, 1977);

(g) the light-regulated Na^+ channels in ROS can be blocked by Ca^{2+} (Wormington and Cone, 1978).

With reference to the hypothesis advanced above and the suggestions given below, the following properties of ROS are of interest:

(a) Light-activated phosphorylation of the photoreceptor membranes has been observed, and inhibitors of the phosphorylation affect the light-induced permeability change of the ROS plasma membrane. In the presence of these inhibitors, small amounts of light produce greater changes in P_{Na} (Miller, Paulsen and Bownds, 1977);

(b) Isolated rod discs contain a Ca^{2+}-ATPase, the activity of which can be modified by the state of the rhodopsin (Ostwald and Heller, 1972).

Recent studies on the control of the ciliary beat reveal how the transducer mechanism of the retinal rods might well have evolved. A mechanical stimulus at the anterior end of *Paramecium* causes an increase in calcium permeability, with a consequent depolarization which further activates the Ca^{2+}-channels in the membrane and depolarization therefore develops regeneratively. The resultant rise in $[Ca^{2+}]_i$ causes a reversal of the ciliary beat together with an increase in frequency (Naitoh, 1974; Eckert, Naitoh and Machemer, 1976). A depolarization produced by raising extracellular Na^+ or K^+ also causes ciliary reversal, and measurements with $^{45}Ca^{2+}$ confirm an associated rise in Ca^{2+}-influx (Browning, Nelson and Hansma, 1976). A stimulus at the posterior end of *Paramecium*, however, activates K^+-channels in the membrane, causing hyperpolarization and, again, an increase in the frequency of ciliary beat (Naitoh, 1974; Eckert *et al.*, 1976). Mutants of *P. aurelia* with modified locomotor behaviour (named "Pawn") have been isolated (Kung, 1971) which fail to reverse their ciliary beat when depolarized. Such mutants show no regenerative Ca^{2+} response (Kung and Eckert, 1972) and no stimulated $^{45}Ca^{2+}$-influx, and it is evident that the Ca^{2+}-gating mechanism is a major component of membrane excitability in *Paramecium* (Browning *et al.*, 1976).

When *Paramecium* is deciliated by treatment with chloral hydrate, the animals retain their hyperpolarizing response to posterior stimulation and the normal resting membrane potential is unaffected. However, deciliated *Paramecium* do not show a depolarizing response to anterior stimulation. The cilia regenerate in the absence of chloral hydrate in 6–8 h and the reciliated *Paramecium* once more responds to anterior stimulation with depolarization (Ogura and Takahashi, 1976; Dunlap, 1977). These experiments confirm that deciliation eliminates the "calcium response" to depolarizing current whilst regrowth restores the normal response (Dunlap, 1976; Dunlap and Eckert, 1976) and strongly suggest that the Ca^{2+}-channels are localized on the ciliary membrane, whereas the K^+-channels are not (Ogura and Takahashi, 1976; Machemer and Ogura, 1979).

Thus, the Ca^{2+}-gating mechanism of the transduction process of the mechanosensory response of *Paramecium* cilia provides circumstantial evidence for the existence of Ca^{2+}-permeability changes in the response of vertebrate photoreceptors since they are developed from modified cilia. Studies on the sensory response in *Paramecium* also reveal how the transducer mechanism of retinal rods could have evolved. Early photoreceptors could have developed by linking the Ca^{2+} gates on cilia to a photopigment whose photoisomerization caused a modification of Ca^{2+} permeability. The cones, with their infolded membrane, represent an intermediate stage. The formation *and separation* of the characteristic discs in the ROS means that these were equipped with the appropriate Ca^{2+}-gating mechanism together with the vectorially organized Ca^{2+}-transport ATPase which translocates Ca^{2+} into these storage sites rather than to the external medium. It is conceivable that the same Ca^{2+}-ATPase serves both these functions. The separation of the discs means that a second messenger (Ca^{2+}, cGMP or both) is necessary.

It is therefore suggested that the cilia of *Paramecium* may be of interest to sensory physiologists, in particular because components of the membrane can be manipulated genetically as well as biochemically and electrically. The following features may also be of value:

(a) Three genes affect the function of the Ca^{2+} channel (Oertel, Schein and Kung, 1978);

(b) The Ca^{2+}-channel lifetime is 5–8 d (Schein, 1976);

(c) The Ca^{2+}-channel undergoes inactivation as a consequence of Ca^{2+}-entry during depolarization (Brehm and Eckert, 1978); its detailed properties are now known (Satow and Kung, 1979);

(d) Ultrastructural correlates can be detected in the membrane of some mutants (Byrne and Byrne, 1978);

(e) Paramecia can be used to study adaptation; K^+-resistant mutants show little or no adaptation (Shusterman, Thiede and Kung, 1978);

(f) Paramecia can act as a model for chemoreceptors, as well as for mechano- and photoreceptors. They hyperpolarize in attractants and depolarize in repellants (Houten, 1979), and a mutant defective in chemotaxis has been described (Houten, 1977);

(g) Finally, a Ca^{2+}-Mg^{2+}-ATPase, believed to be of membrane origin, has been isolated from cilia from *Paramecium* (Doughty, 1978). Glutaraldehyde (0.14 mM) alters the membrane characteristics but is without effect when the paramecia are also exposed to 10^{-6} M ruthenium red; Doughty and Dodd (1978) conclude that both agents act at the Ca^{2+}-channel of the Ca^{2+}-ATPase of the ciliary membrane, glutaraldehyde preventing critical conformational changes that are responsible for electrogenesis.

It is evident that the sensory responses of *Amoeba* (Duncan, 1967) and of *Paramecium*, both single-celled animals being particularly suitable for detailed investigations, may provide clues concerning the molecular events associated with the transducer mechanism of sense organs. Other significant clues may also be available; the studies concerning the involvement of protein methylation in the chemosensory response of bacteria and leukocytes could well repay closer study (Springer, Goy and Adler, 1979).

Summary

The response of sense organs is a localized change in cation-permeability, the receptor potential. The evidence concerning the involvement of Ca^{2+}-Mg^{2+}-ATPases acting as ionophores in regulating P_{Na} is discussed and suggestions are presented for the ways in which the Ca^{2+}-Mg^{2+}-ATPase could be modified in different sense organs, so effecting a graded change in the permeability of the plasma membrane. It is suggested that model systems are of value; the detailed results concerning the cellular physiology of *Paramecium* cilia are of particular interest to studies on the evolution and physiology of ROS and other sense organs that have developed from cilia.

REFERENCES

Abramson, J. J. and Shamoo, A. E. (1978) Purification and characterization of the 45,000-dalton fragment from tryptic digestion of ($Ca^{2+}+Mg^{2+}$)-adenosine triphosphatase of sarcoplasmic reticulum *J. Memb. Biol.*, **44**, 233–257.

Amphlett, G. W., Vanaman, T. C. and Perry, S. V. (1976) Effect of the troponin C-like protein from bovine brain (brain modulator protein) on the Mg^{2+}-stimulated ATPase of skeletal muscle actomyosin *FEBS Letts.*, **72**, 163–168.

Bownds, D., Gordon-Walker, A., Gaide-Huguenin, A. C. and Robinson, W. (1971) Characterization and analysis of frog photoreceptor membranes *J. Gen. Physiol.*, **58**, 225–237.

Brehm, P. and Eckert, R. (1978) Calcium entry leads to inactivation of calcium channel in *Paramecium Science*, **202**, 1203–1206.

Brostrom, C. O., Huang, Y.-C., Breckenridge, B. M. and Wolff, D. J. (1975) Identification of a calcium-binding protein as a calcium-dependent regulator of brain adenylate cyclase *Proc. Nat. Acad. Sci.*, **72**, 64–68.

Brown, A. M., Baur, P. S. and Tuley, F. H. (1975) Phototransduction in *Aplysia* neurons: calcium release from pigmented granules is essential *Science*, **188**, 157–160.

Brown, J. E. and Blinks, J. R. (1974) Changes in intracellular free calcium concentration during illumination of invertebrate photoreceptors. Detection with aequorin *J. gen. Physiol.*, **64**, 643–665.

Brown, J. E., Coles, J. A. and Pinto, L. H. (1977) Effects of injections of calcium and EGTA into the outer segments of retinal rods of *Bufo marinus J. Physiol.*, **269**, 707–722.

Browning, J. L., Nelson, D. L. and Hansma, H. G. (1976) Ca^{2+} influx across the excitable membrane of behavioural mutants of *Paramecium Nature*, **259**, 491–494.

Byrne, B. J. and Byrne, B. C. (1978) An ultrastructural correlate of the membrane mutant "paranoiac" in *Paramecium Science*, **199**, 1091–1093.

Chaplain, R. A. (1975) Evidence for Ca^{2+} control of the transducer mechanism in crayfish stretch receptor *J. Memb. Biol.*, **21**, 335–351.

Charlemagne, D., Leger, J., Schwartz, K., Geny, B., Zachowski, A. and Lelievre, L. (1980) Involvement of tropomyosin in the sensitivity of $Na^+ + K^+$ ATPase to ouabain *Biochem. Pharm.*, **29**, 297–300.

Dedman, J. R., Potter, J. D. and Means, A. R. (1977) Biological cross-reactivity of rat testis phosphodiesterase activator protein and rabbit skeletal muscle troponin-C *J. Biol. Chem.*, **252**, 2437–2440.

De Robertis, E. (1960) Some observations on the ultrastructure and morphogenesis of photoreceptors *J. Gen. Physiol.*, **43**, 1–13.

Diamond, J., Gray, J. A. B. and Inman, D. R. (1958) The relation between receptor potentials and the concentration of sodium ions *J. Physiol.*, **142**, 382–394.

Doughty, M. J. (1978) Ciliary Ca^{2+}-ATPase from the excitable membrane of *Paramecium*. Some properties and purification by affinity chromatography *Comp. Biochem. Physiol.*, **60B**, 339–345.

Doughty, M. J. and Dodd, G. H. (1978) Chemical modification of the excitable membrane in *Paramecium aurelia*: effect of a cross-linking reagent *Comp. Biochem. Physiol.*, **59C**, 21–31.

Duncan, C. J. (1963) Excitatory mechanisms in chemo- and mechanoreceptors *J. Theoret. Biol.*, **5**, 114–126.

Duncan, C. J. (ed.) (1967) *The Molecular Properties and Evolution of Excitable Cells* Pergamon Press, Oxford.

Duncan, C. J. (1976) Properties of the Ca^{2+}-ATPase activity of mammalian synaptic membrane preparations *J. Neurochem.*, **27**, 1277–1279.

Duncan, C. J. (1977) A note on the evolution of the transducer mechanism of the vertebrate retinal rod *Experientia*, **33**, 1310.

Dunlap, K. (1976) Ca channels in *Paramecium* confined to ciliary membrane *Am. Zool.*, **16**, 185.

Dunlap, K. (1977) Localization of calcium channels in *Paramecium caudatum J. Physiol.*, **271**, 119–133.

Dunlap, K. and Eckert, R. (1976) Ca channels in the ciliary membrane of *Paramecium J. Cell Biol.*, **70**, 245a.

Eckert, R., Naitoh, Y. and Machemer, H. (1976) "Calcium in the bioelectric and motor functions of *Paramecium*" in *Calcium in Biological Systems* Symp. Soc. Exp. Biol. (ed. Duncan, C. J.) Cambridge University Press, Cambridge, 233–255.

Fein, A. and Lisman, J. (1975) Localized desensitization of *Limulus* photoreceptors produced by light or intracellular calcium ion injection *Science*, **187**, 1094–1096.

Granit, R. (1955) *Receptors and Sensory Perception* Yale University Press, New Haven.

Gray, J. A. B. and Sato, M. (1953) Properties of the receptor potential in Pacinian corpuscles *J. Physiol.*, **122**, 610–636.

Hagins, W. A., Penn, R. D. and Yoshikami, S. (1970) Dark current and photocurrent in retinal rods *Biophys. J.*, **10**, 380–412.

Hagins, W. A. and Yoshikami, S. (1974) A role for Ca^{2+} in excitation of retinal rods and cones *Exp. Eye Res.*, **18**, 299–305.

Hendriks, T., Daemen, F. J. M. and Bonting, S. L. (1974) Biochemical aspects of the visual process. XXV. Light-induced calcium movements in isolated frog rod outer segments *Biochim. Biophys. Acta*, **345**, 468–473.

Henkart, M. (1975) Light-induced changes in the structure of pigmented granules in *Aplysia* neurons *Science*, **188**, 155–157.

Houten, J. van (1977) A mutant of *Paramecium* defective in chemotaxis *Science*, **198**, 746–748.

Houten, J. van (1979) Membrane potential changes during chemokinesis in *Paramecium Science*, **204**, 1100–1103.

Hudspeth, A. J. and Jacobs, R. (1979) Stereocilia mediate transduction in vertebrate hair cells *Proc. Nat. Acad. Sci. U.S.A.*, **76**, 1506–1509.

Jarrett, H. W. and Penniston, J. T. (1978) Purification of the Ca^{2+}-stimulated ATPase activator from human erythrocytes *J. Biol. Chem.*, **253**, 4676–4682.

Jilka, R. L. and Martonosi, A. N. (1977) The effect of calcium ion transport ATPase upon the passive calcium ion permeability of phospholipid vesicles *Biochim. Biophys. Acta*, **466**, 57–67.

Katz, B. (1950) Depolarization of sensory terminals and initiation of impulses in the muscle spindle *J. Physiol.*, **111**, 261–282.

Kaupp, U. B. and Junge, W. (1977) Rapid calcium release by passively loaded retinal discs on photoexcitation *FEBS Letts.*, **81**, 229–232.

Kaupp, U. B., Schnetkamp, P. P. M. and Junge, W. (1979) Light-induced calcium release in isolated intact cattle rod outer segments upon photoexcitation of rhodopsin *Biochim. Biophys. Acta*, **552**, 390–403.

Kimura, K. and Beidler, L. M. (1961) Microelectrode study of taste receptors of rat and hamster *J. Cell. Comp. Physiol.*, **58**, 131–140.

Knowles, A. F. and Racker, E. (1975) Formation of adenosine triphosphate from P_i and adenosine diphosphate by purified Ca^{2+}-adenosine triphosphatase *J. Biol. Chem.*, **250**, 1949–1951.

Kukushkina, D. M. and Cherepnov, V. L. (1976) Mg, Ca activation of ATPase of Pacinian corpuscles *Bull. Exp. Biol. Med.*, **81**, 173–175.

Kung, C. (1971) Genic mutants with altered system of excitation in *Paramecium aurelia*. I. Phenotypes of the behavioral mutants *Z. Vergl. Physiol.*, **71**, 142–164.

Kung, C. and Eckert, R. (1972) Genetic modification of electric properties in an excitable membrane *Proc. Nat. Acad. Sci. U.S.A.*, **69**, 93–97.

Larsen, F. L., Raess, B. U., Hinds, T. R. and Vincenzi, F. F. (1978) Modulator binding protein antagonizes activation of $(Ca^{2+}+Mg^{2+})$-ATPase and Ca^{2+} transport of red blood cell membranes *J. Supramolec. Struct.*, **9**, 269–274.

Liebman, P. A. (1974) Light-dependent Ca^{++} content of rod outer segment disc membranes *Invest. Ophthalmol.*, **13**, 700–701.

Loewenstein, W. R. (1961) Excitation and inactivation in a receptor membrane *Ann. N.Y. Acad. Sci.*, **94**, 510–534.

Machemer, H. and Ogura, A. (1979) Ionic conductances of membranes in ciliated and deciliated *Paramecium J. Physiol.*, **296**, 49–60.

MacLennan, D. H. and Holland, P. C. (1975) Calcium transport in sarcoplasmic reticulum *Ann. Rev. Biophys. Bioeng.*, **4**, 377–404.

Mason, W. T., Fager, R. S. and Abrahamson, E. W. (1974) Ion fluxes in disk membranes of retinal rod outer segments *Nature*, **247**, 562–563.

Menevse, A., Dodd, G. and Poynder, T. M. (1977) Evidence for the specific involvement of cyclic AMP in the olfactory transduction mechanism *Biochem. Biophys. Res. Comm.*, **77**, 671–677.

Miller, J. A., Paulsen, R. and Bownds, M. D. (1977) Control of light-activated phosphorylation in frog photoreceptor membranes *Biochemistry*, **16**, 2633–2639.

Miller, W. H. and Nichol, G. D. (1979) Evidence that cyclic GMP regulates membrane potential in rod photoreceptors *Nature*, **280**, 64–66.

Moran, D. T., Varela, F. J. and Rowley, J. C. (1977) Evidence for active role of cilia in sensory transduction *Proc. Nat. Acad. Sci. U.S.A.*, **74**, 793–797.

Naitoh, Y. (1974) Bioelectric basis of behavior in protozoa *Am. Zool.*, **14**, 883–893.

Nathanson, J. A. (1977) Cyclic nucleotides and nervous system function *Physiol. Rev.*, **57**, 157–256.

Oertel, D., Schein, S. J. and Kung, C. (1978) A potassium conductance activated by hyperpolarization in *Paramecium J. Membr. Biol.*, **43**, 169–185.

Ogura, A. and Takahashi, K. (1976) Artificial deciliation causes loss of calcium-dependent responses in *Paramecium Nature*, **264**, 170–172.

Ohnishi, S. T. (1977) "Calcium-binding proteins extracted from erythrocyte membranes" in

Calcium-Binding Proteins and Calcium Function (eds. Wasserman, R. H., Corradino, R. A., Carafoli, E., Kretsinger, R. H., MacLennan, D. H., Siegel, F. L.) North-Holland, New York, 501–503.

Ostwald, T. J. and Heller, J. (1972) Properties of a magnesium- or calcium-dependent adenosine triphosphatase from frog rod photoreceptor outer segment disks and its inhibition by illumination *Biochemistry*, **11**, 4679–4686.

Ottoson, D. (1964) The effect of sodium deficiency on the response of the isolated muscle spindle *J. Physiol.*, **171**, 109–118.

Poo, M. M. and Cone, R. A. (1973) Lateral diffusion of rhodopsin in *Necturus* rods *Exp. Eye Res.*, **17**, 503.

Portzehl, H., Zaoralek, P. and Gaudin, J. (1969) The activation by Ca^{2+} of the ATPase of extracted muscle fibrils with variation of ionic strength, pH and concentration of MgATP *Biochim. Biophys. Acta*, **189**, 440–448.

Post, R. L., Taniguchi, K. and Toda, G. (1974) Synthesis of adenosine triphosphate by Na^+, K^+-ATPase *Ann. N.Y. Acad. Sci.*, **242**, 80–91.

Rossi, J. P. F. C., Garrahan, P. J. and Rega, A. F. (1978) Reversal of the calcium pump in human red cells *J. Membr. Biol.*, **44**, 37–46.

Sack, R. A. and Harris, C. M. (1977) Ca^{2+}-dependent ATPase activity of bovine receptor cell outer segment *Nature*, **265**, 465–466.

Satow, Y. and Kung, C. (1979) Voltage sensitive Ca-channels and the transient inward current in *Paramecium tetraurelia J. Exp. Biol.*, **78**, 149–161.

Scharff, O. (1978) Stimulating effects of monovalent cations on activator-dissociated and activator-associated states of Ca^{2+}-ATPase in human erythrocytes *Biochim. Biophys. Acta*, **512**, 309–317.

Schein, S. J. (1976) Calcium channel stability measured by gradual loss of excitability in pawn mutants of *Paramecium aurelia J. Exp. Biol.*, **65**, 725–736.

Shamoo, A. E. (1978) Ionophorous properties of the 20,000-dalton fragment of $(Ca^{2+} + Mg^{2+})$-ATPase in phosphatidylcholine: cholesterol membranes *J. Membr. Biol.*, **43**, 227–242.

Shamoo, A. E. and Goldstein, D. A. (1977) Isolation of ionophores from ion transport systems and their role in energy transduction *Biochim. Biophys. Acta*, **472**, 13–53.

Shusterman, C. L., Thiede, E. W. and Kung, C. (1978) K^+-resistant mutants and "adaptation" in *Paramecium Proc. Nat. Acad. Sci. U.S.A.*, **75**, 5645–5649.

Smith, H. G., Fager, R. S. and Litman, B. J. (1977) Light-activated calcium release from sonicated bovine retinal rod outer segment disks *Biochemistry*, **16**, 1399–1405.

Springer, M. S., Goy, M. F. and Adler, J. (1979) Protein methylation in behavioural control mechanisms and in signal transduction *Nature*, **280**, 279–284.

Tada, M., Yamamoto, T. and Tonomura, Y. (1978) Molecular mechanism of active calcium transport by sarcoplasmic reticulum *Physiol. Rev.*, **58**, 1–79.

Wang, J. H. and Desai, R. (1977) Modulator binding protein *J. Biol. Chem.*, **252**, 4175–4184.

Wareham, A. C., Duncan, C. J. and Bowler, K. (1974) Electrogenesis in cockroach muscle *Comp. Biochem. Physiol.*, **48A**, 799–813.

Wormington, C. M. and Cone, R. A. (1978) Ionic blockage of the light-regulated sodium channels in isolated rod outer segments *J. Gen. Physiol.*, **71**, 657–681.

Yagi, K., Yazawa, M., Kakiuchi, S., Ohshima, M. and Uenishi, K. (1978) Identification of an activator protein for myosin light chain kinase as the Ca^{2+}-dependent modulator protein *J. Biol. Chem.*, **253**, 1338–1340.

Yoshikami, S. and Hagins, W. A. (1971) Light, calcium and the photocurrent of rods and cones *Biophys. J.*, **11**, 47a.

Zuckerman, R. (1973) Ionic analysis of photoreceptor membrane currents *J. Physiol.*, **235**, 333–354.

CHAPTER EIGHT
STRAIN DETECTION IN THE ARTHROPOD EXOSKELETON

FRIEDRICH G. BARTH

Introduction

Mechanical stresses and strains are as closely related to each other as are the chicken and the egg—one cannot exist without the other. Although they may differ in detail, the forces contained in the stimuli corresponding to the various types of mechanoreceptors will always produce some strain in the receptor structures, even though this may be very small.

The receptors treated in this chapter share this general property; nevertheless they form a particular group of mechanoreceptors. Their distinctive feature is a specific mechanical linkage to the exoskeleton of the arthropod, which enables animals in this group to measure exoskeletal strains resulting from various types of loads. Nothing similar is known in the skeletons of other animals. These sensilla, then, are as typical a feature of arthropods as is the cuticular exoskeleton itself.

Such biological strain gauges are known in insects, arachnids, and crustaceans. Although they vary in morphological detail, basically they are all holes in the cuticle covered by a thin membrane to which the dendrite of a sensory cell is attached. One of the most striking features of the various cuticular auxiliary structures is that their design and arrangement provides for deformation even by small forces. This implies high sensitivity.

Recent years have seen a number of advances in our understanding of these receptors. This review deals mainly with insect campaniform and arachnid slit sensilla. Particular emphasis is given to a number of mechanical aspects which are of particular interest in a mechanoreceptor system. Only a short description of crustacean "cuticular stress detectors" is included, because these were recently reviewed in detail by Clarac (1976).

Receptor structure

As in other sense organs, the stimulus-conducting structures of campaniform and slit sensilla are most closely correlated with the filter action and

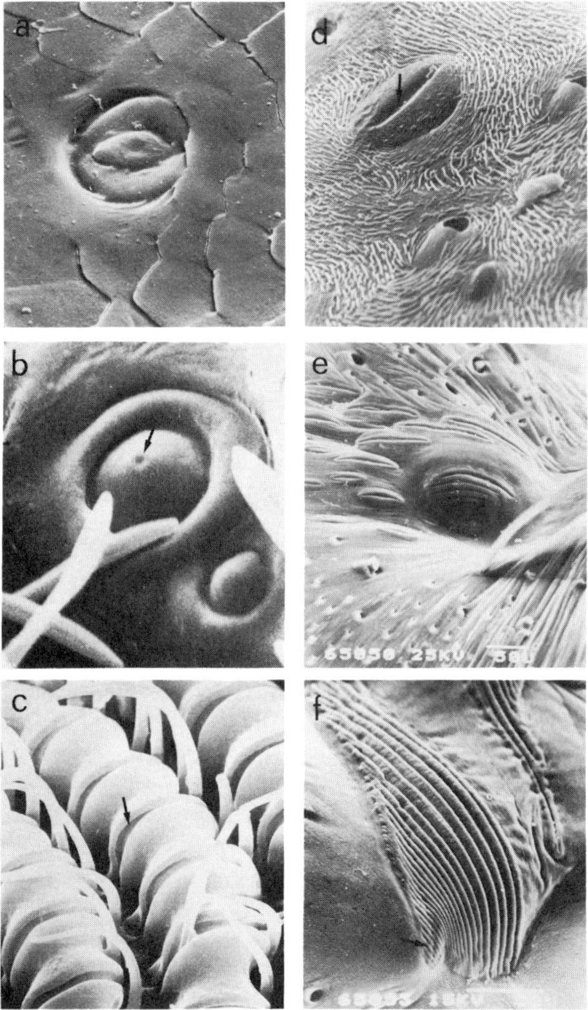

Figure 1 A variety of arthropod strain detectors; a–c, insect campaniform sensilla (courtesy of W. Gnatzy), d–f, spider slit sensilla. a, *Periplaneta americana*, tibia; note ellipsoid cap and horseshoe-shaped cuticular wall surrounding it; × 1800. b, *Gryllus bimaculatus*, close to socket of cercal thread hair (cf. Fig. 2B); note round cap with moulting pore (arrow); × 6300. c, *Calliphora erythrocephala*, haltere base (cf. Fig. 2C); note slit (arrow) between vertebra shaped bulging cuticular thickenings; × 3900. d, *Cupiennius salei*, femur; note dendrite attachment site (arrow) (cf. Fig. 2D); × 1400. e, *C. salei*, trochanter with a group of slits and a compound organ; calibr. 50 μm. f, *C. salei*, patella, lyriform organ; note dendrite attachment sites (arrow); calibr. 50 μm.

specificity of the receptors. They must therefore be reviewed in some detail for later functional interpretation (Figs. 1 and 2).

(a) The *hole* formed by all such receptors in the cuticle may be round or elliptical (as in campaniform sensilla) or strongly elongated (as in the slit sensilla). As a rule, campaniform sensilla are smaller (those found on the butterfly wing (Cartheuser, 1975) with a long axis of 13 μm (cap) are exceptionally large), whereas slit sensilla may be up to 200 μm long but only 1–2 μm wide (Barth and Libera, 1970; Barth, 1971).

(b) The *covering membrane* of the cuticular hole varies among the different sensilla as does the coupling of the dendritic end. While in slit sensilla the covering membrane is about 0.25 μm thick and interpreted as being mainly formed by the epicuticular dense layer (Barth, 1971), it consists of several layers in insect campaniform sensilla (e.g. Chevalier, 1969). In these, an outer layer (L1) can be distinguished from an inner layer (L3) and in the majority of cases a third spongy-looking layer (L2) is found in between. The average thickness of both L1 and L3 is about 0.5 μm. L1 appears non-fibrous in the electron microscope, like the covering membrane of the slit sensillum. It is therefore also considered to be mainly epicuticular. L3 resembles the surrounding cuticle in containing fibrous material. In Fig. 2 an attempt is made to homologize the various layers on the basis of their electron microscopical appearance.

It has been proposed that L1 contains *resilin* (Thurm, 1964; Chevalier, 1969). Histological evidence, such as staining properties and fluorescence, is not sufficient, but Chapman *et al.* (1979) have recently found that campaniform sensilla on the cockroach tibia show resilin-like visco-elasticity for small amplitude cap indentation (max. 20 nm). Some, however, behaved purely elastically, thus outperforming even resilin.

Typically the membranes covering slit sensilla bulge inwards and those of insect campaniform sensilla bulge outwards. Crustacean campaniform sensilla on the dactylopodite are flat (Shelton and Laverack, 1968; Barth, unpubl.) as are some insect campaniform sensilla (Hawke *et al.*, 1973). In contrast, those potential campaniform sensilla on the crustacean antennules (Laverack, 1976) have a conspicuously arched dome.

(c) The *dendritic end* contains a tubular body typical of most arthropod cuticular mechanoreceptors (Thurm, 1964; Barth, 1971; Gaffal and Hansen, 1972). It attaches to the covering membrane by way of a delicate coupling cylinder in the slit sensillum (Fig. 2D) and more simply terminates in L3 (partly in L2) in campaniform sensilla (Fig. 2, A–C). Only parts of the dendrite sheath penetrate into L1 which may have a moulting pore (Moeck, 1968; Schmidt and Gnatzy, 1971; Grünert and Gnatzy, unpubl.).

From about a dozen electron microscopical studies an essentially uniform picture can be drawn of insect campaniform sensilla (Fig. 2, A–C). There are modifications in the general *Bauplan*, however, which are functionally significant. The same applies to slit sensilla. Their fine structural analysis now includes data on spiders (Fig. 2D), a scorpion (Barth, unpubl.), and a harvestman (Fig. 2E; Gnatzy, unpubl.); variation in dendrite coupling is obvious. A common feature in all these arachnids is a second dendrite of unknown function.

The following variations in sensillar fine structure are of interest in this context:
Campaniform sensilla (1) The cap may be slightly arched (Thurm, 1964; Schmidt, 1969) or very much so (Hochreuther, 1912; Zacharuk, 1962). (2) Sensilla may be circular (Gnatzy and Schmidt, 1971) or elliptical (Chevalier, 1969). (3) The cap is often linked to the surrounding cuticular bulge by a softer hinge (Fig. 2B; Chapman *et al.*, 1973) and one or more buttresses (Moran and Rowley III, 1975; Gnatzy and Schmidt, 1971; McIver and Siemicki, 1978). (4) The dendrite tip may be round or strongly bilateral in cross section (Smith, 1969; Thurm *et al.*, 1975). (5) L1 is sometimes reinforced by an amorphous looking (EM) band (Fig. 2C) (Smith, 1969). (6) A cuticular collar may protrude from the ring of raised cuticle surrounding the cap (Fig. 2B, C); L3, which contains the dendrite tip and attaches to it (Chevalier, 1969; Gnatzy and Schmidt, 1971; Moran and Rowley III, 1975; McIver and Siemicki, 1978).
Slit sensilla (1) Harvestman (Gnatzy, unpubl.): apart from orthodox slit sensilla there are some with a solid cuticular cupola bulging on one side. The dendrite tip sharply bends in a plane parallel to the short axis of the slit before it attaches to the covering membrane

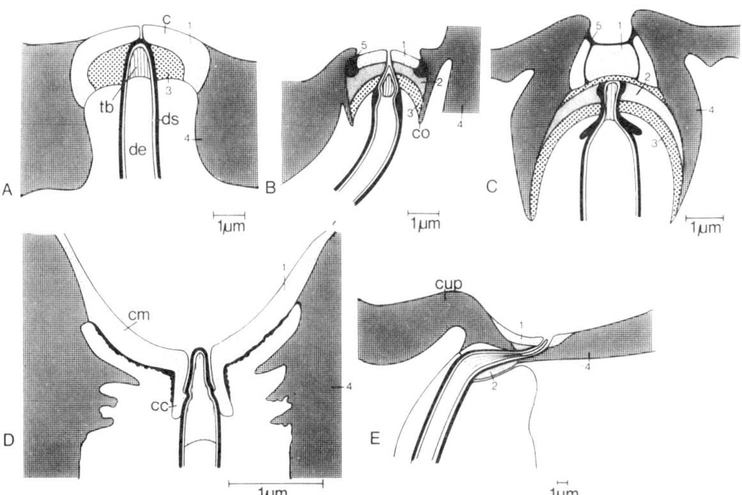

Figure 2 Dendrite attachment sites of various arthropod strain detectors. Cross sections through cuticle parallel to small axis of hole. A–C, insect campaniform sensilla, D–E, arachnid slit sensilla. The various layers (1–5) of the cuticle were identified according to their electron microscopical appearance (standard treatment): L1, homogeneous, most likely epicuticular; L2, spongy; L3, fibrous; L4, general cuticle; L5, very electron dense. *c*, cap; *tb*, tubular body; *de*, dendrite; *ds*, dendrite sheath; *co*, collar; *cm*, covering membrane; *cc*, coupling cylinder; *cup*, cupola. A, *Apis mellifera*, head (modified from Thurm, 1964); B, *Gryllus bimaculatus*, close to socket of cercal thread hair (modified from Gnatzy and Schmidt, 1971); C, *Calliphora erythrocephala*, haltere, dorsal scapal plate (modified from Smith, 1969); D, *Cupiennius salei*, spider leg (modified from Barth, 1971); E, *Opilio ravennae*, leg of harvestman (Gnatzy, in prep.). In D and E a second dendrite ending more proximally is not included in the drawing.

(Fig. 2E). Morphology suggests that the cupola presses the dendrite from above when the sensillum is adequately stimulated by lateral compression of the slit. (2) Scorpion (Barth, unpubl.): here the dendrite tip is also bent, but in a plane parallel to the long axis of the slit. It ends tightly embedded in a covering membrane which is probably equivalent to L3. By contrast to the spider the slit is covered by a rather thick epicuticle (in addition to covering membrane) which is detached from the underlying cuticle above the slit. (3) Supernumerary dendrites: all arachnid cases studied have a second dendrite ending more proximally. In the scorpion there are sometimes still more. For the spider, a number of arguments against a stimulation of the second dendrite by slit compression have been given (Barth, 1971, 1972*a*, *b*). The actual role of all these dendrites, however, is unknown.

Occurrence

1. *Campaniform sensilla of insects*

Campaniform sensilla have been found in a rich variety of insect species (Bullock and Horridge, 1965). Their description started as early as 1857, when Hicks studied the spectacular accumulation on the dipteran haltere which is studded with hundreds of campaniform sensilla arranged in groups and closely in parallel around its base (Pflugstaedt, 1912). Subsequently, campaniform sensilla have been described from all major parts of the adult insect exoskeleton.

Although there is no comprehensive map of the campaniform sensilla of one insect species, maps of various parts of the exoskeleton of different species give a good idea of their widespread occurrence. The reader is particularly referred to the cockroach leg (Pringle, 1938; Krämer and Markl, 1978), the dipteran haltere (Pflugstaedt, 1912; Pringle, 1948), the antenna of the honey bee (Dietz and Humphreys, 1971; Esslen and Kaissling, 1976), the antenna of a saturniid moth (Boeckh, Kaissling and Schneider, 1960), the antenna of the ambrosia beetle (Moeck, 1968), the wing of a grasshopper (Albert *et al.*, 1976), various butterflies and other insects (Vogel, 1911; Pringle, 1957; Cartheuser, 1975), and orthopteran cerci (Siehler, 1924). More details are listed in Table 1.

Like arachnid slit sensilla, insect campaniform sensilla can be classified according to three types of configuration (Fig. 1): isolated (single c.s.), loosely grouped (group of c.s.), and lying closely side by side (compound c.s.).

2. *Campaniform sensilla of Crustacea*

Two types of campaniform sensilla are known in crustaceans. One is found on the dactylopodite of crabs and lobsters and has been identified electrophysiologically as mechanoreceptive (Shelton and Laverack, 1968; Barth, 1980). There are about 200 (5th pereiopod) to 500 (2nd pereiopod) such sensilla on the dactylopodite of a medium-sized shore crab (Barth and Lafaire, unpubl.); the density increases distally and they are parti-

Table 1 Examples of the occurrence of campaniform sensilla in insects

Animal	**Part of body**	**Number**	**Comment**	**Author**
Periplaneta americana (cockroach)	leg	91–100	93 % forming 6 groups on trochanter, femur, and tibia; remainder single sens. on tarsus	Pringle (1938)
Typodendron lineatum (ambrosia beetle)	antenna	26	only single camp. sens. and almost exclusively on 1st and last segment	Moeck (1968)
Apis mellifera (worker bee)	antenna	44–53	mainly on 1st and last segment with 5–8 and 16–18 camp. sens. each	Esslen and Kaissling (1976)
Melanoplus sanguinipes (grasshopper)	wing	fore wing 54 hind wing 124	only on top surface; concentrated along longitudinal veins; on fore wing only single camp. sens., among hind wing sens. 4 groups at base with 20–30 each	Albert *et al.* (1976)
Musca domestica (house fly)	wing	105	mainly on upper side with 72 as groups near base and 4 single; on lower side 27 in groups and 2 single	Melin (1941)
Calliphora erythrocephala (blowfly)	haltere	330	3 large compound organs with ca. 100 each; 2 small compound organs with 17 and 10 sens., respectively	Pflugstaedt (1912) Pringle (1948)

cularly numerous at the epicuticular tip. The diameter of this type is about 5 μm and its cap is flat. The second type is much more conspicuous, with an arched cap sunk into the cuticle. It occurs on the antennules of several decapods (Laverack, 1976) but still awaits fine structural and physiological identification.

3. *Slit sensilla of arachnids*

Among the arachnids, spiders are the best studied group. From detailed surveys we know the number and distribution of slit sensilla in both hunting and web spiders (McIndoo, 1911; Vogel, 1923; Kaston, 1935; Barth and Libera, 1970). The general picture of sensillum distribution is rather uniform and *Cupiennius salei*, the most intensively studied case, will serve as an example here (Barth and Libera, 1970).

The majority of slits can easily be classified into three categories of configuration (Barth and Stagl, 1976): isolated, single slits (distance from closest neighbouring slit $>100\ \mu m$), groups of slits (maximum distance $100\ \mu m$), and compound or lyriform organs (close side-by-side arrangement with typical shortest distance $\leqq 5\ \mu m$) (Fig. 1). Roughly half of the 3300 slits found in *Cupiennius* are either single slits or small groups. The other half forms a total of 144 lyriform organs, each composed of 2 to 29 slits. Whereas single slits are found on all parts of the skeleton, compound organs are restricted to the appendages (134 on legs and pedipalps, 10 on spinnerets and chelicerae). Conspicuous groups occur on the trochanter (Fig. 1), chelicerae, and petiolus.

A wide range of both the richness in total sensillar supply and the relative share contributed to it by the three configuration types was found by a comparison of the walking legs of representatives of 5 arachnid orders (Barth and Stagl, 1976). While spiders have 325 slits on the leg, only 47 and 76 slits were counted on that of a harvestman and whip spider, respectively. Spiders are also unparalleled with respect to the number of lyriform organs. In contrast to the 15 lyriform organs on each of their legs only one or two were counted on the legs of species in the other four arachnid orders.

Mechanical aspects

Much of the refinement and specialization found in the morphology of arthropod strain detectors can be understood in terms of its mechanical significance. This is true at all levels of consideration: the individual receptor, the groups of sensilla and compound organs, and finally the distribution over the exoskeleton. Clearly, an understanding of the potential adequate input parameters is essential at every step of the analysis.

1. *The input*

1.1. *General* The strains measured by slit sensilla and campaniform sensilla result from a variety of loads. Muscular activity is one source and the arrangement of a large number of sensilla suggests a direct proprioceptive measurement of strain induced displacements at and around muscle and tendon attachment sites (single slits on spider leg and opisthosoma; Barth and Libera, 1970). In other cases muscular activity is monitored in a more indirect way, when the sensilla (e.g. lyriform organs on spider leg) are placed close to hinge lines and articular condyli at joints where the forces generated are transferred from one leg segment to the next. In addition, the sensilla may be found far away from both muscle attachment sites and articulations, and may for instance monitor bending and twisting of wings far out in their periphery (Vogel, 1911; Pringle, 1957; Albert *et al.*, 1976). In spiders, hemolymph pressure (which is used to extend the leg at some joints lacking extensor muscles) is another potential input (Stewart and Martin, 1974; Blickhan and Barth, 1979; Blickhan, in prep.).

In a few cases arthropod exoskeletal strain detectors are not dealing with proprio-, but exteroreception. Vibration of the substratum is the adequate input to some campaniform sensilla (Markl, 1970; Schnorbus, 1971; Shelton and Laverack, 1968; Barth, 1980) and slit sensilla (Walcott and van der Kloot, 1959; Liesenfeld, 1961; Barth, in press). Campaniform sensilla on the cricket eye are stimulated by dirt particles and involved in eliciting eye cleaning behaviour (Honegger *et al.*, 1979). Campaniform sensilla at the socket of thread hairs on the cricket cercus (Fig. 1b) are stimulated whenever the hair movement is strong enough to touch and slightly deform the socket (Dumpert and Gnatzy, 1977).

In view of this variety of possibilities for adequate load application it is important to realize that the *surface* of the exoskeleton is of particular interest. In all sensilla of concern here the dendrite is coupled to a covering membrane attached to the outermost layers of the cuticle and for a number of good reasons its very tip is considered the site of transduction. No matter what type of load is applied—the exoskeleton may be stretched, compressed, sheared, bent, buckled or twisted—the same applies to the surface in all cases (except if loaded directly): there are strains only in its plane, tension in one direction and compression perpendicular to it (Barth, 1972*a*). It follows that adequate stimulation, i.e. compression of the cuticular hole perpendicular to its long axis, does not depend on one type of load application alone, but may result from all of them.

1.2. *A word on definitions* Three different effects of load may be distinguished when forces pertinent to situations like those mentioned above act on the exoskeleton (Barth, 1972*b*). (1) Stress (N/mm^2) is the force per unit area generated in the material under the external force and resisting it. (2) Strain ($\varepsilon = \Delta l/l_0$) is the relative change in length of a unit volume in a given direction under load. (3) Displacement (ω) of a specific point or line of the material under load is to be distinguished from strain of a unit volume. In a bar under tension (monoaxial stress) it is the integral of strains of all unit volumes in between the site of load application and that particular point: $\omega = \int_0^s \varepsilon\, ds$. Sites of greatest strain (stress) and displacement are not identical. Even in the simple case of the bar under tension, displacement increases with length of the bar whereas strain (stress) is constant all along its axis. In case of multiaxial stresses the situation is much more complex.

When discussing strain reception it is important to realize that strain is the *relative* change in length. The sensilla do not measure relative change in length, but absolute change of length which is the sum of many unit strains, i.e. *displacement*. The ease of deformability of the auxiliary structures and the lack of spatial closeness of the dendrite tip to the areas of particularly high stresses along the circumference of the cuticular hole emphasize the importance of displacement (Barth, 1972*b*, 1976).

The holes formed by the sensilla in the exoskeleton are sources of stress concentration, i.e. localized high stresses as they occur at grooves, shoulders, notches, holes, etc. If closeness of the dendrite tip to areas of high stress were crucial, it would be best placed in cuticle areas at the long ends of the hole or—in one case of a round hole—close to the ends of the diameter perpendicular to the direction of stress in the undisturbed cuticle (Peterson, 1974). No such arrangement is found.

Stress concentration is given by the stress concentration factor $K_{tg} = \sigma_{max}/\sigma$, i.e. the ratio of maximum stress to applied stress distant from the hole. For circular holes, K measures between 3 and 5 for $a/w \leqq 0.6$ (a, diameter of hole; w, width of disc). At the edge of an elliptical hole, K mainly depends on the ratio of the long (b) to the short axis (a). Typical values are between 3 and 18 for $1 \leqq b/a \leqq 10$ in an infinite disc and may be even higher in finite width (w) discs provided $0.5 \leqq b/w \leqq 1.0$. In slits such as those of slit sensilla K-factors as high as 20 can be expected (Peterson, 1974; Barth, 1972*b*).

1.3. *Measurement in vivo* There are no published data on the stresses, strains, and displacements actually occurring in the arthropod exoskeleton *in vivo*. We have now succeeded in applying miniature strain gauges to the cuticle of large spiders and have monitored strains during locomotion (Blickhan and Barth, 1979; Blickhan, in prep.). Typical values for strain are in the range of 20 $\mu\varepsilon$, but peak values may be four times as large. At the site of the tibial lyriform organ HS8, compressional strains are found when the leg touches the ground during locomotion. Tensional strains, most likely due to hemolymph pressure, accompany the other parts of the movement cycle.

2. *Cuticular auxiliary structures*

Adequate stimulation of campaniform and slit sensilla invariably includes a transformation of the input on its way from the general cuticle to the dendrite. Deformation of the cuticular hole is transferred to the covering membrane and from there to the dendrite tip. Both the shape of the hole and of the covering membrane have an important influence on these processes and consequently on receptor sensitivity. Fig. 3 summarizes the basic effects of the most important morphological features of the sensillar design on deformability (sensitivity). All these parameters vary, and it is this variation which to a large extent is the basis for the adaptive radiation found. The effects to be expected can be readily demonstrated by model

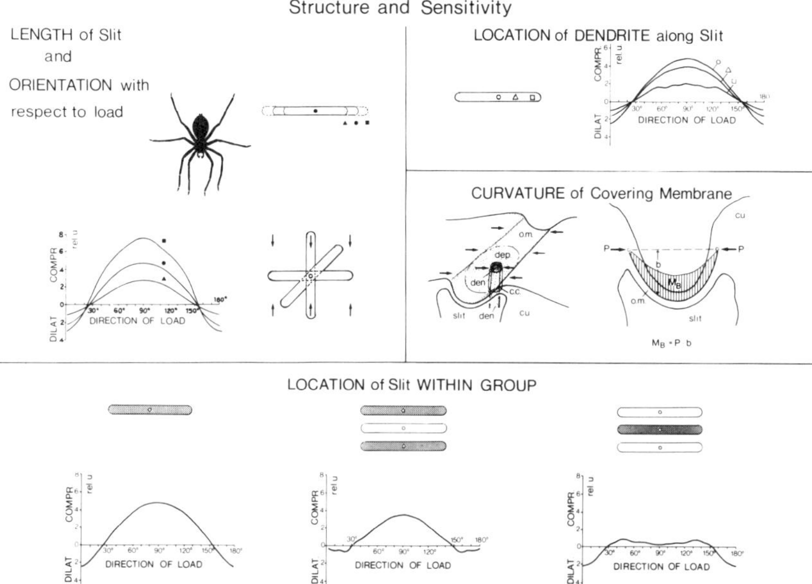

Figure 3 Morphological parameters which determine deformability and thus sensitivity of arthropod strain detectors as shown for spider slit sensilla. Graphs present results of model studies with slits cut into araldite discs (load applied in their plane). *Dilat.*, dilatation of slit; *compr.*, compression of slit; *rel. u.*, relative units for displacement; *Mb*, bending moment; *P*, force; *b*, depth of covering membrane (*o.m.*). Graphs at bottom refer to shaded slit in respective drawings above.

experiments (Pringle, 1938; Barth, 1972*a*, *b*; Barth and Pickelmann, 1975; Barth, in prep.).

2.1. *The hole* Whereas campaniform sensilla are round or (more often) elliptical, with maximum ratios of the axes rarely exceeding 3 : 1 (Pringle, 1955), slit sensilla have length-to-width ratios from about 4 to 100.

Both the absolute amount of deformation and its directionality increase with increasing length-to-width ratio (surrounding material loaded in its plane). Elongated slits are much more easily deformed by forces perpendicular to their long axis than by forces in parallel with it and their deformation rapidly increases with increasing absolute length (Fig. 3).

2.2. *The covering membrane* A prominent feature of the cuticular membrane covering both the slit and campaniform sensillum is its curvature. Even in most of those cases of campaniform sensilla where L1 is flat, L3, which takes up the dendrite tip, is arched (Chevalier, 1969; Moran and Rowley III, 1975). The depth-to-width ratio of the arch seen in cross section of the covering membrane may reach 1.

This curvature increases the bending moment resulting from lateral forces when the sensillar hole is deformed by strains in the cuticle. It therefore decreases the forces necessary to deform the covering membrane. The effect of outward (in campaniform sensilla) and inward (slit sensilla) bulging on deformability is mechanically equivalent.

Taking a trough-like covering membrane such as that of a slit sensillum, the ease with which deformation is produced by *lateral* forces is underlined by considering bending by forces *parallel* to its long axis. The membrane is stiffer for bending along its long axis for the same geometrical reason.

The bending moment (M_b) of such an arched structure if loaded by a pair of lateral forces (P) is given as $M_b = P \times b$ (b, depth or height of arch). M_b increases with the amount of prebending. Additional bending of the membrane increases accordingly (Barth, 1972*a*). When calculating the amount of displacement along the arch as a function of the amount of prebending, to study the effect of a constant displacement of its ends on purely geometrical grounds is not sufficient. The force necessary to produce such constant displacement depends on the amount of prebending. Application of the theorems of Castigliano (Mönch, 1971; Marwitz and Barth, unpubl.) enable one to determine displacements as a function of prebending and location along the cross-section at a constant applied force. Both the vertical and horizontal displacement components rapidly increase with increasing depth (b) to width (a) ratio.

2.3. *Adequate stimulation and dendrite deformation* Knowledge of the various geometrical and morphological features of the cuticular auxiliary structures now allows us to draw a picture of the sequence of mechanical events occurring during adequate stimulation. A number of similarities again emerge for slit and campaniform sensilla (Fig. 4).

Slit sensilla

According to model studies performed in combination with microscopical and electrophysiological observations of the original slit sensilla (Barth, 1972*a*, *b*, 1973*a*; Barth and Pickelmann, 1975; Barth, 1976) the various cuticular structures conducting the stimulus are designed and arranged so as to provide for high deformability. Therefore an analysis of the stimulus at this level clearly favours displacement and deformation as the most important factor, and not stress or strain proper. The specificity, selectivity, and sensitivity of the receptor explain themselves to a large extent as a consequence of this feature.

A sequence of four events focuses the stimulus on to less than 1 μm^2 of dendrite area (Barth, 1972*b*). (1) The slit is compressed by forces roughly perpendicular to its long axis. This direction most effectively deforms the slit due to the mechanical filter action, which results from its elongated shape. Dilatation of the slit is not effective physiologically. (2) The covering membrane is most effectively further bent by slit compression due to its arched cross-section and thinness (Fig. 4). (3) The coupling cylinder attached to the covering membrane in an area of maximum bending moment is then in turn deformed by this bending. The main

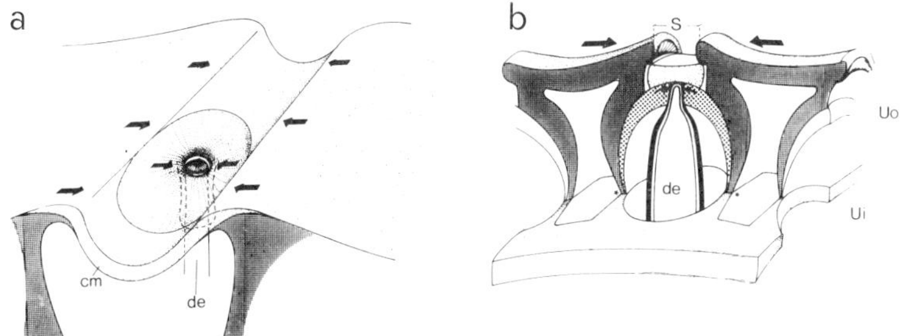

Figure 4 Adequate deformation of a slit (a) and a campaniform (b) sensillum. Arrows indicate direction of compressional forces which finally lead to a deformation of the dendrite tip. a, spider (modified from Barth, 1972*b*); b, fly haltere (modified from Thurm *et al.*, 1975). S decreases by up to 0.3 μm if circumference Ui flattens during adequate stimulation.

component contained in this deformation is argued to be the compressional deformation of its outer cross-section perpendicular to the slit's long axis. According to our model studies there is no amplification of the displacement on its way to the dendrite. (4) The final event is a deformation of the dendrite tip in the coupling cylinder by monoaxial compressional forces. The essential aspect here, as in other mechanoreceptors, is the non-uniformity of the forces applied which inevitably leads to a non-uniform deformation. This in turn implies both pressure and tension (Barth, 1972*b*, 1976) which in a mechanically homogeneous cylinder would be oriented perpendicular and parallel to its long axis, respectively.

Stretching the dendrite in the gross morphological sense of earlier hypotheses (Pringle, 1955) is not effective (Barth, 1972*a*, *b*, 1976). Arguments against the importance of shear movements parallel to the slit's outer border and also against the importance of deformation at the inner opening of the slit are found in the literature (Barth, 1972*a*, *b*, 1976). The same applies to the inner end of the coupling cylinder.

Campaniform sensilla of insects

Due to their structural similarity, many of the findings on the slit sensilla also apply to insect campaniform sensilla.

In elliptical sensilla the mechanical directionality again favours deformation by forces perpendicular to the long axis. This contradicts the hypothesis developed by Pringle (1938) that stretching the dendrite by an outward bulging of the long axis of the cap due to forces parallel to it is the essential effect. In addition to the arguments derived from the study of slit sensilla (Barth, 1972*b*) direct evidence has now accumulated which supports the first alternative and implies dendrite deformation by monoaxial compressional forces (Fig. 4; Spinola and Chapman, 1975; Thurm *et al.*, 1975). This can also be deduced from other studies like that of Heinzel and Gewecke (1979) on campaniform sensilla on the locust antenna.

A number of additional arguments all derived from structural features fit well into this picture. (1) In many cases the arching of the covering membrane along its short axis exceeds that along its long axis. (2) Even more important is the fact that the dendrite proper with its tubular body ends in L3 (and L2, if present) and not in L1 (Fig. 2). L3 is often if not always much more arched than L1 (e.g. Chevalier, 1969; Moran and Rowley III, 1975) which again favours deformation as described above. (3) The importance of L3 for the uptake of lateral forces and deformation of the dendrite is stressed by a ring of softer cuticle (L5) which couples the cap (L1) to the surrounding exocuticle (L4). (4) The dendrite was found to flatten at its tip in bilateral sensilla. The long axis of such a dendritic fan is oriented parallel to that of the cuticular hole (Chevalier, 1969; Smith, 1969; Moran *et al.*, 1971). The area exposed to lateral compressional forces is thereby increased.

The arguments given by Spinola and Chapman (1975) to show that proprioceptive stimuli indent rather than bulge the cap are not wholly satisfactory. While it is not surprising that an indentation of the cap with an experimental probe stimulates the sensillum, it is difficult to understand how such indentation can result from compression perpendicular to the long cap axis, which at the same time is considered the natural input by these authors. For the same reason the amplification of cap indentation suggested to occur due to the arched geometry of L3 (Moran *et al.*, 1976) seems of doubtful significance.

3. *Groups and compound organs*

A prominent feature of both the arachnid slit sensilla and insect campaniform sensilla is their tendency to form groups and compound organs. If we wish to understand the physiological implications of such grouping we have first of all to determine its mechanical consequences. These were studied both in models and in original organs and found to have a dramatic effect on (1) deformability and hence sensitivity distribution within the group, (2) distribution of the sites of maximum deformation, and (3) directionality.

(1) Deformability of a slit is drastically reduced by the presence of neighbouring slits closely arranged in parallel (Fig. 3; Barth and Pickelmann, 1975). Peripheral slits take up more load than the intermediate ones, and in large groups (e.g. 5 slits) they may even be more deformed than an isolated slit of the same dimension. Maximum values of compression found in a group of seven slits arranged to model the tibial lyriform organ HS8 varied by a factor of 41 (Barth and Pickelmann, 1975). Spider lyriform organs can be classified as five basic types of arrangement differing in length distribution among the slits and their lateral spread. Fig. 5 depicts two extreme cases: one impresses with the uniformity of the deformation found in its slits due to their constant length and lateral shift, the other demonstrates the complex effects variations in both parameters may have.

(2) In lyriform organs the dendrite tip often does not end midway along the slit (Barth and Libera, 1970). Model experiments suggest that in general the attachment site coincides with the area of maximum compression. As a rule compression is greatest with pressure loads applied at an angle of 60° to 105° to the organ's long axis (Figs. 3 and 5).

(3) Change in load direction in general does not alter the distribution

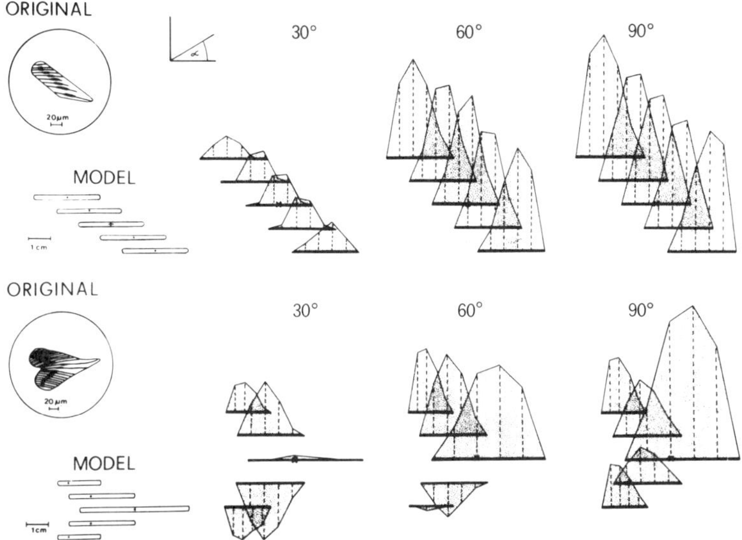

Figure 5 Model experiments to show mechanical effects of various types of close parallel slit arrangement. Slits were cut into araldite discs according to the patterns derived from two different lyriform slit sense organs (left). Models loaded in their plane from varying angles and deformation of slits measured with sensitive strain gauge device. Baseline of graphs gives length of slit; deformation plotted in relative units at the respective site along slit (compression upwards, dilatation downwards). Load direction given above graph. Note dependence of deformation on type of slit arrangement, loading angle, and position of slit within group.

of the sites of maximum compression by much if it is between 75° and 105°. At other angles, changes as small as 15° or less may result in a considerable shift (Fig. 5). In theory this shift could be used for an analysis of load direction, as does the divergence of slit direction found in other cases (Barth and Stagl, 1976). Load direction would then be reflected in the pattern of relative excitation of the slits within the group (despite their parallel arrangement). Whether load direction does indeed change at any one site under natural conditions we do not know. A gradation in threshold sensitivity as predicted by (1) was shown directly in physiological experiments (see below).

The distinction between more loosely arranged "groups" of slits and lyriform organs was originally made purely on morphological grounds (Barth and Stagl, 1976). The more significant question concerns the minimum distance at which slits do not influence each other mechanically. According to model studies with slits of equal length l the critical distance is roughly $2 \times l$, which coincides with values established technologically (Ficker, pers. comm.).

4. *Topography of sensilla*

Looking at the multitude of sites where slit and campaniform sensilla are found in many different species it seems too ambitious to explain their varying topography by a relatively limited set of rules. It is evident that they occur at sites on the exoskeleton which are subject to loads. However, it is hard to think of a piece of exoskeleton *not* subject to load. The widespread occurrence of the sensilla on practically all parts of the skeleton is an expression of this. In the spider the slit sensilla are found not only in stiff cuticle but also (even though in much smaller numbers) embedded in the soft cuticle of the opisthosoma.

The main question is: what is the direction and amplitude of stresses and strains at the sites of the sensilla under naturally occurring load conditions, and how does the location, orientation, sensitivity, and directionality correlate with them both mechanically and physiologically? Answers come from both an experimental approach and comparative studies of sensillar topography.

Experimental data Only one case studied in some detail will be quoted: the lyriform organ HS8 on the spider leg tibia is typical of a large proportion of lyriform organs in its location laterally on the leg and close to the distal end of the leg segment, and in the orientation of its slits roughly parallel to the long leg axis (Barth and Libera, 1970). According to tension optical experiments with model legs, under load conditions simulating muscular activity, the lines of principal stresses are indeed compression lines at the site of the sense organ. Furthermore they take a course close to perpendicular to the organ. Both results were predicted by reason of the directional properties of slit deformation (Barth and Pickelmann, 1975). They also agree with electrophysiological studies on the sensitivity of the organ to compressional forces (Barth, 1972*b*; Barth and Bohnenberger, 1978). The most recent in a series of experiments gave us a measure of the strains actually occurring at the organ site during locomotion. 20 $\mu\varepsilon$ is a typical value and it is compressional strain when the leg touches the ground. However, considerably more information on the origin and distribution of strains in the exoskeleton is needed if we are to understand fully the sensory system measuring them.

Comparative topography Since all the variations of load application (tension, bending, torsion etc.) as well as their combinations will result in tension and compression at the surface, they are all potentially effective stimuli. An accordingly broad spectrum of topographical features should be expected and does indeed exist. Unifying features are most likely to emerge from comparative studies like those on the leg (Barth and Stagl, 1976) and wing (Pringle, 1957) sensilla. Bilateral symmetry of a sensillum is particularly helpful because the directionality implied is an indication of the effective load direction to be expected.

Organs on the leg are taken as an example. In spiders they account for more than 80% of the total number of slit sensilla present. The following rules on their topography apply at least to a large proportion of them.

(*1*) Both the insect campaniform sensilla (Pringle, 1938) and the arachnid slit sensilla (Barth and Stagl, 1976) on a leg are massively concentrated on the proximal segments, in particular on the trochanter. This is paralleled by a concentration of musculature proximally in the leg which offers a plausible explanation. It is here that the main amplitudes of return and power strokes are produced during locomotion and the contraction of the muscles introduces loads into the skeleton at the sites of their origin and insertion.

(*2*) A location laterally on the leg and close to a joint and with the slits oriented roughly parallel to the long leg axis (as found for lyriform organ HS8) is also characteristic of other organs. This applies not only to the spider leg, but to legs of other arachnids as well. The experimental results provided for HS8 are in essence also applicable to these cases.

(*3*) A proximity to joints is a prominent feature of many slits and insect campaniform sensilla on the leg. Their closeness to the joint is relative, however. Some are found right behind the load-bearing surface which would seem to be a good place for a strain detector. Others are clearly not in the immediate neighbourhood of condyli or hinges, even though they are at the end of the leg segment. This underlines the previous statement that neither stress nor strain proper are the important input parameters at the level of the sensory hole, but displacement. Displacement may very well increase up to some distance from the points of load transfer. Furthermore, compressional forces transferred across the joints are likely to cause bending of the cuticle. This again must preferably occur at some distance from the thickened and stiff structures of the joint proper.

(*4*) Single slit sensilla on the spider leg are usually found far from joints but often close to muscle attachment sites.

Physiological properties

1. *Absolute sensitivity*

The following data on sensitivities are presented to illustrate the functional refinement found in arthropod strain detectors. A direct comparison among the various cases is difficult due to differences in shape of skeletal parts, cuticle stiffness, structure of joints, and the like.

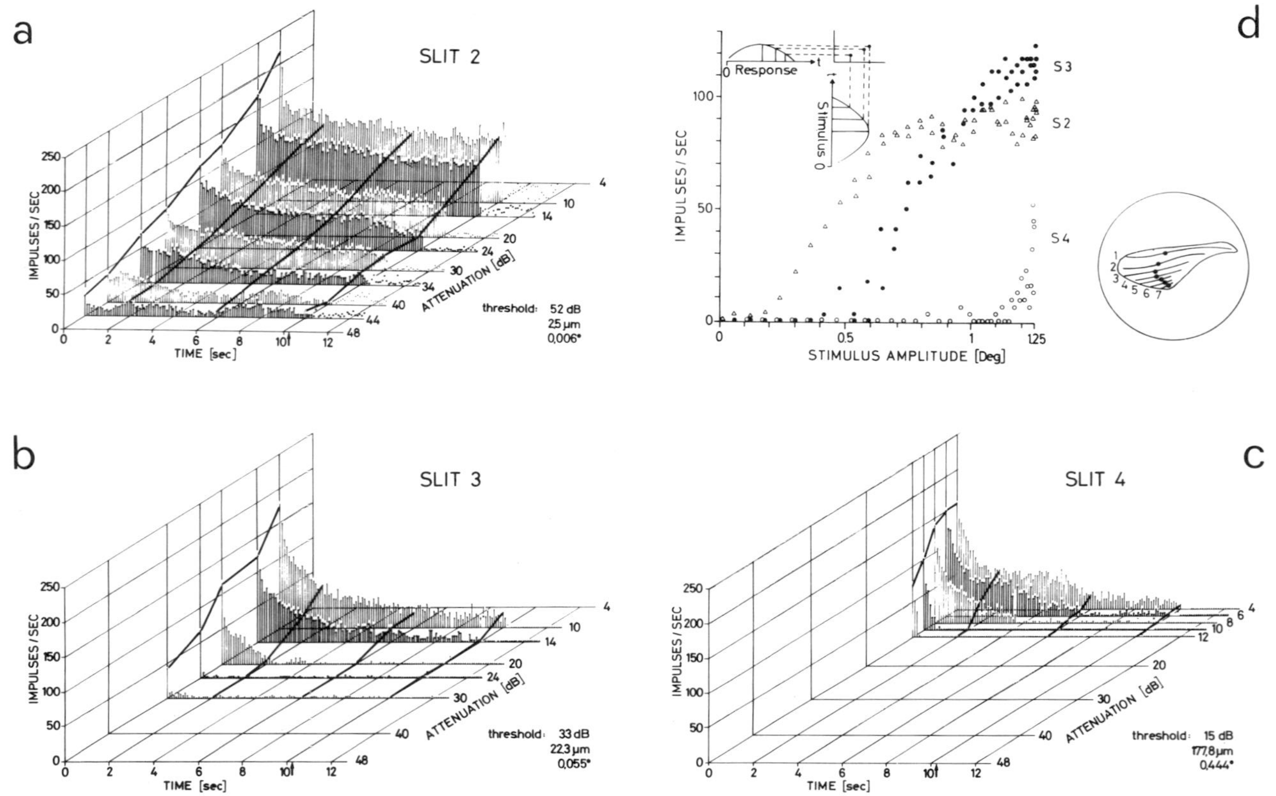
a
SLIT 2
IMPULSES / SEC
TIME [sec]
ATTENUATION [dB]
threshold: 52 dB
25 µm
0,006°
d
IMPULSES / SEC
STIMULUS AMPLITUDE [Deg]
Response
Stimulus
S3
S2
S4
b
SLIT 3
IMPULSES / SEC
TIME [sec]
ATTENUATION [dB]
threshold: 33 dB
22,3 µm
0,055°
c
SLIT 4
IMPULSES / SEC
TIME [sec]
ATTENUATION [dB]
threshold: 15 dB
177,8 µm
0,444°

Proprioceptive

Lyriform organ HS8 on the posterior aspect of the tibia is stimulated by a backward deflection of the metatarsus. Starting from a position in which the articular surfaces just touch each other, angular movements necessary to stimulate 5 of its 7 slits vary from 0.01° to 0.92° (ramp stimuli; Barth and Bohnenberger, 1978). With sinusoidal stimuli, threshold values measured as little as 0.006° at 100 Hz (Fig. 7; Bohnenberger, 1979). The forces necessary to produce a deflection of 0.25° were 1.32 mN, and about 40 μN for 0.006°.

Group 6 campaniform sensilla on the cockroach tibia (Fig. 1a) were extensively studied by Chapman and associates. Their standard experimental stimulus is indentation of the cap (Chapman *et al.*, 1973). Minimum thresholds for indentation at 3 Hz are 10 to 20 nm. The forces necessary to produce them are about 100 to 200 μN.

In *fly haltere* campaniform sensilla the width of the cap as seen from above (Figs. 1c and 2c) narrows by roughly 0.2 μm with maximal stimulation produced by a dorsal deflection of the haltere by ca. 15° (ventral scapal receptor field, haltere base immobilized) (Thurm *et al.*, 1975). A change in dendrite diameter of the same order of magnitude may result. This is close to the maximum of 0.1 μm found for an insect hair receptor (Thurm, 1965).

Exteroceptive

A *single slit* on the tarsus of a spider responds to airborne sound in the far field. In its best frequency range (0.3 to 0.7 kHz) the lowest thresholds are about 40dB SPL (0.02 μbar) (Barth, 1967).

The metatarsal lyriform organ of the spider is vibration sensitive. Threshold vibration amplitudes are minimal between 1 and 5 kHz where they measured consistently from 10^{-3} to 10^{-2} μm in different species (Walcott and van der Kloot, 1959; Liesenfeld, 1961; Geetha Bali and Barth, in prep.). Minimal acceleration was found as low as 2×10^{-3} cm/sec^2 (0.1 Hz).

Figure 6 The effects of a close parallel arrangement of slits in lyriform organs studied electrophysiologically by recording from individual slits. The example given is lyriform organ HS8 (Barth and Libera, 1970) on the spider tibia (s. inset in d). (a), (b), and (c) give the working ranges of slits 2, 3, and 4. Note difference in threshold and overlap. Ramp and hold stimulation by sideways movement of metatarsus. (d) gives the instantaneous impulse frequency plotted in phase with sinusoidal stimulus (0.01 Hz). Note that linear parts (great increment sensitivity) of the dynamic response curves of the three slits complement each other. (a–c, from Barth and Bohnenberger, 1978; d, from Bohnenberger, in prep.).

Campaniform sensilla between trochanter and femur are substrate vibration sensitive in leaf cutting ants. Typically minimum displacement of the substrate at threshold is between 10^{-2} and 10^{-3} μm (1 to 3 kHz) and smallest acceleration is 5 cm/sec^2 (100 to 1500 Hz) (Markl, 1970).

Campaniform sensilla on the crab dactylopodite respond to touch and vibration. When vibrating the cuticle directly with a fine probe, ampli-

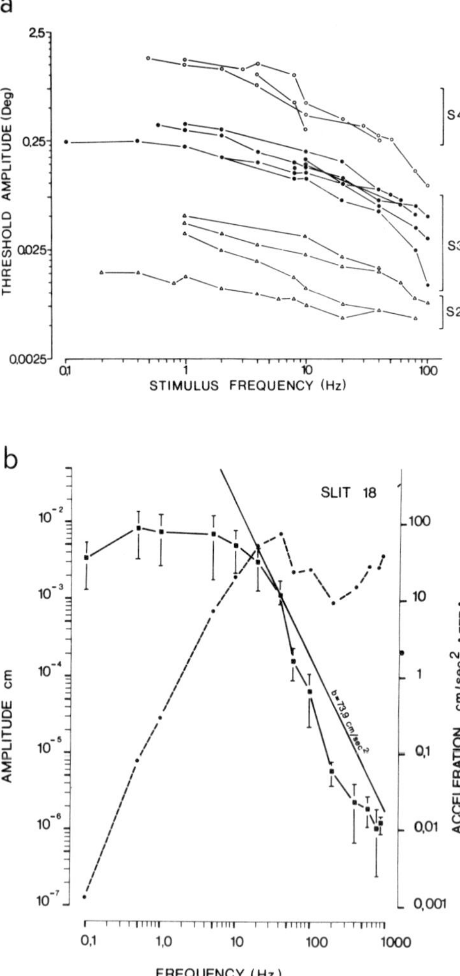

Figure 7 Tuning curves of individual slits in spider lyriform organs. (a) slits 2, 3, and 4 of lyriform organ HS8 (cf. Fig. 6); stimulation by sinusoidal sideways movement. (b), slit of the metatarsal lyriform organ which is sensitive to substrate vibration; stimulus given as displacement (pp; N = 10; standard deviation given) and acceleration. (a, from Bohnenberger, in prep.; b, from Geetha Bali and Barth, in prep.).

tudes as small as 4×10^{-1} μm are effective between 100 and 130 Hz. Smallest acceleration is 0.02 cm/sec^2 at 1 Hz (Barth, 1980).

2. *The significance of grouping*

There is only one compound organ which has been studied for the physiological consequences of a close arrangement of individual sensilla. Again it is the lyriform organ HS8 of the spider leg tibia. What can the compound organ do more or better than the single sensillum? What is the functional difference between the slits? The main answers are given in Figs. 6 and 7.

(*1*) The differences in *threshold* sensitivity predicted from model studies for the different slits in a group could indeed be confirmed in the electrophysiological experiment. Threshold deflection of the metatarsus varied by about 40dB among 5 of the 7 slits, not even including the most and the least sensitive which are difficult to handle experimentally.

(*2*) The stimulus *amplitude ranges* covered by the slits show much overlap. Apart from differences in threshold there is no range fractionation. The 45dB range covered by slit 2 also encloses the ranges of slits 3, 4 and 5.

(*3*) The instantaneous impulse frequency during sinusoidal stimulation (Fig. 6d) discloses, however, that the *linear parts* of the working ranges do to a large extent complement each other with only little overlap. Taking the organ as a whole, its linear range and range of high absolute increment sensitivity is much increased compared to the individual slit whose absolute increment sensitivity drops markedly only 10dB or even less above threshold.

(*4*) *The largest of the slits* (no. 1) differs from the rest by its much lower threshold and it is the only one normally spontaneously active and with a strictly phasic response.

(*5*) The question of whether there is *tuning* of the slits to different frequencies is posed by the variation of slit length in the lyriform organs. The answer comes from electrophysiological experiments with lyriform organ HS8 and the metatarsal lyriform organ (Fig. 7). In both cases examined, tuning curves were determined for the component slits individually (HS8: 0.005 Hz to 1 kHz, Bohnenberger, 1979; metatarsal organ: 0.1 Hz to 1.0 kHz, Geetha Bali and Barth, in prep.). No marked tuning was found, nor significant differences among the slits. The slits do behave like high pass filters, however, and the tuning curve of the slits in the metatarsal vibration receptor declines steeply beyond about 20 Hz (Fig. 7). A shift of the lower frequency end below 0.1 Hz towards higher values is found comparing slits of decreasing threshold sensitivity in HS8. This is also reflected by differences in adaptation rate (Fig. 6).

Lyriform organ HS8 is involved in idiothetic (kinesthetic) orientation behaviour (Barth and Seyfarth, 1971; Seyfarth and Barth, 1972) and in a synergic leg reflex (Seyfarth, 1978*a*, *b*) which clearly places it among proprioceptors. Both its stimulus amplitude range, which is small as compared to long distance exteroreceptors like the eye and ear, its response to low frequencies, and the extension of the range of high increment sensitivity by the grouping of slits agree well with its proprioceptive function. Like other proprioceptors, this organ is considered to be part of a feedback system and to monitor relatively small deviations to bring the system back to the desired state.

3. *Transduction and encoding*

3.1. *Receptor current* In their studies on the primary processes in insect epithelial receptors, Thurm and his associates have largely used campaniform sensilla on the fly haltere (Thurm, 1974, 1977; Thurm and Wessel, 1979).

The crucial aspect of their theory is the existence of a potential difference across the epithelium, the *transepithelial potential* difference (TEP), at the receptor site. This TEP usually lies between 20 and 80 mV, with the cuticular side positive. It decreases with adequate receptor stimulation.

TEPs were found in many insect species and a terrestrial isopod. They are not a special feature of mechanoreceptors but also found with chemoreceptors. Dependence of the TEP on oxidative metabolism is readily demonstrated by anoxia. Its very quick recovery (up to 58 mV/s) after resupply of oxygen indicates that the underlying mechanism is an electrogenic ion (cation) transport and not mere diffusion. The site of such active transport is suggested to be the microvillous apical membrane of the *tormogen cell*, which is one of the sheath cells of the dendrite (Fig. 8). A number of its fine structural details resemble insect epithelia known to secrete potassium. It is potassium which is considered the main cation transported across the membrane. Accordingly the receptor lymph space of fly haltere campaniform sensilla does indeed contain as much as thirteen times the K^+-concentration found in the hemolymph (Küppers, 1974).

The potential difference generated by the non-neural tormogen cell is closely linked to the generation of the *receptor current*. Its polarity results in an increase of the receptor current which is also driven by other, neural batteries (Fig. 8). This situation is reminiscent of the role attributed to the non-neural battery of the *stria vascularis* in the inner ear (Davis, 1965; Thurm, 1974).

Similar to the hair cells of the inner ear, the *sensor region* of the dendrite is interpreted as a variable resistance and its adequate deformation assumed to increase its conductivity. The change in TEP found with receptor stimulation is taken to signal an increase of the current through

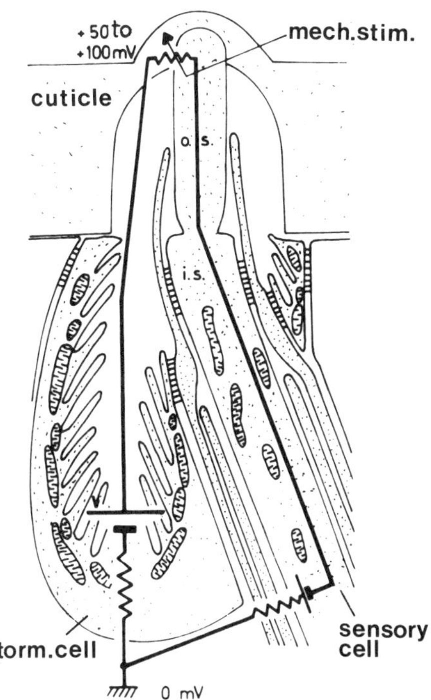

Figure 8 Schematic representation of the receptor current in a campaniform sensillum (from Thurm, 1977). Note non-neural battery located in apical membrane of tormogen cell (*torm. cell*) and variable resistance at site of adequate dendrite deformation (*mech. stim.*).

the sensory cell, which in turn would generate impulses by depolarizing more proximal regions of the dendritic membrane. In campaniform sensilla of the fly haltere sensitivity does indeed increase (or decrease) if the TEP is increased (or decreased) experimentally during mechanical stimulation. However, in other mechanoreceptors experimental results are different and more difficult to interpret (Erler and Thurm, 1978).

Several data point to a significant difference between insects and spiders (Barth, 1976) despite the general equivalence of types and arrangement of the cells making up their sensilla. No TEP can be recorded in the spider (Barth, 1976; Thurm and Wessel, 1979) and there is no such structural similarity between the apical membrane of the tormogen cell and insect epithelia known to actively secrete K^+ as in insect campaniform sensilla (Barth, 1971). Even stronger evidence against the existence of an electrogenic K^+-pump in slit sensilla comes from X-ray microanalysis of their receptor lymph. It contains high concentrations of Na and Cl, but almost no K (Rick *et al.*, 1976). In conclusion then, there is no evidence for a participation of non-neural cells in the generation of the receptor current in spiders.

3.2. *Transfer functions* Both slit and insect campaniform sensilla exhibit thresholds and rectifying properties with respect to dilatation. For that reason alone they are not strictly linear systems. Within limits, however, both do behave nearly linearly (output directly proportional to input: superposition law holds; input frequency preserved in output) and linear systems analysis has been applied successfully to the low amplitude and low frequency part of their working range. When subjected to a ramp and hold stimulus the response of both slit and campaniform sensilla in general exhibits a phasic initial peak and a subsequent, rather slow decline (Chapman and Smith, 1963; Schlegel, 1970; Barth, 1967, 1972*b*; Thurm *et al.*, 1975; Heinzel and Gewecke, 1979).

A strictly phasic slit was found in the lyriform organ HS8 on the tibia (Barth and Bohnenberger, 1978) and the metatarsal lyriform organ contains such slits, too (Geetha Bali and Barth, in prep.). These are exceptions, however.

The time course of this decline follows a *power law function* of the form

$$\mathrm{Y(t)} = \mathrm{d} \cdot \mathrm{A} \cdot \mathrm{t}^{-k}$$

where Y(t) = impulse frequency, d = receptor constant indicating gain, A = stimulus amplitude, t = time, and k = constant determining the slope of the decay (straight line on double logarithmic plot) (Chapman and Smith, 1963; Mann and Chapman, 1975; Chapman *et al.*, 1979; Barth, 1967; Bohnenberger, 1978 and in prep.). This type of step response is typical of a large number of receptors responding to different stimulus modalities and in various animal groups (Thorson and Biederman-Thorson, 1974).

The absolute values for the power coefficient k range from about 0.2 to 0.7 for the slits of the lyriform organ HS8 (stimulus: lateral deflection of metatarsus) and about 0.5 for campaniform sensilla on the cockroach tibia (stimulus: cap indentation). Such values are characteristic of the many receptors known with a response type between that of a frequency independent amplitude receptor ($k = 0$) and that of a velocity receptor ($k = 1$). Accordingly the phase shift ($\varphi = k \cdot 90°$) as expressed in the Bode plot indicates a lead of the response by about 30° to 40° in both cases. Within lyriform organ HS8, k values increase for slits with higher thresholds. Accordingly, their high pass characteristic (decreasing bandwidth, i.e. higher low frequency limit) increases in the same direction. This is also reflected by their different speeds of adaptation to ramp stimuli (Fig. 6).

A remarkable feature of both the slit and campaniform sensilla is their wide *frequency range* covering about 5 powers of ten and starting at about 5 mHz (Bohnenberger, 1979; Chapman *et al.*, 1979).

In campaniform sensilla of the cockroach tibia, Chapman and his associates successfully separated various *component mechanisms* respon-

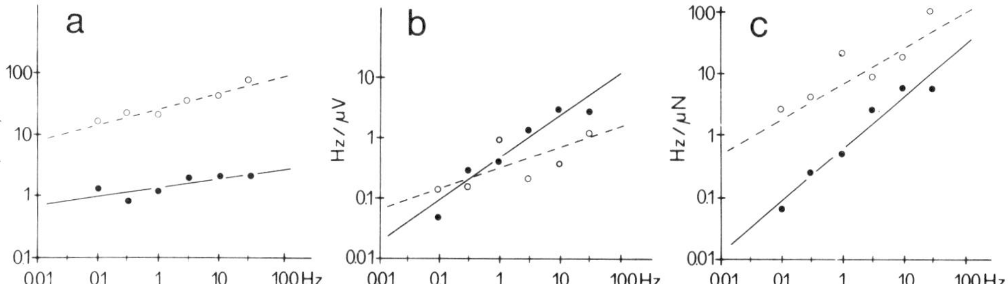

Figure 9 Bode plots of sensitivity for a campaniform sensillum on the cockroach tibia. (a) for the combined coupling and transduction mechanisms (μV/μN; receptor potential/applied force); (b), for the encoding mechanism (Hz/μV; impulse frequency/receptor potential); (c), for the receptor throughput (Hz/μN; impulse frequency/applied force). Open circles: low mean force ($F_0 = -5 \pm 20\ \mu$N); solid circles: high mean force ($F_0 = 170 \pm 20\ \mu$N). Stimulation by direct indentation of sensillar cap with experimental probe (redrawn from Mann and Chapman, 1975).

sible for the input–output relationship. Using punctate stimulation they established linear transfer functions for coupling and transduction (receptor potential, i.e. TEP/force, μV/μN), encoding (Imp. frequ./Rec. pot. Hz/μV) and throughput (Imp. frequ./force, Hz/μN) separately (Fig. 9) (Mann and Chapman, 1975).

Coupling and transduction exhibits non-linear, time independent range compression; sensitivity decreases with high mean force. Encoding, on the other hand, mainly shows a nonlinear increase in adaptation with high mean force. Coupling and transduction are thought to be mainly responsible for throughput sensitivity, and encoding for throughput "adaptation". Linear transfer functions (0.003 Hz–100 Hz) have been determined for cap compliance (nm/μN), cap indentation sensitivity (Hz/nm), and force sensitivity (Hz/μN) (Chapman *et al.*, 1979). Most sensilla behave viscoelastically, i.e. they stiffen as a power of frequency. Rate sensitivity is greater for indentation (sensitivity) than for force (sensitivity). A mild "filtering action" throughout the entire time course in "adaptation" is attributed to cap compliance. Its effect, however, is rather small and for adaptation to force even in the wrong direction, i.e. opposing it. Furthermore, there are some sensilla which do "adapt" but do not show time-dependent cap compliance and instead behave purely elastically. The amount of time-dependence shown by the transducer and in particular for the spike discharge (Fig. 9) suggests a major source of "adaptation" somewhere in between the cap and the afferent axon.

Despite the importance and precision of these studies a note of caution should be added as to whether cap indentation really represents the natural stimulus situation. The hinge membrane (L5) coupling the cap (L1) to the cuticular wall (L4) is likely to exert a different influence on the coupling mechanics in case of laterally introduced forces (normal proprioceptive input. Contrasting the indentation case it would lie in series with proprioceptive input. In addition the arched layer (L3), which eventually pinches the dendrite, may behave differently if deformed by lateral forces.

A different case

The attention of the reader is finally drawn to quite a different type of receptor, the crustacean "cuticular stress detectors", CSD1 and CSD2, which are found in the basi–ischiopodite of the walking legs close to the breakage plane in reptantian decapods. These receptors are chordotonal sensilla. Their strands, however, do not span a joint nor attach to a muscle or a tendon. Instead they are linked to small patches of soft cuticle in the exoskeleton. Up to about 60 bipolar cells project their dendrites into the organs' respective strands (Wales *et al.*, 1971).

CSDs are easily stimulated by pressure applied to the basi–ischiopodite cuticle and direct deformation of the soft patch of cuticle (Clarac *et al.*, 1971). They also respond to imposed joint movement and to increased tension in the coxo–basipodite joint muscles, in particular to isometric contractions of the anterior levator muscle which is the main autotomizer.

More details are given in a recent comprehensive review by Clarac (1976). The reader is also referred to a later paper by Findlay (1978) on the complex role played by one of these receptors in locomotion and limb autotomy.

Conclusion

Our attempt to understand the principles underlying strain detection in the arthropod exoskeleton must give particular attention to mechanical aspects. Model studies have been very helpful in elucidating a number of basic mechanical features both of the fine structure of the sensilla, their arrangement as groups and compound organs, and their distribution in the exoskeleton. A good proportion of these features could be verified directly by observing the original sensilla by microscopical and electrophysiological methods.

The main deficiency in our knowledge is the lack of a detailed analysis of stresses, strains, and displacements actually occurring at the specific sites of the sensilla. Again, tension optical model studies like the one carried out with the spider leg tibia will be helpful, but even more important now is a direct measurement of these parameters in the exoskeleton of live animals. This certainly is a difficult task but it can successfully be attempted at selected sites of at least the larger arthropods, as shown by the experiments currently under way in our laboratory. Can we always take the orientation of the bilateral sensilla as an indication of the direction of principal stresses which would be roughly perpendicular to their long axis? What are the absolute values of the mechanical input at the various sites and in various behavioural situations? Do the strain directions change at particular sites as suggested by the spread of slit orientation found in some receptor arrangements and by the potential of a directional analysis predicted from model studies for slit arrangements found in some lyriform organs?

The answers to such questions will also inform us about the mechanical design of whole skeletal parts which as yet has received almost no quantifying attention.

The picture available of the fine structure of insect campaniform sensilla now seems complete. Much, however, has still to be learned about that of crustacean campaniform sensilla, and the recent studies on the slit sensilla of a harvestman and a scorpion both show that the arachnids still offer surprises. The function of the supernumerary dendrites invariably present in arachnid slit sensilla is still unknown. Essentially the same applies to the tubular body of both insect and arachnid strain detectors. A unified picture has now emerged of the adequate dendrite deformation, but we still do not have any detailed information on the events leading to an increased conductivity of the dendritic membrane at the molecular level.

From a comparative point of view the difference in primary processes between insect campaniform sensilla and spider slit sensilla is surprising, because the basic structure of the dendrite and the arrangement of non-neural auxiliary cells are so similar. No trans-epithelial-potential difference could be recorded in the spider; nothing is known of the receptor potential either, which is likely to be independent of non-neural batteries. Clearly we need intracellular recordings from the sensory cells.

Thus our present knowledge of "strain" detection in the arthropod skeleton is far from being complete. Apart from our general interest in mechanoreception a particular incentive to fill the gaps should come from the close association of this sensory system with the exoskeleton, the most typical structure of the arthropods, which has certainly been particularly important in making the impressive story of evolutionary success of this animal group come true.

Acknowledgements

Research done in the author's laboratory was generously supported by the Deutsche Forschungsgemeinschaft. I am grateful to Prof. Dr W. Gnatzy for providing Figs. 1, a–c and the data for Fig. 2E and to Dr J. Bohnenberger for providing Figs. 6d and 7a. Dr E. A. Seyfarth made a number of much appreciated comments on the manuscript; also Prof. Gnatzy and Dr Bohnenberger kindly read parts of it. Thanks are due to Springer Verlag, Heidelberg, and Elsevier Sci. Publ. Co., Amsterdam, for permission to use previously published illustrations.

REFERENCES

Albert, P. J., Zacharuk, R. Y. and Wong, L. (1976) Structure, innervation, and distribution of sensilla on the wings of a grasshopper. *Can. J. Zool.*, **54**, 1542–1553.

Barth, F. G. (1967) Ein einzelnes Spaltsinnesorgan auf dem Spinnentarsus: seine Erregung in Abhängigkeit von den Parametern des Luftschallreizes *Z. vergl. Physiol.*, **55**, 407–449.

Barth, F. G. (1971) Der sensorische Apparat der Spaltsinnesorgane (*Cupiennius salei* Keys., Araneae) *Z. Zellforsch. mikrosk. Anat.*, **112**, 212–246.

Barth, F. G. (1972*a*) Die Physiologie der Spaltsinnesorgane, I. Modellversuche zur Rolle des cuticularen Spaltes beim Reiztransport *J. comp. Physiol.*, **78**, 315–336.

Barth, F. G. (1972*b*) Die Physiologie der Spaltsinnesorgane, II. Funktionelle Morphologie eines Mechanoreceptors *J. comp. Physiol.*, **81**, 159–186.

Barth, F. G. (1973*a*) Bauprinzipien und adäquater Reiz bei einem Mechanorezeptor *Verh. Dtsch. Zool. Ges.*, **66**, 25–30.

Barth, F. G. (1976) "Sensory information from strains in the exoskeleton" in *The Insect Integument* (ed. Hepburn, H. R.) Elsevier Sci. Publ. Co., Amsterdam, 445–473.

Barth, F. G. (1978) Slit sense organs: "Strain gauges" in the arachnid exoskeleton *Symp. zool. Soc. Lond.*, **42**, 439–448.

Barth, F. G. (1980) Campaniform sensilla: another vibration receptor in the crab leg *Naturwiss.*, **67**, 201.

Barth, F. G. and Bohnenberger, J. (1978) Lyriform slit sense organ: thresholds and stimulus amplitude ranges in a multi-unit mechanoreceptor *J. comp. Physiol.*, **125**, 37–43.

Barth, F. G. and Libera, W. (1970) Ein Atlas der Spaltsinnesorgane von *Cupiennius salei* Keys. Chelicerata (Araneae) *Z. Morph. Ökol. Tiere*, **68**, 343–369.

Barth, F. G. and Pickelmann, H. P. (1975) Lyriform slit sense organs in spiders. Modelling an arthropod mechanoreceptor *J. comp. Physiol.*, **103**, 39–54.

Barth, F. G. and Seyfarth, E. A. (1971) Slit sense organs and kinesthetic orientation *Z. vergl. Physiol.*, **74**, 326–328.

Barth, F. G. and Stagl, J. (1976) The slit sense organs of arachnids. A comparative study of their topography on the walking legs (*Chelicerata, Arachnida*) *Zoomorph.*, **86**, 1–23.

Blickhan, R. and Barth, F. G. (1979) *Dehnungen und Spannungen im Außenskelett von Arthropoden.* GESA-Symp. Braunschweig.

Boeckh, J., Kaissling, K.-E. und Schneider, D. (1960) Sensillen und Bau der Antennengeißel von *Telea polyphemus* (Vergleiche mit weiteren Saturniden: *Antheraea*, *Platysamia* und *Philosamia*) *Zool. Jb. Anat.*, **78**, 559–584.

Bohnenberger, J. (1978) On the transfer characteristics of a lyriform slit sense organ *Symp. zool. Soc. Lond.*, **42**, 449–455.

Bohnenberger, J. (1979) *Das Übertragungsverhalten eines zusammengesetzten Spaltsinnesorgans auf dem Spinnenbein* Dissertation, Universität Frankfurt.

Bullock, Th. H. and Horridge, G. A. (1965) *Structure and Function in the Nervous System of Invertebrates* Freeman, San Francisco and London.

Cartheuser, C. F. (1975) *Bau und Meßleistung einzelner Sensilla campaniformia auf den Flügeln von Tag-Schmetterlingen* Dissertation, Universität Braunschweig.

Chapman, K. M. and Smith, R. S. (1963) A linear transfer function underlying impulse frequency modulation in a cockroach mechanoreceptor *Nature*, **197**, 699–701.

Chapman, K. M., Duckrow, R. B. and Moran, D. T. (1973) Form and role of deformation in excitation of an insect mechanoreceptor *Nature*, **244**, 453–454.

Chapman, K. M., Mosinger, J. L. and Duckrow, R. B. (1979) The role of distributed viscoelastic coupling in sensory adaptation in an insect mechanoreceptor *J. comp. Physiol.*, **131**, 1–12.

Chevalier, R. L. (1969) The fine structure of the campaniform sensilla on the halteres of *Drosophila melanogaster J. Morph.*, **128**, 443–463.

Clarac, F. (1976) "Crustacean cuticular stress detectors" in *Structure and Function of Proprioreceptors in the Invertebrates* (ed. Mill, P. J.) Chapman and Hall, London, 299–321.

Clarac, F., Wales, W. and Laverack, M. S. (1971) Stress detection at the autotomy plane in decapod Crustacea. II. The function of the receptors associated with the cuticle of the basi–ischiopodite *Z. vergl. Physiol.*, **73**, 383–407.

Davis, H. (1965) A model for transducer action in the cochlea *Cold Spring Harb. Symp. quant. Biol.*, **30**, 181–190.

Dietz, A. and Humphreys, W. J. (1971) Scanning electron microscopic studies of antennal receptors of the worker honeybee, including sensilla campaniformia *Ann. Entomol. Soc. Am.*, **64**, 4.

Dumpert, K. and Gnatzy, W. (1977) Cricket combined mechanoreceptors and kicking response *J. comp. Physiol.*, **122**, 9–25.

Erler, G. and Thurm, U. (1978) The impulse response of epithelial receptor cells as a function of the transepithelial potential difference *Verh. Dtsch. Zool. Ges.*, 1978, 279.

Esslen, J. and Kaissling, K.-E. (1976) Zahl und Verteilung antennaler Sensillen bei der Honigbiene (*Apis mellifera* L.) *Zoomorph.*, **83**, 227–251.

Findlay, J. (1978) The role of the cuticular stress detector, CSD_1, in locomotion and limb autotomy in the crab *Carcinus maenas J. comp. Physiol.*, **125**, 79–90.

Gaffal, K. P. and Hansen, K. (1972) Mechanoreceptive Strukturen der antennalen Haarsensillen der Baumwollwanze *Dysdercus intermedius Dist. Z. Zellforsch. mikrosk. Anat.*, **132**, 78–94.

Gnatzy, W. and Schmidt, K. (1971) Die Feinstruktur der Sinneshaare auf den Cerci von *Gryllus bimaculatus* Deg. I. Faden- und Keulenhaare *Z. Zellforsch. mikrosk. Anat.*, **122**, 190–209.

Hawke, S. D., Farley, R. D. and Greany, P. D. (1973) The fine structure of sense organs in the ovipositor of the parasitic wasp, *Orgilus lepidus* Muesebeck *Tissue & Cell*, **5**, 171–184.

Heinzel, H.-G. and Gewecke, M. (1979) Directional sensitivity of the antennal campaniform sensilla in locusts *Naturwiss.*, **66**, 212.

Hicks, J. B. (1857) On a new organ in insects *J. Proc. Linn. Soc. (Zool.)*, **1**, 136–140.

Hochreuther, R. (1912) Die Hautsinnesorgane von *Dytiscus marginalis* L., ihr Bau und ihre Verteilung am Körper *Z. wiss. Zool.*, **103**, 1–114.

Honegger, H.-W., Reif, H. and Müller, W. (1979) Sensory mechanism of eye cleaning behavior in the cricket *Gryllus campestris. J. comp. Physiol.*, **129**, 247–256.

Kaston, B. J. (1935) The slit sense organs of spiders *J. Morph.*, **58**, 189–209.

Krämer, K. and Markl, H. (1978) Flight inhibition on ground contact in the American cockroach, *Periplaneta americana.* I. Contact receptors and a model for their central connections *J. Insect Physiol.*, **24**, 577–586.

Küppers, J. (1974) "Measurements of the ionic milieu of the receptor terminal in mechanoreceptive sensilla of insects" in *Mechanoreception* (ed. Schwartzkopff, J.) Rhein.-Westf. Akad. Wiss., **53**, 387–394.

Laverack, M. S. (1976) "External proprioceptors" in *Structure and Function of Proprioceptors in the Invertebrates* (ed. Mill, P. J.) Chapman and Hall, London, 1–63.

Liesenfeld, F. J. (1961) Über Leistung und Sitz des Erschütterungssinnes von Netzspinnen *Biol. Zbl.*, **80**, 465–475.

Mann, D. W. and Chapman, K. M. (1975) Component mechanism of sensitivity and adaptation in an insect mechanoreceptor *Brain Res.*, **97**, 331–336.

Markl, H. (1970) Die Verständigung durch Stridulationssignale bei Blattschneiderameisen. III. Die Empfindlichkeit für Substratvibrationen *Z. vergl. Physiol.*, **69**, 6–37.

McIndoo, N. E. (1911) The lyriform organs and tactile hairs of araneids *Proc. Acad. natl. Sci. Philad.*, **63**, 375–418.

McIver, S. and Siemicki, R. (1978) Fine structure of tarsal sensilla of *Aedes aegypti* (L.) (Diptera: Culicidae) *J. Morph.*, **155**, 137–156.

Melin, D. (1941) Contributions to the knowledge of the flight of insects, especially of the function of the campaniform organs and halteres *Uppsala Univ. Arsskrift*, **4**, 1–247.

Moeck, H. A. (1968) Electron microscopic studies of antennal sensilla in the ambrosia beetle *Trypodendron lineatum* (Olivier) (Scolytidae) *Can. J. Zool.*, **46**, 521–556.

Moran, D. T., Carter Rowley, J. C. III, Zill, S. N. and Varela, F. G. (1976) The mechanism of sensory transduction in a mechanoreceptor. Functional stages in campaniform sensilla during the molting cycle *J. Cell Biol.*, **71**, 832–847.

Moran, D. T., Chapman, K. M. and Ellis, R. A. (1971) The fine structure of cockroach campaniform sensilla *J. Cell Biol.*, **48**, 155–173.

Moran, D. T. and Rowley, J. C. III (1975) High voltage and scanning electron microscopy of the site of stimulus reception of an insect mechanoreceptor *J. Ultrastructure Res.*, **50**, 38–46.

Mönch, E. (1971) *Technische Mechanik* R. Oldenbourg, München und Wien.

Peterson, R. E. (1974) *Stress Concentration Factors* John Wiley & Sons, Inc., New York-London-Sydney-Toronto.

Pflugstaedt, H. (1912) Die Halteren der Dipteren *Z. wiss. Zool.*, **100**, 1–59.

Pringle, J. W. S. (1938) Proprioception in insects. II. The action of the campaniform sensilla on the legs *J. exp. Biol.*, **15**, 114–131.

Pringle, J. W. S. (1948) The gyroscopic mechanism of the halteres of Diptera *Phil. Trans. R. Soc.*, **233**, B 602, 347–384.

Pringle, J. W. S. (1955) The function of the lyriform organs of arachnids *J. exp. Biol.*, **32**, 270–278.

Pringle, J. W. S. (1957) *Insect flight* Cambridge University Press, Cambridge.

Rick, R., Barth, F. G. and von Pawel, A. (1976) X-ray microanalysis of receptor lymph in a cuticular arthropod sensillum *J. comp. Physiol.*, **110**, 89–95.

Schlegel, P. (1970) Die Leistungen eines Gelenkreceptors der Antenne von *Calliphora* für die Perzeption von Luftströmungen. Elektrophysiologische Untersuchungen *Z. vergl. Physiol.*, **66**, 45–77.

Schmidt, K. (1969) Die campaniformen Sensillen im Pedicellus der Florfliege (*Chrysopa, Planipennia*) *Z. Zellforsch. mikrosk. Anat.*, **96**, 478–489.

Schmidt, K. and Gnatzy, W. (1971) Die Feinstruktur der Sinneshaare auf den Cerci von *Gryllus bimaculatus* Deg. II. Die Häutung der Faden- und Keulenhaare *Z. Zellforsch. mikrosk. Anat.*, **122**, 210–226.

Schnorbus, H. (1971) Die subgenualen Sinnesorgane von *Periplaneta americana*: Histologie und Vibrationsschwellen *Z. vergl. Physiol.*, **71**, 14–48.

Seyfarth, E.-A. (1978*a*) Lyriform slit sense organs and muscle reflexes in the spider leg *J. comp. Physiol.*, **125**, 45–57.

Seyfarth, E.-A. (1978*b*) Mechanoreceptors and proprioreceptive reflexes: lyriform organs in the spider leg *Symp. zool. Soc. Lond.*, **42**, 457–467.

Seyfarth, E.-A. and Barth, F. G. (1972) Compound slit sense organs on the spider leg: mechanoreceptors involved in kinesthetic orientation *J. comp. Physiol.*, **78**, 176–191.

Shelton, R. G. J. and Laverack, M. S. (1968) Observations on a redescribed crustacean cuticular sense organ *Comp. Biochem. Physiol.*, **25**. 1049–1059.

Siehler, H. (1924) Die Sinnesorgane an den Cerci der Insekten *Zool. Jahrb. Abt. Anat. Ontag. Tiere*, **45**, 519–580.

Smith, D. S. (1969) The fine structure of haltere sensilla in the blowfly, *Calliphora erythrocephala* (Meig.) with scanning electron microscopic observations on the haltere surface *Tissue & Cell*, **1**, 443–484.

Spinola, S. M. and Chapman, K. M. (1975) Proprioceptive indentation of the campaniform sensilla of cockroach legs *J. comp. Physiol.*, **96**, 257–272.

Stewart, D. M. and Martin, D. W. (1974) Blood pressure in the tarantula *Dugesiella hentzi. J. comp. Physiol.*, **80**, 141–172.

Thorson, J. and Biederman-Thorson, M. (1974) Distributed relaxation processes in sensory adaptation *Science*, **183**, 161–172.

Thurm, U. (1964) Mechanoreceptors in the cuticle of the honeybee. Fine structure and stimulus mechanism *Science*, **145**, 1063–1065.

Thurm, U. (1965) An insect mechanoreceptor. I. Fine structure and adequate stimulus *Cold Spring Harbor Symp. Quant. Biol.*, **30**, 75–82.

Thurm, U. (1974) "Basics of the generation of receptor potentials in epidermal mechanoreceptors in insects" in *Mechanoreception* (ed. Schwartzkopff, J.) Rhein. Westf. Akad. Wiss., **53**, 355–385.

Thurm, U. (1977) "Sensorische Transduktionsprozesse" in *Biophysik Ein Lehrbuch* (eds. Hoppe, W. *et al.*) Springer Verlag, Berlin-Heidelberg, 391–402.

Thurm, U., Stedtler, A. and Foelix, R. (1975) Reizwirksame Verformungen der Terminalstrukturen eines Mechanorezeptors *Verh. Dtsch. Zool. Ges.*, **67**, 37–41.

Thurm, U. and Wessel, G. (1979) Metabolism-dependent transepithelial potential differences at epidermal receptors of arthropods: I Comparative data *J. comp. Physiol.*, **134**, 119–130.

Vogel, R. (1911) Über die Innervierung der Schmetterlingsflügel und über den Bau und die Verbreitung der Sinnesorgane auf demselben *Z. wiss. Zool.*, **98**, 68–134.

Vogel, H. (1923) Über die Spaltsinnesorgane der Radnetzspinnen *Jena Z. Med. Naturw.*, **59**, 171–208.

Walcott, Ch. and van der Kloot, W. G. (1959) The physiology of the spider vibration receptor *J. exp. Zool.*, **141**, 191–244.

Wales, W., Clarac, F. and Laverack, M. S. (1971) Stress detection at the autotomy plane in decapod Crustacea. I. Comparative anatomy of the receptors of the basi–ischiopodite region *Z. vergl. Physiol.*, **73**, 357–382.

Zacharuk, R. Y. (1962) Sense organs on the head of larvae of some Elateridae (Coleoptera): Their distribution, structure and innervation *J. Morph.*, **111**, 1–33.

CHAPTER NINE

BISTABLE AND PHOTOSTABLE PIGMENTS IN MICROVILLAR PHOTORECEPTORS

KUNO KIRSCHFELD

Introduction

Visual pigments in both vertebrates and invertebrates are chromoproteins. In the invertebrates investigated so far the chromophore is 11-*cis* retinal, the same as that of vertebrate rhodopsin. Hence invertebrate visual pigments are also called "rhodopsin" (R) (see review by Hamdorf, 1979). A quantum of light, if absorbed by the visual pigment molecule, isomerizes the chromophore from 11-*cis* into the all-*trans* conformation, and with high probability leads to an excitation of the receptor, that is, a "receptor potential".

There is a striking difference between vertebrates and invertebrates inasmuch as only in vertebrates quantum absorption leads to "bleaching" of the visual pigment, i.e. a separation of the all-*trans* chromophore from the protein. In contrast, in many invertebrates the metarhodopsin (with the chromophore still attached to the protein) is thermostable. Reisomerization primarily occurs also by means of absorbed light quanta (see reviews by Goldsmith, 1972; Hamdorf, 1979). This "bistability" of invertebrate visual pigments has several functional consequences. As we shall see, this special property can also be used as a tool to analyse the transduction process.

In addition to the bistable visual pigments, photostable pigments have also been found in invertebrates. These pigments considerably modify the properties of photoreceptors by reducing their sensitivity in special spectral ranges or at special *e*-vector orientations due to an optical filter effect; there is also evidence that photostable pigments are capable of enhancing the spectral sensitivity in special wavelength regions due to sensitization. Finally, photostable pigments might help to protect rhabdomeres against photo-oxidation (see review by Kirschfeld, 1979).

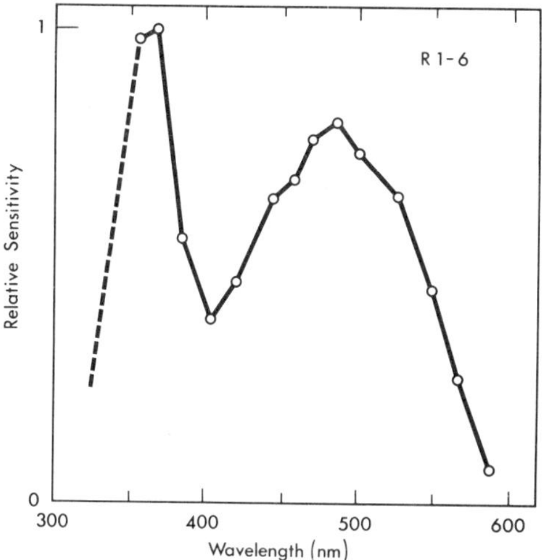

Figure 1 Spectral sensitivity of a receptor type R1–6 of the housefly, *Musca*, with the two maxima. Dashed part of the curve is extrapolated according to known spectra from other species. (Courtesy of Dr R. Hardie, MPI für biologische Kybernetik, Tübingen.)

We will first discuss some properties of photostable pigments, and then deal with bistable visual pigments and the problem of transduction.

Photostable pigments

Ultraviolet (UV) sensitivity in photoreceptors

Whereas there are only few examples of UV sensitivity in vertebrates (e.g. pigeons and hummingbirds; see Goldsmith, 1980), UV-sensitivity seems to be almost universal in the invertebrates (see review by Menzel, 1979). Two different types of spectral sensitivities of photoreceptors have been described: in one type there is only a single peak of sensitivity in the UV; whereas in the other there is, besides the UV-maximum, a second maximum at longer wavelengths.

A representative of the first case is the neuropter *Ascalaphus*. Spectral sensitivity, as measured in the so-called "frontal eye", has one maximum at 345 nm. This sensitivity is due to a rhodopsin, R 345, which is converted by light into a metarhodopsin, M 475 (see review by Hamdorf, 1979).

A typical example of the second type are receptors 1–6 (R1–6, see inset Fig. 2) in the ommatidia of flies. These receptors have one sensitivity maximum close to 500 nm, and, in addition, another at 360 nm (Burkhardt, 1962) (Fig. 1). Dual-peak spectral sensitivity of this type cannot be explained on the basis of extinction spectra of known rhodopsins, since such pigments have only a small peak at shorter wavelengths (a β-peak about 25 % of the maximum).

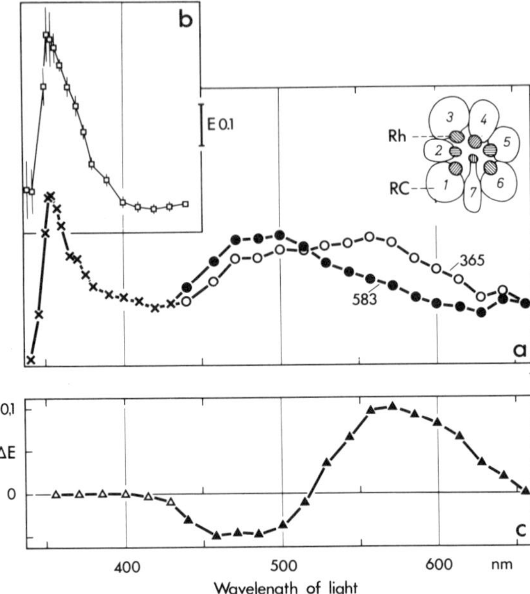

Figure 2 (a) Extinction spectrum of rhabdomeres type R1–6 of *Musca* as measured in a microspectrophotometer. During the measurement the preparation at regular intervals was either illuminated with strong orange ($\lambda = 583$ nm) light, in order to shift most of the pigment into the rhodopsin state, or with ultraviolet ($\lambda = 365$ nm) light, in order to shift some rhodopsin into metarhodopsin. Inset: cross-section through ommatidium, indicating receptor cells RC and rhabdomeres Rh.
(b) Mean extinction spectrum in the ultraviolet of 6 ommatidia.
(c) Difference spectrum of (a).
Redrawn from Kirschfeld *et al.* (1977).

Suggested explanations for this dual peak spectral sensitivity have been, amongst others, two different visual pigments in the same photoreceptor, waveguide effects, or electrical coupling between different receptors with UV and 500 nm sensitivity. All these hypotheses which attempt to explain the high UV-sensitivity can, however, be excluded experimentally (see review by Kirschfeld, 1979).

Evidence for a sensitizing pigment

Microspectrophotometrically it can be shown (Fig. 4) that in fly photoreceptors 1–6 there is extinction in the visible range due to the rhodopsin–metarhodopsin system (Hamdorf *et al.*, 1973; Stavenga *et al.*, 1973). Depending upon the wavelength of the pre-illumination more of either R or M is measured. In addition, there is extinction in the UV. The absorption spectrum in the UV, in contrast to that in the visible part, cannot be modified by pre-illumination with light of different wave-

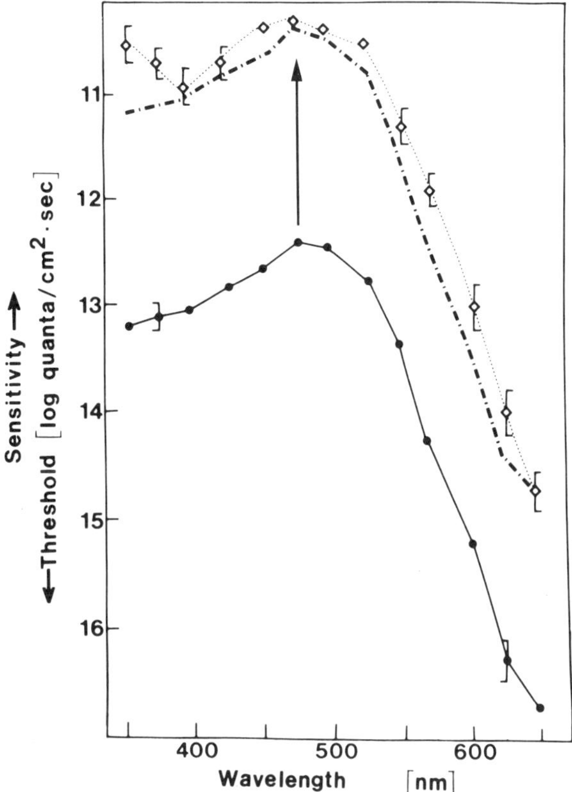

Figure 3 Spectral sensitivity of the compound eye of *Drosophila*, measured in a white eye mutant by means of the electroretinogram. Diamonds represent the sensitivity of normal flies, points that of flies raised on a vitamin A deprived medium. For a convenient shape comparison, the curve for vitamin A-deprived flies was also plotted near the curve of the normal flies. Redrawn from Stark *et al.* (1976).

lengths. Consequently the difference spectrum differs from zero only at wavelengths longer than 400 nm (Fig. 2). On the other hand, it can be shown that UV light induces formation of the same metarhodopsin as blue light. These observations fit the concept that the UV extinction is due to a photostable pigment that acts as a sensitizer for rhodopsin according to the following process: due to absorption of a light quantum the photostable (sensitizer) molecule is converted into the excited state. In a secondary process it then may interact with a R-molecule by transferring its energy to R. R then is changed into M as if it had absorbed a quantum of light itself (Kirschfeld *et al.*, 1977). A similar interpretation was given by Stark *et al.* (1977).

If the energy transfer occurs by means of the well known dipole–dipole

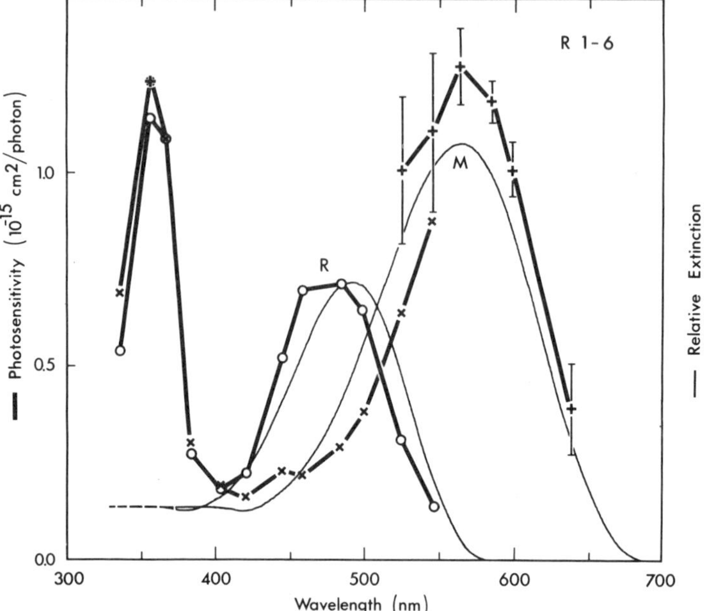

Figure 4 Photosensitivity spectra of fly receptor type R1–6 (*Calliphora*) rhodopsin (○) and metarhodopsin (×, +). The methods used to derive the spectra measure the efficiency with which rhodopsin and metarhodopsin are interconverted, depending upon the wavelength and intensity of light. Therefore instead of absorption spectra, photosensitivity spectra are derived, which include effects of sensitizing pigments. Thin lines: extinction spectra of rhodopsin (R) and metarhodopsin (M) (Hamdorf, Schlecht and Täuber, pers. comm.) as derived from the difference spectrum of *Calliphora* receptors R1–6. Redrawn from Minke and Kirschfeld (1979).

interaction according to Förster's (1951) theory several conditions must be fulfilled.

1. The donor (= sensitizing) molecule should be close to the acceptor (= sensitized) molecule. Estimates show that distances should be not much larger than 5 nm.
2. The absorption spectrum of the acceptor molecule should overlap sufficiently with the fluorescence spectrum of the donor molecule.
3. The dipoles of both molecules should be nearly parallel (the efficiency is proportional to the cosine of the angle between the dipoles).

The conditions for the efficiency of energy transfer as formulated above can be used for predictions that can be checked experimentally. Experiments that test the sensitizing pigment concept are the following.

The R and M concentrations in the microvilli can be considerably reduced (to less than 10%) by growing flies on vitamin A-deprived media (see Hamdorf, 1979). The distance in the microvillar membrane between donor and acceptor molecules can be expected to increase in these conditions. According to condition 1 we should expect that the sensitivity of receptors 1–6 in these flies should be selectively reduced in the UV. Fig. 3 shows that such a reduction does indeed occur.

According to condition 2 the photosensitivity not only of R, but also of M, should be high. This conclusion follows from the fact that the absorption spectra of R and M overlap considerably (Fig. 4). Hence the fluorescence spectrum of the sensitizing pigment should overlap not only with the absorption spectrum of R but also with that of M. We found that the photosensitivity of M in the UV is very high indeed, and furthermore that the shapes of the UV photosensitivity spectra of R and M are practically identical, as is to be expected if both spectra are created by the same sensitizing pigment (Fig. 4) (Minke and Kirschfeld, 1979). The fluorescence excitation spectrum of a UV-photostable substance as measured by Stark *et al.* (1979) also fits the sensitizing pigment concept.

As far as polarization sensitivity is concerned, we found no dichroic absorption in the UV using the microspectrophotometer. Polarization sensitivity of receptors 1–6, measured electrophysiologically, is also confined to the visible part of the spectrum (Smola and Kuo, pers. comm.). This observation indicates that the dipoles responsible for the UV-sensitivity are different from those causing the sensitivity peak in the green region at 500 nm.

All observations made to date are in agreement with the sensitizing pigment concept. However, it has not yet been possible to isolate the UV pigment chemically nor to identify it (Paulsen and Schwemer, 1979). So far we have thus no direct proof of its existence. Paulsen and Schwemer discuss the possibility that the UV-sensitivity could also be due to unusual absorbance properties of the rhodopsin itself when densely packed. No mechanism to explain such a hypothesis is however known.

Photostable pigments as colour and polarization filters

In special photoreceptors of the fly (no. 7y—see Fig. 2), there is a photostable pigment with high extinction in the blue spectral range (review by Kirschfeld, 1979). Since this rhabdomere is in front of another one, no. 8, the photostable pigment acts as a colour filter for the latter.

Fig. 5 shows the spectral sensitivity of receptor no. 8 as determined in a *Drosophila* mutant, which has this receptor only. The figure also shows the extinction spectrum of the photostable pigment as well as the spectral sensitivity of the receptor no. 8 as predicted. The spectral sensitivity as measured in a receptor R8 (*Calliphora*) is also shown. In both cases maximal sensitivity is shifted to longer wavelengths. Furthermore the sensitivity spectrum is more narrow than expected from absorption by pure rhodopsin.

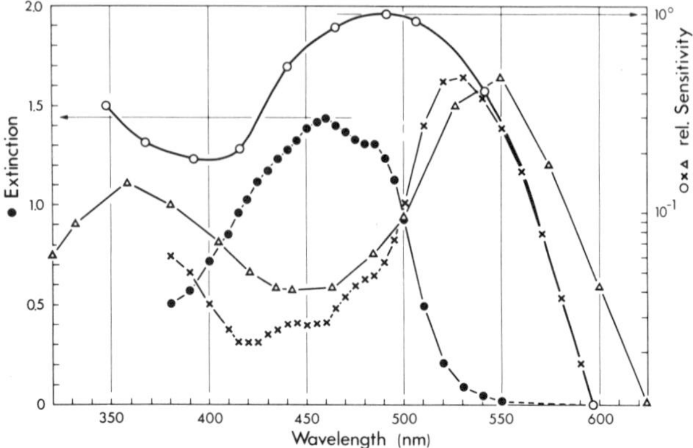

Figure 5 The effect of the photostable pigment from rhabdomeres R7y (●) on the spectral sensitivity of receptors R8. Open circles represent spectral sensitivity of receptors R8 as measured in a *Drosophila* mutant, lacking all receptors except no. 8, and hence also lacking the screening effect of rhabdomere R7 (Harris *et al.*, 1976). Crosses: predicted spectral sensitivity of receptors R8 if the screening effect of R7y is taken into account. For comparison, the spectral sensitivity of an identified receptor R8 (*Calliphora*) is also drawn (Hardie, 1977). From Kirschfeld *et al.* (1978*a*).

Since the photostable pigment also absorbs dichroically, the polarization sensitivity (PS) of R7 and R8 is modified. Fig. 6 shows an example of how PS in receptor no. 7 varies with the wavelength of light due to the screening effect of the photostable pigment in R7.

Bistable pigments

The time sequence of events in photoreceptors

Since the work of Hecht, Shlaer and Pirenne (1942) and Bouman and Van der Velden (1948) it has been obvious that photoreceptor sensitivity is not limited by properties of the biological system (e.g. receptor noise) but by physics, since photoreceptors are capable of detecting single light quanta. This conclusion was drawn from psychophysical experiments. The first observation of events obviously ascribable to effects of single quanta in photoreceptors was published by Yeandle (1958): individual light quanta in dark adapted photoreceptors of *Limulus* lead to discrete potential transients, called "bumps". These have an amplitude in the range of millivolts, which is far above the noise level of the receptor membrane. Single photon responses have now also been demonstrated directly in retinal rods (Baylor *et al.*, 1979). Between the isomerization of the chromophore of the visual pigment and the occurrence of a "bump", or at higher light intensity levels of the receptor potential, several intermediate steps ("dark reactions") are interposed. Known steps are indicated in Fig.

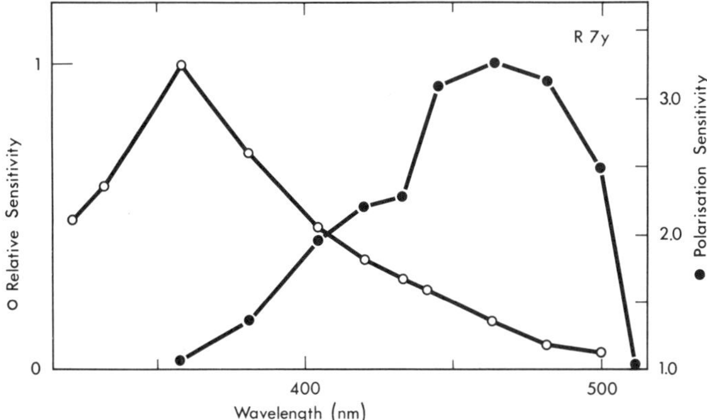

Figure 6 Spectral- and polarization sensitivity of receptors R7y (*Calliphora*). Redrawn from Hardie *et al.* (1979).

7 (time scale shown for vertebrate rods). From the fact that the late receptor potential (LRP) occurs approximately simultaneously with metarhodopsin II, it can be concluded that all reactions up to and including the formation of metarhodopsin II are possible sources of the excitation of the membrane. To decide which of the reactions is the important one has not yet been possible.

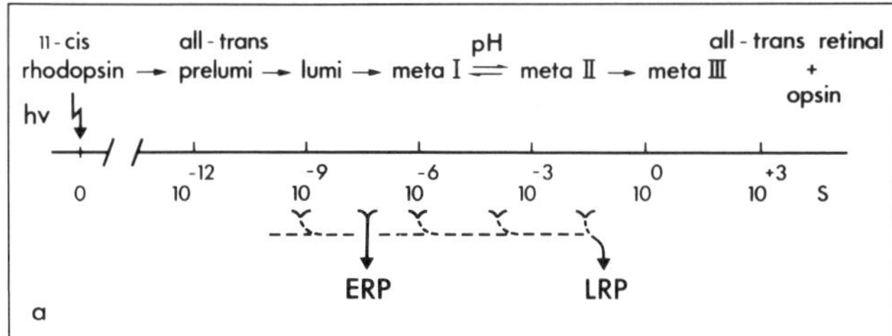

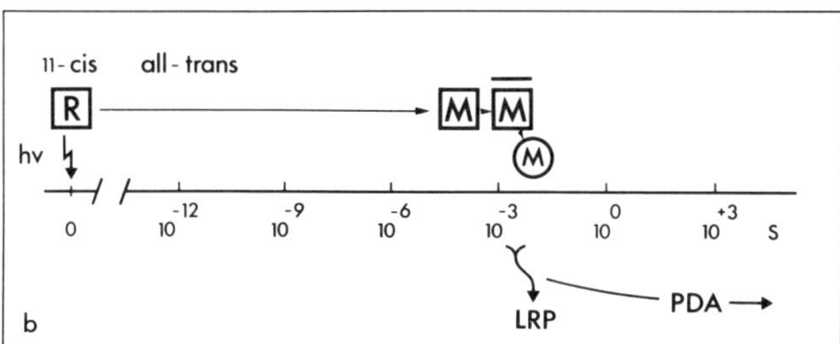

Figure 7 Sequence of events following light absorption in bovine rhodopsin (a, after several authors, redrawn from Stieve, 1974) and in rhodopsin of the receptors R1–6 of the fly (b). ERP: early receptor potential, LRP: late receptor potential, PDA: prolonged depolarizing afterpotential. Explanation of symbols in the text.

It is difficult to understand why such a considerable latency elapses between absorption of a light-quantum and the appearance of the LRP. In the fly for instance the "bump" latency is in the order of 30 ms (room temperature); with increasing intensity the latency shortens considerably but is never less than 3–5 ms. Surprisingly, this is much longer than the time necessary for conductance changes mediated by chemical transmitters in, for example, membranes of neurones or of muscles, where fractions of a millisecond are sufficient. In other vertebrate and invertebrate photoreceptors latency is usually still considerably longer.

There are several hypotheses available to explain the long photoreceptor latency. It may for instance be due to properties of the visual pigment molecules, properties of transport processes, or to the time needed to produce and accumulate chemical substances. Several different experimental approaches allow us to specify in more detail which one of the different possible components actually contributes to the latency.

The following sections describe experiments carried out on photoreceptors R1–6 of the fly. These photoreceptors are especially suitable for spectrophotometry: the rhabdomeres are isolated from each other and not fused. They are relatively long (> 100 μm) and have a nearly constant diameter over their entire length. The bistability of the visual pigments allows shifting the pigments back and forth and makes it unnecessary to

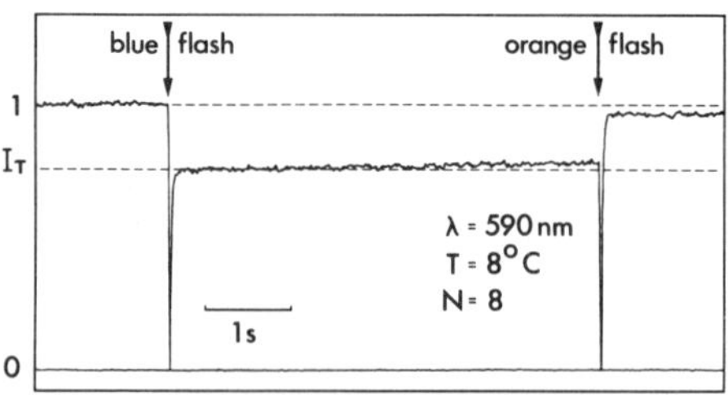

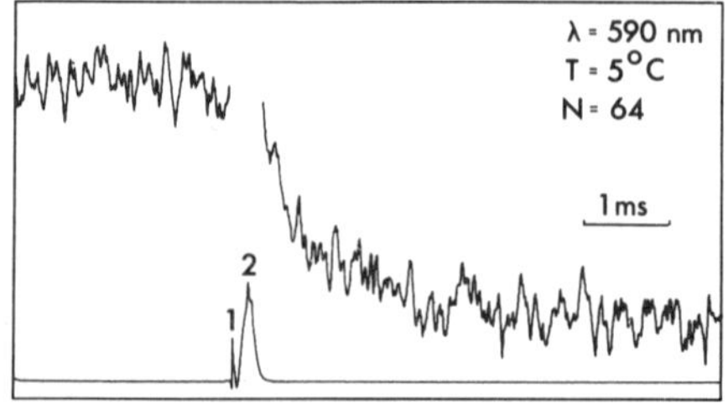

Figure 8 Top: formation and decomposition of metarhodopsin in *Drosophila* photoreceptors after blue and orange flashes, respectively, as monitored by means of orange ($\lambda = 590$ nm) measuring light (ordinate: transmitted intensity I_T). Bottom: formation of metarhodopsin after a blue flash on a fast time scale. Temperature: 8 and 5°C; N = 8 and N = 64 readings were averaged, respectively. Redrawn from Kirschfeld *et al.* (1978*b*).

use infrared light combined with a IR-converter for the adjustment of the preparation in the photometer. A disadvantage is that the cells are not very easily accessible for electrophysiological recording. Voltage-clamp experiments such as those performed in *Limulus* ventral photoreceptors (Millecchia and Mauro, 1969) have not yet been possible.

Kinetics of the R → M transition

It is possible to measure the extinction of rhabdomeres in living flies by using the technique of "antidromic" illumination, combined with the "deep pseudopupil" technique (see Franceschini, 1975). In the experiment, the visual pigment is first shifted by means of orange light (compare spectra in Fig. 4) into R, then a blue flash is given to the eye, and the decrease in transmission at 590 nm—indicating the formation of M—is measured.

Since the kinetics of the formation of M are rather fast, the present measurements were done primarily at low temperatures. At 5°C the time constant of the transition in *Drosophila* was found to be 500 μs (Fig. 8); extrapolation to room temperature yields approximately 100 μs, a figure confirmed by Stark *et al.*, 1979. This result shows that the R–M transition is fast compared to the occurrence of the late receptor potential and cannot account for the long latency of this potential.

Additional changes at the visual pigment molecule

The second question that we may ask is whether the response of the receptor is due to light quantum hits at R, or rather to the number of M molecules remaining after the stimulus. In other words, must M exist for some time in order to trigger the response? The bistability of the invertebrate visual pigment offers an opportunity to answer this question. We are able first to stimulate the receptor by means of a blue flash that converts R into M, then, within the latency of the response, M can be reconverted into R by means of an orange flash. The question is whether a receptor potential is induced even if M has disappeared before the occurrence of the LRP. It was found that the occurrence of the LRP can be stopped by the second flash if this flash is given 3 to 5 ms after the first one (Hamdorf and Kirschfeld, 1980*a*). For practical reasons the reduction of the response is not "all or none" as might be expected in an ideal case. In fact the response is only *reduced* by the second flash (Fig. 9), but, nevertheless, more light gives a smaller response! The response cannot be cancelled completely because (1) not all M molecules, created by the first flash, can be reconverted into R by the second flash, and (2) the second flash itself, due to the overlap of the absorption spectra of R and M (Fig. 4) also converts some R into M. Quantitative estimates show that the

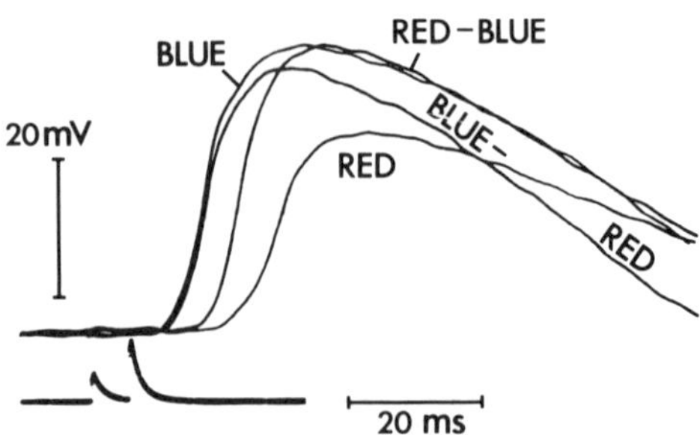

Figure 9 Intracellularly recorded responses of a photoreceptor type R1–6 of *Calliphora* to light flashes (monitor: lower trace). Either a blue flash, a red flash, or two flashes with a delay of 5 ms in the sequence blue–red or red–blue, respectively, were given. The response to the sequence blue–red is significantly smaller than that to a blue flash alone. Note that the longer latency of the sequence red–blue is due to the fact that the blue flash occurs second. Temperature 10°C. Redrawn from Hamdorf and Kirschfeld (1980*b*).

reduced response amplitude corresponds to a reduction of the stimulus intensity to some 25%. Parallel spectrophotometric measurements have shown that some 25% of the M remains after the second flash. Hence the amplitude reduction corresponds to that expected.

This result shows that, following the conversion of R into M, there remains a period of 3 to 5 ms during which reconversion of M to R more or less completely abolishes the effect of the initial R to M conversion. During this period no irreversible transmitter release or chemical chain reaction can have been initiated. The M formed must exist for a few milliseconds in order to trigger the response.

Photometry shows that after a blue flash, M is formed within a fraction of a millisecond. What happens to the visual pigment molecule during the next few milliseconds is not directly detectable in the microspectrophotometer within the absorption range of metarhodopsin. The double flash experiment shows nevertheless that a time-consuming process that remains localized at the pigment molecule must happen before a response can be triggered. This process could be a conformational change of the molecule, which might take place apart from the chromophore and hence is not affecting its absorption.

The consequences of double flashes such as those described above for the later parts of the receptor potential have been analysed by Muijser and Stavenga (1979).

The latency of the LRP

The latency distribution of "bumps" induced by short flashes in most receptors is rather extended: histograms of excentric cells of the *Limulus* compound eye extend from 0.5 to 4 seconds at 7°C (Fuortes and Yeandle,

1964), those of *Limulus* ventral nerve photoreceptor from 0 to more than 1 second at 18°C (Yeandle and Spiegler, 1973) and those from the locust are between 0 and 140 ms (18–20°C) (Lillywhite, 1977). ("0" of course does not mean that there are bumps without latency. The first bar of the histograms includes all bumps with latencies starting from 0 seconds.) The LRP in rhabdomeric photoreceptors to stronger light stimuli is considered a superposition of individual "bumps", whereby each "bump" is triggered by the absorption of a single light-quantum (Dodge *et al.*, 1968; Wu and Pak, 1978).

The LRP-latency shortens considerably with increasing stimulus intensities. On the basis of the "bump"-superposition concept this shortening can be interpreted in the following way: strong stimuli trigger large numbers of "bumps", and therefore (with a high probability) also "bumps" with short latency. A difficulty with the concept of "bump"-superposition, as far as latency of the LRP is concerned, arises from the following fact. The bump latency histogram of receptors R1–6 of flies is—in contrast to those mentioned above—rather narrow. Bumps occur with a mean latency of 60 ms ± 20 ms (10°C). The latency of the LRP to strong stimuli is reduced to 5 to 7 ms, a latency that is never reached by individual bumps. Hence an acceleration of the system must occur if many quanta are absorbed in a rhabdomere at the same time. This acceleration must develop *before* any receptor potential can be detected (Hamdorf and Kirschfeld, 1980*b*).

We found that 30 to 300 quanta have to be absorbed within a rhabdomere in order merely to reduce the latency. Within each rhabdomere there are 10^8 rhodopsin molecules and 1.5×10^5 microvilli (see Hamdorf, 1979). From these figures, double hits at R-molecules can be excluded as the cause for the reduction in latency: application of Poisson statistics shows that double hits at R-molecules need more than 10^4 absorbed quanta per flash. In order to score double hits at individual microvilli at least 440 quanta have to be absorbed. Double hits at directly neighbouring microvilli occur if in the mean only 125 quanta are absorbed.

These numbers indicate that the most probable reason for the shortening in latency is double hits on neighbouring microvilli. However, because of some uncertainty in the estimates of the mean number of absorbed quanta, double hits on one microvillus cannot yet be excluded with certainty.

Irrespective of whether the reduction in latency is due to double hits on neighbouring or individual microvilli, we expect that the *shortening could occur in a discrete manner* since double hits are qualitatively different from single hits.

A shortening of the latency in a discrete manner actually could be demonstrated. In Fig. 10 at relative intensity (I) 10^{-8}, "all-or-nothing"

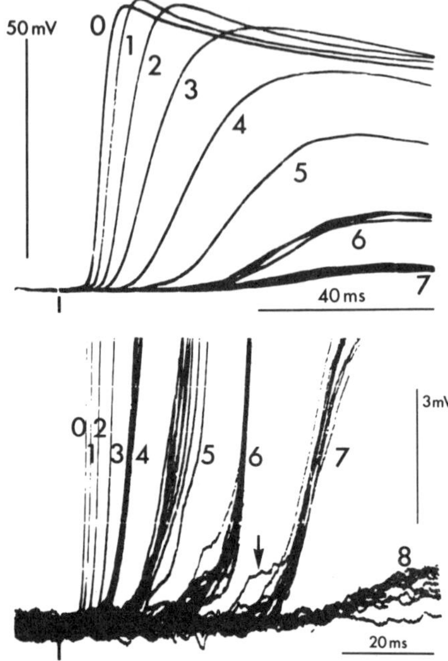

Figure 10 Intracellularly recorded receptor potentials of a receptor type R1–6 of *Calliphora* in response to blue flashes (vertical bar indicates onset of flash). The latency of the response varies between 6 and 40 ms depending upon the stimulus intensity (10°C). Numbers indicate the negative logarithm of the relative stimulus intensities. In the top figure the whole amplitude of the response is shown, in the lower one the onset of the receptor potential was recorded at a high gain in order to show the occurrence of "prebumps" (arrow). Several traces to stimuli of the same intensity have been superimposed at most of the stimulus intensities in order to illustrate the variability of the responses. Redrawn from Hamdorf and Kirschfeld (1980*a*).

bumps were recorded. At $I = 10^{-7}$ the amplitude of the response is increased. The latency remains constant, however, in 9 of 10 traces. In one trace, in addition to the normal response, a "prebump" (arrow) can clearly be seen. This "prebump" has a shorter latency, and an amplitude of approximately one millivolt, similar to the single "bumps". Increasing I to 10^{-6} shortened the latency since at this intensity many double hits occur. In addition, a class of still faster "prebumps" was discriminated. Calculation showed that these "prebumps" should be due to triple hits, and so on.

The structural basis of excitation in microvillar photoreceptors

The ion channels of the photoreceptor that are opened by light absorption are arranged in the plasma membrane that separates the intra- and

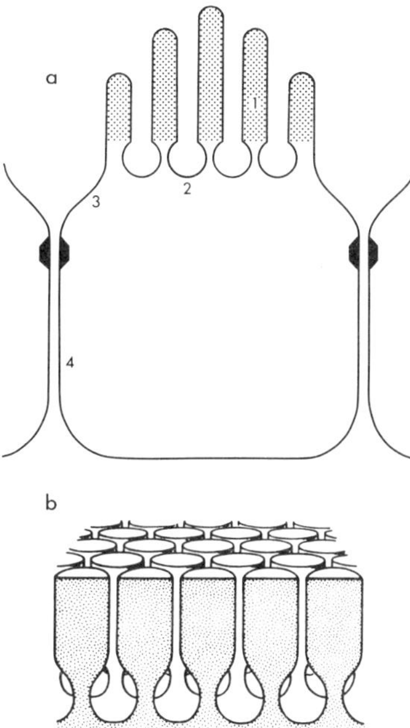

Figure 11 (a) Cross-section of a photoreceptor type R1–6 of the fly (schematic). Numbers indicate the possible location of channels that are opened during excitation. Stippled: microvilli.
(b) Schematic drawing of rhabdomere tubule attachment. (Redrawn from Boschek, 1971.)

extracellular spaces. The structure of the photoreceptor (Fig. 11) suggests the following sites (Hamdorf and Kirschfeld, 1980*a*): (1) the microvillus; (2) the "bubbles" at the basis of the microvilli (the "bubbles" appear as such only in section; actually they are part of a complicated three-dimensional structure, as shown in the inset of Fig. 11); (3), (4) an area of the plasma membrane separate from the rhabdomere. The third location seems unlikely due to the close proximity within a rhabdomere needed for two absorbed light quanta to reduce the latency (see page 153). If the channel system were located far from the microvilli, interaction between quanta absorbed much further apart than one microvillus are to be expected.

The results have shown that the reduction in latency is caused by double hits either at neighbouring or single microvilli. To distinguish between these two cases seems to be of particular interest: if double hits at neighbouring microvilli are sufficient it does not seem unlikely that the channel system is located at the "bubbles", because precisely this membrane area is accessible from neighbouring microvilli. In the (less likely) case that double hits at microvilli are necessary for the latency reduction, it would seem possible that channels might be localized within the microvillar membrane.

A model of the function of the visual pigment system

Many microvillar photoreceptors exhibit a phenomenon described first in the photoreceptor of the median ocellus of *Limulus* (Nolte and Brown, 1972; Minke *et al.*, 1973). After a stimulus that converts a large fraction of R to M, the cell remains depolarized for a long time (many minutes) even after cessation of the light. This "prolonged depolarizing afterpotential" (PDA) can be abolished if a light flash is given that shifts the M produced by the first flash back into R. The rules, common to all microvillar photoreceptors investigated so far, according to which a PDA is created or abolished have been summarized by Hillman (1977). These general rules have been used in order to devise "models" which are intended primarily to aid in memorizing the rather complicated phenomenology, but which, it is hoped, will also reflect some of the processes that underlie

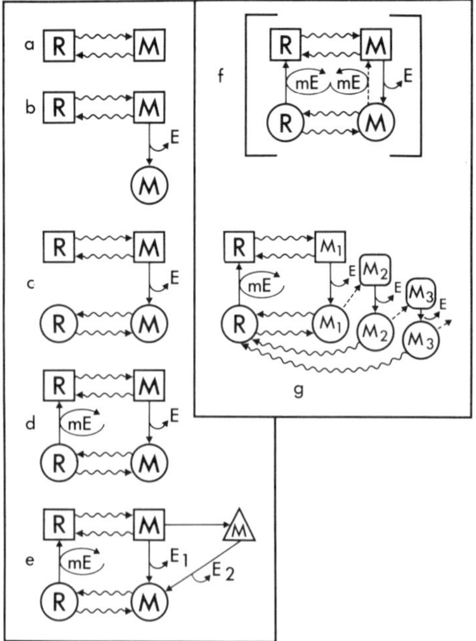

Figure 12 (a)–(e) A schematic model of the coupling of photopigment states to excitation in invertebrate photoreceptors. (Redrawn from Hamdorf and Razmjoo, 1977.)
(f), (g) A modified version of the above model; details are discussed in the text. Square symbols represent "energy-rich" forms, circular symbols "energy-poor" forms. Triangular symbol represents slowly-transforming form.

the transduction process in these receptors. Furthermore, such models should allow predictions on the behaviour of photoreceptors under conditions which can be verified experimentally.

One of the models is the excitor/inhibitor model as suggested by Hochstein *et al.* (1973); another has been presented by Hamdorf and Razmjoo (1977, 1979). It seems at present as if the latter model can more completely describe the phenomena as observed under varying experimental conditions (Razmjoo and Hamdorf, 1980), and the properties of the latter will therefore be described.

In Fig. 12a the conversion of R into M by absorption of light is schematically indicated. M is created in 100 μs, and it then triggers the excitation (E) of the membrane (Fig. 12b). After the excitation, M is still present (as can be shown by its absorption, Fig. 8) but it is no longer able to excite the membrane. Therefore it is called "energy-poor" (circled symbols) in contrast to the "energy-rich", newly-created M (square symbols). If "energy-poor" M absorbs a quantum of light it is re-isomerized into R (Fig. 12c, circled symbol), as manifested by a change in absorption. This circled R is not identical with the initial R, since if it absorbs a quantum of light, it does not lead to excitation but only to the formation of energy-poor M. This is shown by the phenomenon of the "anti-PDA" (see e.g. Minke, 1979): in order to obtain a full response, including a PDA, by giving a flash to R, a recovery time in the dark (several seconds to minutes) is needed. During this time the energy-poor R is believed to be raised (by means of metabolic energy mE) to the energy-rich state of the R molecule (Fig. 12d).

Besides this phenomenology of the kinetics of pigments and LRP, the model has to take into account the PDA. In order to do so it is assumed that besides the transition from energy-rich M to energy-poor M which leads to the normal LRP, there is a transition of energy-rich M to another form (triangular symbol), which is transformed at a low rate to energy-poor M, whereby the PDA is induced (E_2) (Fig. 12e). This is the model as originally presented by Hamdorf and Razmjoo. In order to explain the fact that a significant PDA is induced only if a considerable amount of R is converted into M (in contrast to the normal LRP, where fractions of a per cent of the transition of R to M are already saturating the response), one has to assume that a significant amount of the slowly-transforming form of M is created only if large amounts of R have been shifted to M. It is only under these conditions that an "overflow" of energy-rich M to "slowly-transforming" M takes place.

In fact there are several different possibilities which could explain the PDA. In Fig. 12f a modification of the Hamdorf–Razmjoo model is shown with a different argument for the occurrence of the PDA. As illustrated in Fig. 12e, in order to reconvert energy-poor R to the original energy-rich R, metabolic energy is required. We may ask why such energy does not also convert energy-poor M into energy-rich M, since M is a molecule very similar to R.

Under physiological conditions, this transformation does of course not happen regularly. Otherwise excitation, once M is formed, would never stop. One might expect, however, that under non-physiological conditions, at a high M-concentration and if only a few R molecules are present, M might also be reactivated by metabolism. This reasoning results in the model shown in Fig. 12f. This model is inadequate as it stands as it does not predict a decline of the PDA, once a high concentration of M is present. One might imagine, however, that the reactivation of M by metabolism is not an ideal one, but leads only to a state M_2, which is not identical to M_1 but less "energy-rich". M_2 then becomes M_3, etc. (Fig. 12g). The number of cycles that can be undergone by M is limited, and the PDA has a limited life-time. A cyclic model has also been suggested by Horridge and Tsukahara (1978).

The difference between the models shown in Fig. 12e and g is that in the latter, one absorbed quantum is able to lead to more than one "bump" (hence can create extremely long PDA's), and also that metabolic energy is required to generate the PDA. Only the fact that both models can be discriminated experimentally justifies the discussion.

It has been shown that the PDA, like the LRP, is composed of individual "bumps" (Tsukahara and Horridge, 1977). There is, however, a significant difference between light-induced depolarization and PDA-depolarization: the noise in light-induced depolarization (at the same mean depolarization) is significantly higher (Hamdorf and Razmjoo, 1979). This result shows that the bumps that form the PDA are smaller than the bumps induced directly by light. This means also that either E_2 leads to smaller bumps than E_1 (Fig. 12e), or that the dynamic properties of the system are different as long as the slowly-transforming form of M (or M_1, M_2, M_3, etc.) are present. The presence of energy-poor M seems not to be the reason for the difference, since individual PDA "bumps" that are recorded at the end of the decline of a PDA seem to be indistinguishable (at least in the locust), from "bumps" triggered by light in a dark adapted photoreceptor (Horridge and Tsukahara, 1978). Since responses to short light-flashes superimposed during a PDA are shorter than those superimposed on a light-induced depolarization (Kirschfeld *et al.*, in prep.) the system is obviously altered during the PDA: E acting on a light-induced depolarization leads to a different signal than during a PDA. The reason for this change, in molecular terms, is still unclear.

What sense do stable and bistable pigments make in visual cells?

As far as stable pigments are concerned, it is obvious that knowledge of their existence helps to interpret many complicated phenomena, particularly the deviation of sensitivities (absolute, spectral, polarization) of photoreceptors from behaviour expected on the basis of classical visual pigment properties. The bistability of visual pigments in invertebrates and its use as an experimental tool also offers some additional insight into the transduction process.

1. It is clear that part of the latency of the LRP (a few ms) is due to changes that take place at, or close to, the visual pigment molecule. In the vertebrate rod we do not know where, on its way from prebump to metarhodopsin II, the causal chain leading to excitation is branching off (Fig. 7a). It is clear for fly receptors that M must exist for some time in order to trigger a response (Fig. 7b).

2. It has been demonstrated that the latency of the LRP is shortened in a qualitative manner (Fig. 10) if double-hits occur in the rhabdomere close enough to each other. This finding excludes for fly photoreceptors all models of function in which the latency is unaffected by the strength of the response. This is the case for instance in the model by Hodgkin and Fuortes (see review by Fuortes and O'Bryan, 1972), which well describes the LRP in *Limulus* photoreceptors. Nonlinearity affecting the amplitude of the response in this model is introduced by a feedback from the response. In the fly the shortening of the latency develops, however, *before* any LRP can be detected. Nonlinearity by a feedback from the response is hence excluded as an explanation.

3. There are some hints as to the likely locus of the channels that increase the permeability during excitation (Fig. 11: 1, 2).

Besides these additional statements, however, much basic knowledge is lacking. Why, for instance, do the bumps vary so much between individual photoreceptors in amplitude, latency and scatter of latency? One might suspect that this variation has to do with different sizes of microvilli, but this obviously is not the case: in the *Limulus* ventral photoreceptors, and the locust and *Calliphora* photoreceptors, the amplitude of the bumps decreases from a mean of 12 mV (Yeandle and Spiegler, 1973) over 3 mV (Lillywhite, 1977) to 1.5 mV (Hamdorf and Kirschfeld, 1980*a*). The size of the microvilli is respectively 1.8 μm, 0–1 μm and 0.5–2 μm, that is, they are not related to the "bump" amplitude. There is however, a strict correlation between amplitude and the mean (dark-adapted) latency of the "bump". The amplitude decreases from 150 over 50 to 20 ms (at 18–25°C). This correlation indicates that there may be a common parameter, such as the state of adaptation, that governs transduction in all three cases, but which is quantitatively different in each of them.

Furthermore, we do not know at all which steps are interposed between what we have called $\overline{\text{M}}$ (Fig. 7b) and the change of permeability, nor whether there exists an intracellular diffusable transmitter, or a kind of "chemical wave" as discussed by Brown *et al.* (1979), which transmits the information from the rhodopsin molecule to the channels. Which of these problems can be solved by use of bistable visual pigments will be shown in the future.

Acknowledgments

I thank Professor K. Hamdorf and Dr B. Minke for stimulating collaboration, Dr K. Vogt for discussion and Professor G. Höglund for reading the English manuscript.

REFERENCES

Baylor, D. A., Lamb, T. D. and Yau, K. W. (1979) Responses of retinal rods to single photons *J. Physiol.*, **288**, 613–634.

Boschek, C. B. (1971) On the fine structure of the peripheral retina and ganglionaris of the fly, *Musca domestica Z. Zellforsch.*, **118**, 369–409.

Bouman, M. A. and van der Velden, H. A. (1948) The two quanta hypothesis as a general explanation for the behavior of threshold values and visual acuity for the several receptors of the human eye *J. opt. Soc. Amer.*, **38**, 570–581.

Brown, J., Brown, H. M., Hess, B., Mueller, P., Oesterhelt, D., Parson, W., Rüppel, H., Sperling, W. and Stieve, H. (1979) "Rhodopsin Mediated Processes Group Report" in *Light-Induced Charge Separation in Biology and Chemistry* (eds. Gerischer, H., Katz, J. J.) Dahlem Konferenzen, Berlin, 525–551.

Burkhardt, D. (1962) Spectral sensitivity and other response characteristics of single visual cells in the arthropod eye *Symp. Soc. exp. Biol.*, **16**, 86.

Dodge, F. A. Jr., Knight, B. W. and Toyoda, J. (1968) Voltage noise in *Limulus* visual cells *Science*, **160**, 88–90.

Förster, T. (ed.) (1951) *Fluoreszenz organischer Verbindungen* Vandenhoeck und Ruprecht, Göttingen.

Franceschini, N. (1975) "Sampling of the visual environment by the compound eye of the fly: Fundamentals and applications" in *Photoreceptor Optics* (eds. Snyder, A. W., Menzel, R.) Springer, Berlin-Heidelberg-New York, 98–125.

Fuortes, M. G. F. and O'Bryan, P. M. (1972) "Generator potentials in invertebrate photoreceptors" in *Handbook of Sensory Physiology* (ed. Fuortes, M. G. F.) Vol. VII/2, Springer, Berlin-Heidelberg-New York, 279–338.

Fuortes, M. G. F. and Yeandle, S. (1964) Probability of occurrence of discrete potential waves in the eye of *Limulus J. Gen. Physiol.*, **47**, 443–463.

Goldsmith, T. H. (1972) "The natural history of invertebrate visual pigments" in *Handbook of Sensory Physiology* (ed. Dartnall, H. J. A.), Vol. VII/1, Springer, Berlin-Heidelberg-New York, 685–719.

Goldsmith, T. H. (1980) Hummingbirds see near ultraviolet light *Science*, **207**, 786–788.

Hamdorf, K. (1979) "The Physiology of Invertebrate Visual Pigments" in *Handbook of Sensory Physiology* (ed. Autrum, H.) Vol. VII/6A, Springer, Berlin-Heidelberg-New York, 145–224.

Hamdorf, K., Paulsen, R. and Schwemer, J. (1973) "Photoregeneration and sensitivity control of photoreceptors of invertebrates" in *Biochemistry and Physiology of Visual Pigments* (ed. Langer, H.) Springer, Berlin-Heidelberg-New York, 155–166.

Hamdorf, K. and Razmjoo, S. (1977) The prolonged depolarising afterpotential and its contribution to the understanding of photoreceptor function *Biophys. Struct. Mech.*, **3**, 163–170.

Hamdorf, K. and Razmjoo, S. (1979) Photoconvertible pigment states and excitation in *Calliphora*: the induction and properties of the prolonged depolarising afterpotential *Biophys. Struct. Mech.*, **5**, 137–161.

Hamdorf, K. and Kirschfeld, K. (1980*a*) "Prebumps": Evidence for double hits at functional subunits in a rhabdomeric photoreceptor *Z. Naturforsch.*, **35c**, 173–174.
Hamdorf, K. and Kirschfeld, K. (1980*b*) Reversible events in the transduction process of photoreceptors *Nature*, **283**, 859–860.
Hardie, R. C. (1977) Electrophysiological properties of R7 and R8 in Dipteran retina *Z. Naturforsch.*, **32c**, 887–889.
Hardie, R. C., Franceschini, N. and McIntyre, P. D. (1979) Electrophysiological analysis of fly retina. II. Spectral and polarisation sensitivity in R7 and R8 *J. Comp. Physiol.*, **133**, 23–39.
Harris, W. A., Stark, W. S. and Walker, J. A. (1976) Genetic dissection of the photoreceptor system in the compound eye of *Drosophila melanogaster J. Physiol.* (*Lond*), **256**, 415–439.
Hecht, S., Shlaer, S. and Pirenne, M. H. (1942) Energy quanta and vision *J. Gen. Physiol.*, **25**, 819–840.
Hillman, P. (1977) Discussion of selected topics about the transduction mechanism in photoreceptors *Biophys. Struct. Mech.*, **3**, 183–189.
Hochstein, S., Minke, B. and Hillman, P. (1973) Antagonistic components of the late receptor potential in the barnacle photoreceptor arising from different stages of the pigment process *J. Gen. Physiol.*, **62**, 105–128.
Horridge, G. A. and Tsukahara, Y. (1978) The distribution of bumps in the tail of the locust photoreceptor afterpotential *J. exp. Biol.*, **73**, 1–14.
Kirschfeld, K., Franceschini, N. and Minke, B. (1977) Evidence for a sensitising pigment in fly photoreceptors *Nature*, **269**, 386–390.
Kirschfeld, K., Feiler, R. and Franceschini, N. (1978*a*) A photostable pigment within the rhabdomere of fly photoreceptors no. 7 *J. Comp. Physiol.*, **125**, 275–284.
Kirschfeld, K., Feiler, R. and Minke, B. (1978*b*) The kinetics of formation of metarhodopsin in intact photoreceptors of the fly *Z. Naturforsch.*, **33c**, 1009–1010.
Kirschfeld, K. (1979) The function of photostable pigments in fly photoreceptors *Biophys. Struct. Mech.*, **5**, 117–128.
Lillywhite, P. G. (1977) Single photon signals and transduction in an insect eye *J. Comp. Physiol.*, **122**, 189–200.
Menzel, R. (1979) "Spectral sensitivity and color vision in invertebrates" in *Handbook of Sensory Physiology* (ed. Autrum, H.) Vol. VII/6A Springer, Berlin-Heidelberg-New York, 503–580.
Millecchia, R. and Mauro, A. (1969) The ventral photoreceptor cells of *Limulus*. III. A voltage-clamp study *J. Gen. Physiol.*, **54**, 331–351.
Minke, B., Hochstein, S. and Hillman, P. (1973) Antagonistic process as source of visible-light suppression of afterpotential in *Limulus* UV photoreceptors *J. Gen. Physiol.*, **62**, 787–791.
Minke, B. (1979) Transduction in photoreceptors with bistable pigments: intermediate processes *Biophys. Struct. Mech.*, **5**, 163–174.
Minke, B. and Kirschfeld, K. (1979) The contribution of a sensitizing pigment to the photosensitivity spectra of fly rhodopsin and metarhodopsin *J. Gen. Physiol.*, **73**, 517–540.
Muijser, H. and Stavenga, D. G. (1979) Rapid photopigment conversions in blowfly visual sense cells. Consequences for receptor potential and pupillary response *Biophys. Struct. Mech.*, **5**, 187–196.
Nolte, J. and Brown, J. E. (1972) UV-induced sensitivity to visible light in UV receptors of *Limulus J. Gen. Physiol.*, **59**, 186–200.
Paulsen, R. and Schwemer, J. (1979) Vitamin A deficiency reduces the concentration of visual pigment protein within blowfly photoreceptor membranes *Biochimica et Biophysica Acta*, **557**, 385–390.
Razmjoo, S. and Hamdorf, K. (1980) In support of the "photopigment model" of vision in invertebrates *J. Comp. Physiol.*, **135**, 209–215.
Stark, W. S., Ivanyshyn, A. M. and Hu, K. G. (1976) Spectral sensitivities and photopigments in adaptation of fly visual receptors *Naturwiss.*, **63**, 513–518.
Stark, W. S., Ivanyshyn, A. M. and Greenberg, R. M. (1977) Sensitivity and photopigments of R1–6, a two-peaked photoreceptor, in *Drosophila, Calliphora* and *Musca J. Comp. Physiol.*, **121**, 289–305.
Stark, W. S., Stavenga, D. G. and Kruizinga, B. (1979) Fly photoreceptor fluorescence is related to UV sensitivity *Nature*, **280**, 581–583.

Stavenga, D. G., Zantema, A. and Kuiper, J. W. (1973) "Rhodopsin process and the function of the pupil mechanism in flies" in *Biochemistry and Physiology of Visual Pigments* (ed. Langer, H.) Springer, Berlin-Heidelberg-New York, 175–180.

Stieve, H. (1974) Mechanismen der Erregung von Lichtsinneszellen *Naturwiss. Rundschau*, **27**, 45–56.

Tsukahara, Y. and Horridge, G. A. (1977) Miniature potentials, light adaptation and afterpotentials in locust retinula cells *J. exp. Biol.*, **68**, 137–149.

Wu, Ch.-F. and Pak, W. L. (1978) Light-induced voltage noise in the photoreceptor of *Drosophila melanogaster J. Gen. Physiol.*, **71**, 249–268.

Yeandle, S. (1958) Electrophysiology of the visual system. Discussion *Amer. J. Ophthalmol.*, **46**, 82–87.

Yeandle, S. and Spiegler, J. B. (1973) Light-evoked and spontaneous discrete waves in the ventral nerve photoreceptor of *Limulus J. Gen. Physiol.*, **61**, 552–571.

CHAPTER TEN

ROLES OF CALCIUM IN VISUAL TRANSDUCTION IN INVERTEBRATES

H. STIEVE

Introduction

The membrane voltage (i.e. the potential difference which is measured between the inside and outside of the photoreceptor cell) is mainly a diffusion potential due to ion gradients across the cell membrane and its selective ion (specific) permeability. Active ion transport mechanisms consuming metabolic energy restore the ion gradients. There is also a certain contribution to the membrane voltage by electrogenic active transport processes.

Illumination induces a transient, graded change in ion selectivity of the photoreceptor membrane, thus causing a transient change in membrane voltage. Successful light absorption by the visual pigment triggers a delayed transient opening (invertebrates) or closing (vertebrates) of specific ion channels. The transduction mechanisms of invertebrate and vertebrate photoreceptors therefore show essential differences.

Invertebrate photoreceptors

Fig. 1 shows a general scheme of the visual transduction mechanism of a photoreceptor cell of an invertebrate, e.g. an arthropod. Most of the facts described in the following about the transduction mechanism of invertebrates will be taken from experiments with *Limulus* or barnacle photoreceptors. Many of the characteristics described, however, can also be applied to most other species.

It is reasonably certain that the ion specificity of the visual cell membrane is based upon the existence of discrete ion channels bridging the cell membranes. According to this model, the photoreceptor membrane contains several types of ion channels:

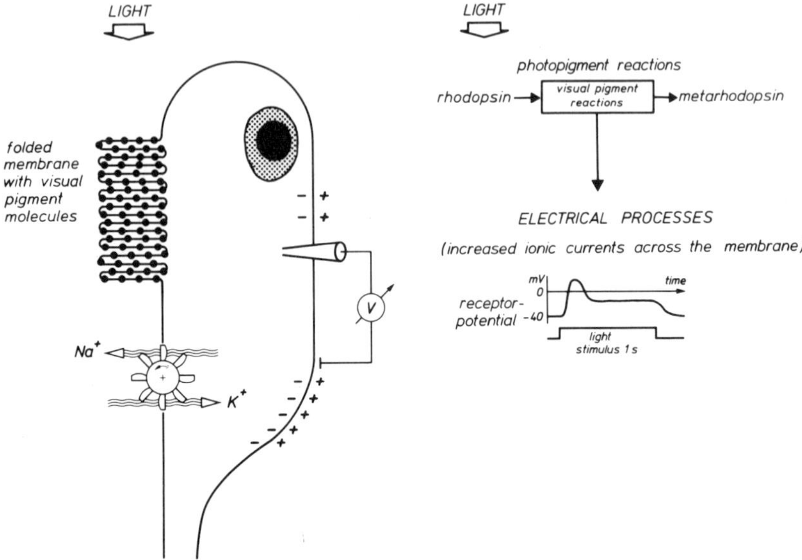

Figure 1 Functional mechanism of a visual cell of an invertebrate (rhodopsin contained in microvillar membrane, i.e. finger-like exfoldings of the cell membrane). The pump symbol indicates active ion transport mechanism.

(1) dark-channels, which are permanently open in the dark and during illumination;
(2) light-activated channels (or light channels) which are only transiently opened following light absorption, "directly" triggered by light-induced rhodopsin reactions (i.e. not by a change in membrane voltage) via a not yet understood trigger mechanism;
(3) additional voltage-sensitive ion channels which can be activated by changes in membrane voltage.

The dark channels have a preference for K^+-ions, thus the membrane potential in resting dark conditions is close to the Nernst potential for potassium according to the concentration gradient of potassium ions across the cell membrane, ca. -50 mV (inside negative against outside) (H. M. Brown, 1976; Stieve, 1974, 1977). The light channels, however, have a preference for Na^+ over K^+ of ca. 2 : 1 (H. M. Brown, 1976). They overbalance the dark channels so that, if many of them are activated, the membrane potential reaches values of $+10$ to $+20$ mV.

The depolarization due to the opening of the light-activated channels causes, in turn, the opening of voltage-sensitive channels; firstly, calcium channels which allow the influx of Ca^{2+} and so tend to augment the depolarization of the cell (Fein and Lisman, pers. comm.), and also K^+-

channels which tend to repolarize the cell membrane and thus cause a faster decay of the receptor potential (Pepose and Lisman, 1978).

(4) In barnacle photoreceptors there is an additional K^+-channel type which is activated by the rise in intracellular Ca^{2+} concentration (Hanani and Shaw, 1977).

Different areas of the cell membrane differ in their properties. The rhodopsin-containing photosensory membrane which is greatly enlarged by folding (in invertebrates forming microvilli) can amount to 90% of the total surface membrane area of the visual cell. It is not known at present in which area of the cell membrane the different ion channels are located nor where the ion pumps are located. According to measurements of Fioravanti and Fuortes (1972) in the photoreceptors of the leech, the light-induced conductance change occurs in (or close to) the microvillar membrane. It is, however, not known whether the whole photosensory membrane undergoes the light induced conductance changes or whether certain areas in, or close to, the photosensory membrane exclusively contain the light activated channels. Hamdorf and Kirschfeld (1980) presented data suggesting that the light-activated channels may be at the basis of the microvilli. It may be that the other channel types (dark channels and voltage-sensitive channels), as well as the membrane-bound enzymes responsible for active ion transport, are not in the rhodopsin-containing membrane areas.

Calcium ions play an important role in the transduction process of the invertebrate photoreceptor cells in at least four important functions:

(a) current transmission through the cell membrane
(b) control of membrane conductance
(c) adaptation (control of amplification)
(d) coupling between rhodopsin reactions and membrane conductance change (quantum efficiency).

These will be discussed in turn in the following account.

(a) *Current transmission*

In barnacle and squid photoreceptor Ca-ions can carry charge into the cell during the light response due to a light-induced increase in Ca-permeability (H. M. Brown *et al.*, 1970; Duncan and Pynsent, 1979; Clark and Duncan, 1978; Meech, 1978). In *Limulus* photoreceptors the voltage-sensitive Ca-channels mentioned above allow a charge transport through the cell membrane by an influx of Ca^{2+} during the light response. Whether there is an additional Ca^{2+}-influx via other pathways is not yet known. There may also be an electroneutral Ca^{2+}-influx into the cell via a Ca^{2+}/Na^+ antiport exchange mechanism (Maaz and Stieve, 1980) as observed in nerve membrane (Baker and Glitsch, 1975).

(b) *Conductance control*

If the concentration of the divalent cations Ca^{2+} and Mg^{2+} in the saline superfusing a ventral nerve photoreceptor is reduced to very low values (< 1 μmol/l, e.g. by adding EDTA to the superfusate) the photoreceptor

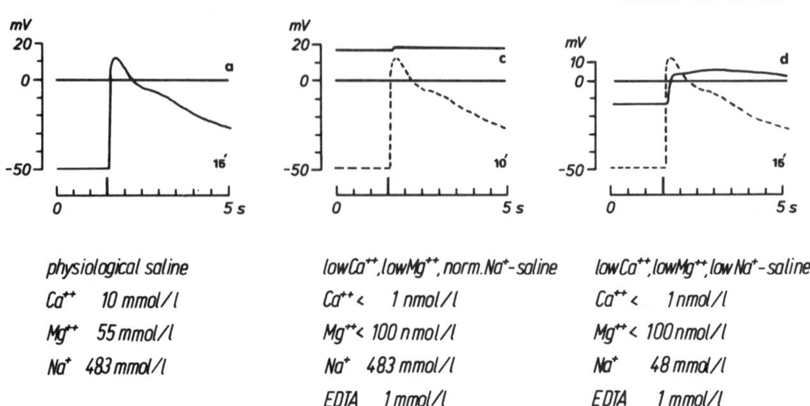

Figure 2 Receptor potentials of *Limulus* ventral nerve photoreceptor in salines containing very low concentrations of divalent cations (Me^{2+}) and normal or low sodium concentration (choline is used as Na^+ substitute).

(a) reference light response in physiological saline,

(c) light response after the photoreceptor had spent 10 min in a saline with very low Me^{2+} concentration. The prestimulus membrane potential (PMP) is +18 mV, and the light response is almost abolished. If the period in this saline was prolonged by a few minutes, the light response disappeared entirely.

(d) light response 15 min later than (c), after 15 min in saline whose Ca^{2+} and Mg^{2+} concentration is low, as in (c), and with the Na^+ concentration lowered to 10% of the normal value. Response height saturating 20 ms white light flash; I equivalent to ca. 4×10^{17} 550 nm photons $cm^{-2}\,s^{-1}$; 15°C.

The reference response of (a) is represented by a broken line in (c) and (d). During the period (b) between (a) and (c), the receptor was superfused by the same saline as in (d).

cell depolarizes in the dark, and the membrane potential reaches a positive value about equal to that reached by the transient of the receptor potential following an amplitude-saturating light stimulus (Fig. 2a, c). At the same time the light response is gradually reduced and finally abolished (Stieve, 1965). The simplest explanation for these findings is to assume that the light channels are opened due to the reduction of the extracellular concentration of divalent cations (Stieve, 1974; Stieve and Bruns, 1978). Lowering the external Na^+-concentration, to only ca. 50 mmol/l (e.g. replacing Na^+ by choline) in a saline already low in divalent cations, causes a recovery both of the dark potential as well as of the receptor potential to a certain degree (Fig. 2d). This led us to propose a Ca^{2+}/Na^+ antagonism with the two ion species competing for the same negative binding sites on the external surface of the visual cell membrane (Stieve and Bruns, 1978) (Fig. 3). The ratio of bound Ca^{2+}/Na^+ somehow controls whether the light channels are opened or closed (Fig. 3 shows a possible hypothetical scheme). Binding of calcium ions could cause the light channels to close, whereas a replacement of the bound Ca^{2+} by binding of Na^+ could cause opening. Light could cause a transient affinity

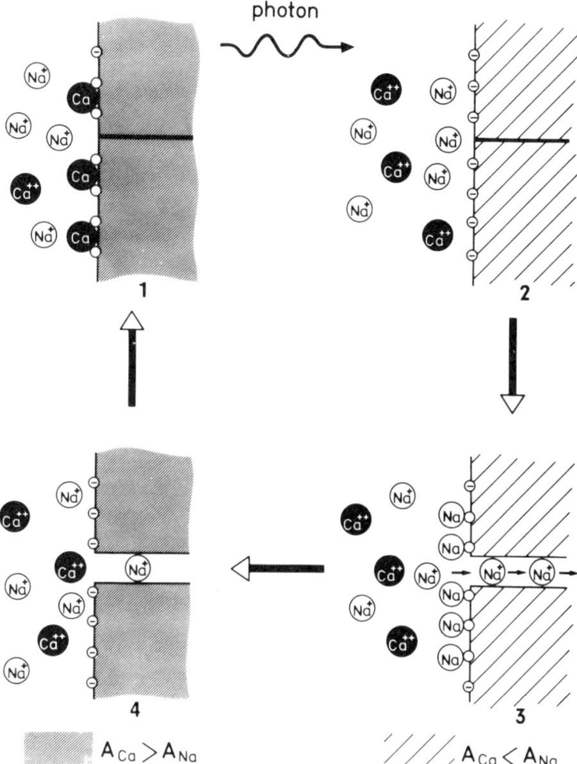

Figure 3 Hypothesis of sodium–calcium binding competition for negatively charged binding sites which control opening and closing of light-activated ion channels in the *Limulus* photosensory membrane. Light channel is closed when calcium is bound, and opened when sodium is bound instead. A_{Ca}: affinity for calcium, A_{Na}: affinity for sodium.

(1) Strong affinity for calcium in the dark, channel closed.

(2) Photon absorption induces transient affinity change, raising the relative affinity for sodium; calcium and sodium compete for binding sites.

(3) Under normal conditions the extracellular sodium concentration is much higher than that of calcium, so that sodium is bound and the channel opens.

(4) The affinity changes back spontaneously in favour of calcium; under normal conditions calcium is bound (1) and the channel closes again (from H. Stieve, 1977 and Stieve and Bruns, 1978).

change of the binding sites resulting in a transient reduction of the preference of Ca^{2+} over Na^{+} and this in turn could cause a transient opening of the light channels.

Voltage clamp measurements under similar conditions are in agreement with this interpretation (Stieve and Pflaum, 1978*b*) (Figs. 4 and 5a, b). Sufficient lowering of the divalent cation concentration abolishes the light-induced conductance increase, and shifts the reversal potential of the dark current to nearly the same voltage (ca. +10 to +20 mV) as that of

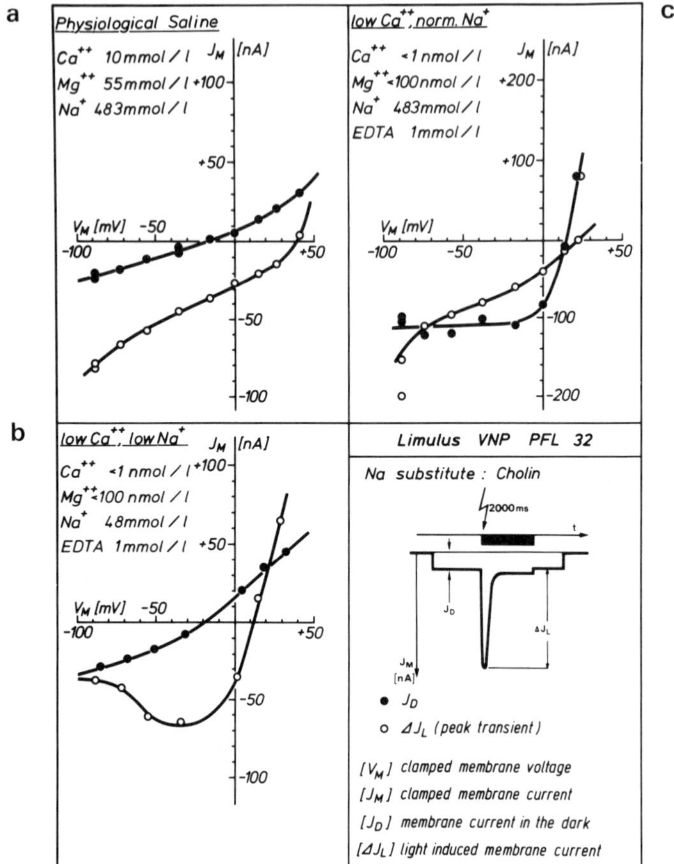

Figure 4 Membrane current *vs* voltage curves for *Limulus* ventral nerve photoreceptor in different Me^{2+}, Na^+ salines (choline is used as Na substitute). *Abscissa*: clamped membrane voltage V_M; *ordinate*: membrane current J_M (see inset). Photoreceptor superfused by

(a) physiological saline (upper left)

(b) saline very low in Me^{2+} and low (10% of normal) in Na^+ concentration (lower left) and

(c) very low in Me^{2+} and normal Na^+ concentration (upper right). Here a light response could still be evoked (light induced current ΔJ_L was still measurable, which would have disappeared after longer in this saline. Receptor potential transient saturating white 2 s illumination: I ca. 6×10^{15} 550 nm photons $cm^{-2}\,s^{-1}$; 15°C.

the saturated maximum of the receptor potential in physiological saline. These observations are in agreement with an increase in membrane conductivity which is caused by reduction in divalent cation concentration and which has the same ion selectivity as that of the light channels. Due to the reduction of the divalent ion concentration the dark, membrane conductance is increased progressively in time, while the light-

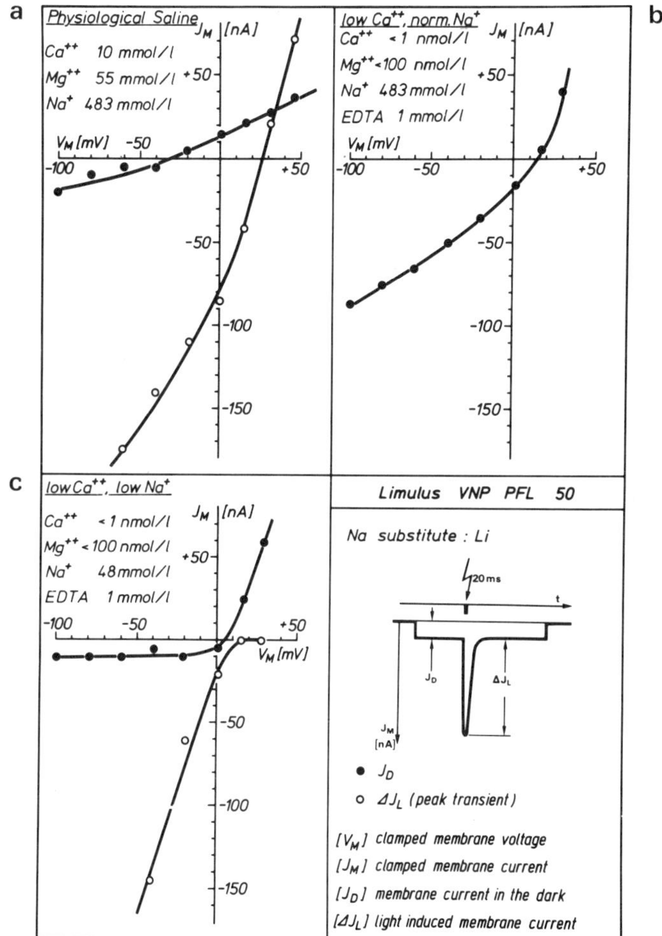

Figure 5 Membrane current *vs* voltage curves of *Limulus* ventral nerve photoreceptor in different Me^{2+}, Na^+ salines. Lithium is used as sodium substitute. Receptor potential transient saturating white 20 ms light flash; remainder as in Fig. 4. Upper right: The light response has already disappeared; no light-induced current ΔJ_L is measurable.

induced conductance increase is progressively diminished, and after 10–20 min is abolished altogether.

The lowering of both the Na^+-concentration to 50 mmol/l (substituted by choline$^+$, Fig. 4) in the superfusate, simultaneously with the strong reduction in the divalent cation concentration, causes only a small increase in membrane dark conductance and the light-induced conductance increase stays higher than at normal Na^+ concentrations (about 500 mmol/l). The light induced membrane current *vs* voltage curve shows, under these conditions, a region with negative slope (Fig. 4b). The reversal potential of both the dark current and the light-induced current are only slightly decreased (by 5–10 mV). This is consistent with the assumption that only a fraction of the light channels are open in the dark, when Na^+ is additionally reduced in a saline low in divalent cation concentration, and that the remaining closed light channels can still be activated by light.

The antagonistic effect of lowering external sodium is smaller if lithium is used as sodium substitute instead of choline (Fig. 5). Lithium ions can partially replace sodium-ions in this Ca^{2+}/Na^+ antagonism with a weaker action. When sodium is lowered to 50 mmol/l in the superfusate which is depleted of divalent cations and Li^+ is used as Na^+ substitute, the reversal potential of the dark current is slightly positive (0–5 mV), the ability for light-induced conductance change is sustained, and the light-induced current is high (and no outward current is seen, Fig. 5c).

What is the action of magnesium-ions in comparison to that of calcium-ions in the effects described? If the *Limulus* photoreceptor is superfused by a saline containing 1 nmol/l Ca^{2+} and normal Na^+-concentration, and the Mg^{2+}-concentration is raised to 100 mmol/l after a prior sojourn of the photoreceptor in a saline in which both divalent cations were strongly reduced (Fig. 6), the dark potential as well as the peak amplitude of the receptor potential are recovered by between one-half and two-thirds (Table 1). Mg^{2+} can substitute for Ca^{2+} in this Ca^{2+}/Na^+ antagonism of

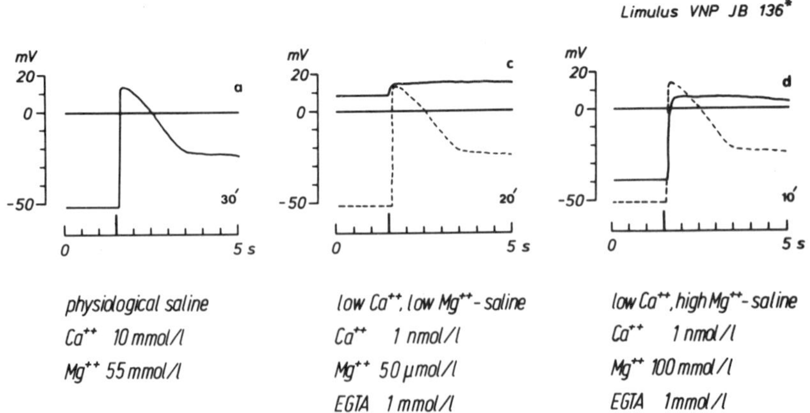

Figure 6 Receptor potentials of *Limulus* ventral nerve photoreceptor in salines containing very low Ca^{2+} concentration and very low or high (100 mmol/l) Mg^{2+} concentration.

(a) reference light response in physiological saline,

(c) light response after 20 min in a saline with very low Ca^{2+} and Mg^{2+} concentration. As in Fig. 2(c), the light response has already almost disappeared.

(d) light response 10 min later than (c), after 10 min in saline whose Ca^{2+} concentration is still low as in (c) but whose Mg^{2+} concentration has been raised to 100 mmol/l. I ca. 1.5×10^{17} 550 nm photons $cm^{-2} s^{-1}$. Remainder as in Fig. 2.

membrane conductance control, but with a definitely weaker action. This is evidence that the action of calcium is by binding to the membrane rather than by a screening effect. Probably the Ca^{2+}/Na^{+} binding competition reaction described occurs at the external surface of the photoreceptor cell membrane, since the effect begins when the extracellular Ca^{2+}-concentration is lowered to values which are still higher than the estimated intracellular Ca^{2+}-concentration (Stieve and Bruns, 1978).

Our model, apart from the calcium-antagonistic role of sodium, has several features in common with the model proposed by Weeks and Duncan (1974), based on their findings in the cephalopod retina. A Ca^{2+}/Na^{+} antagonism was also observed by H. M. Brown *et al.* (1970) in the barnacle photoreceptor. Aside from some striking similarities between their model and ours, there is an important difference: our assumption that light channels are opened in the dark due to a lowering of the external concentration of divalent cations. This is derived from observations with much lower divalent ion concentrations than those used by other authors.

Brown and Ottoson (1976) observed that extracellular K^{+}-ions counteract the action of extracellular calcium in suppressing the light-induced increase of membrane conductance in the barnacle photoreceptor. Omission of potassium from the bathing saline abolished the

Table 1 Membrane potential and height and shape of receptor potential of *Limulus* ventral nerve photoreceptor depending upon extracellular Ca^{2+}, Mg^{2+} and Na^{+} concentration. PMP: prestimulus membrane potential; H_{max}: height of maximum of receptor potential; H_N/H_{max}: shape quotient (where H_N is the height of the receptor potential 500 ms after the maximum), i.e. a measure of the decline of the receptor potential 500 ms after the maximum. In physiological saline it is about 0.5. The slower the decline, the more closely H_N/H_{max} approaches 1. Lowering the divalent cation concentration causes a decrease of PMP and H_{max} and an increase of H_N/H_{max}. PMP and H_{max} are partially restored by lowering external Na^{+} concentration or by raising external Mg^{2+} concentration. However the shape quotient H_N/H_{max} stays large under these two conditions.

Intracellular recording; mean ± S.E.; number *n* of experiments used for average given in parentheses; 15°C (see Fig. 2 and Fig. 6).

Ca^{2+} (mol/l)	Mg^{2+} (mol/l)	buffer (mol/l)	Na^{+} (mol/l)	PMP (mV)	H_{max} (mV)	H_N/H_{max}
				(n = 15)		
10^{-2}	5.5×10^{-2}	—	5.4×10^{-1}	-43 ± 2.7	56 ± 2.2	0.54 ± 0.06
				(4)		
5×10^{-5}	5×10^{-5}	—	5.4×10^{-1}	$+0.4 \pm 3.8$	8 ± 4.0	0.86 ± 0.01
			3.8×10^{-2}	-21 ± 3.9	16 ± 5.0	0.89 ± 0.05
				(4)		
10^{-9}	5×10^{-5}	EGTA 10^{-3}	5.7×10^{-1}	-0.04 ± 5.7	10 ± 3.8	0.92 ± 0.02
	10^{-1}		4.2×10^{-1}	-29 ± 4.7	29 ± 7.2	0.99 ± 0.07

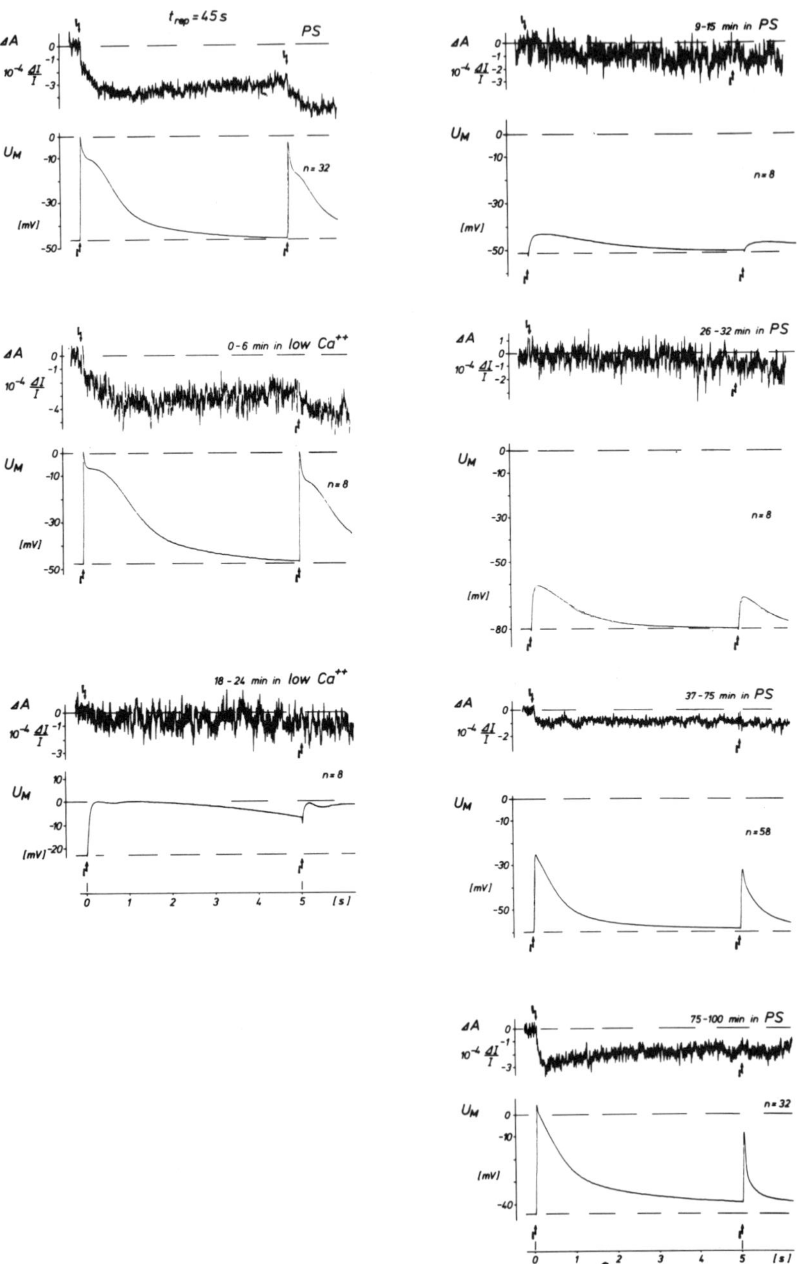

Figure 7 Simultaneous recordings of receptor potentials (lower curves) and absorption changes ΔA of intracellular injected calcium indicator arsenazo III (upper curves) in *Limulus* ventral nerve photoreceptor cell. The receptor cell was stimulated by pairs of 10 ms response height saturating flashes I ca. 3×10^{16} 550 nm photons $cm^{-2} s^{-1}$ repeated every 45 s. A

light response, and additional reduction of calcium caused recovery of excitability. We could not confirm this Ca^{2+}/K^+ antagonism in *Limulus* and crayfish photoreceptors. Both photoreceptors showed no reduction in light response during 90 min in saline which contained no added potassium. Additional reduction in external calcium caused a diminution rather than an increase in light response amplitude (Stieve, Bruns and Claßen-Linke, unpublished).

Fig. 6 shows, however, another conspicuous feature: whereas in low Ca^{2+}-concentration saline a high Mg^{2+}-concentration can restore the prestimulus membrane potential and h_{max}, it does not improve the repolarizing phase of the receptor potential, which is strongly retarded in low Ca^{2+}-concentration. The same is true for the effect of lowering Na^+-concentration (Fig. 3), which partially restores PMP and h_{max} after lowering Ca^{2+} and Mg^{2+}. The repolarizing decay of receptor potential is not restored by low Na^+. The rate of repolarization can be characterized by the quotient H_N/H_{max}, which is close to 0.5 in a normal receptor potential in physiological saline following an amplitude-saturating short light flash. Table 1 compares the effect of lowering Na^+, or raising Mg^{2+} concentration in a superfusate after previously lowering both Mg^{2+} and Ca^{2+} concentration, on PMP, H_{max} and H_N/H_{max}. This effect of Ca^{2+} on the repolarization rate of the receptor potential is obviously a different action of Ca^{2+}. It is not characterized by a Ca^{2+}/Na^+ antagonism and this Ca^{2+} action cannot even partially be fulfilled by Mg^{2+}. We have several indications that the repolarization rate of the receptor potential is strongly influenced by light adaptation (see e.g. Kramer, 1975). This however brings us to the third action of Ca^{2+} in the invertebrate photoreceptor.

(c) *Sensitivity control* (*adaptation*)

Lisman and J. E. Brown (1972, 1975*b*) showed that injection of Ca^{2+} into the *Limulus* ventral nerve photoreceptor cell mimics the effect of light adaptation to desensitize the receptor. Moreover, injection of the Ca^{2+}-buffer EGTA* into the cell results in opposing light adaptation. These workers proposed that a transient light-induced rise in intracellular Ca^{2+} concentration is the cause of the desensitization of the photo-

* ethyleneglycol -bis (β-amino-ethyl ether) -N,N′-tetra-acetic acid.

---

downward deflection of the upper (ΔA) curve (arsenazo-response) indicates an increase in intracellular concentration of free calcium ions. *Upper left*: Reference responses in physiological saline containing 10 mmol/l Ca^{2+}. The superfusion of the ventral nerve is switched to a low calcium (ca. 40 μmol/l) saline, and after 30 min back to physiological saline. Curves are *n* averaged responses as indicated, and the responses were recorded during the indicated time intervals.

In low external calcium the arsenazo response gradually disappears and the repolarization phase of the receptor potential is slowed down tremendously. The recovery in physiological saline (*right row*) takes a considerable time, but the decline of the receptor potential is accelerated immediately (20°C) (from Maaz and Stieve, 1980).

receptor in light adaptation (Lisman and J. E. Brown, 1972). J. E. Brown and Blinks (1974) demonstrated a transient light-induced Ca^{2+}-increase by injecting the Ca^{2+}-indicator aequorin into the *Limulus* photoreceptor cell. Later, J. E. Brown *et al.* (1977) and Maaz and Stieve (1980) showed similar results by the use of the intracellular injected Ca^{2+}-indicator arsenazo III. The light-induced increase in intracellular Ca^{2+} is delayed, compared to the light-induced change of the conductance of the cell membrane (Fig. 7).

Light adaptation develops more slowly than the light response (Lisman and J. E. Brown, 1975*a*). The decrease from transient to steady state of the electrical light response is interpreted as an expression of light adaptation. The increase in intracellular Ca^{2+} concentration roughly coincides with this decrease. However, during sustained illumination the electrical light response reaches a steady-state value which is often not accompanied by a stable intracellular Ca^{2+}-concentration but by a continuous decrease in Ca^{2+} concentration (J. E. Brown and Blinks, 1974; Maaz and Stieve, unpublished).

Hagins, Zonana and Adams (1962) and Hamdorf (1970) have shown that light adaptation by a small light spot in the squid retina and in the fly retinula is localized in the area of the photoreceptor cell which has been illuminated. Fein and Lisman (1975) and Fein and Charlton (1977*a* and 1977*b*) confirmed this finding in the *Limulus* ventral nerve photoreceptor and could show that micro-injection of Ca^{2+} into this photoreceptor has the same localized desensitizing effect as illumination by a light spot. The spread of free Ca^{2+} ions in the photoreceptor cytoplasm is obviously slow, and Ca^{2+} is sequestered intracellularly before it can diffuse over greater distances.

Injection of sodium into the *Limulus* ventral nerve photoreceptor cell also transiently desensitizes the cell (Lisman and J. E. Brown, 1972; Fein and Charlton, 1977*a*) in a somewhat different way. Presumably the sodium acts intracellularly mainly by causing an increase of intracellular Ca^{2+} concentration. How sodium brings about this effect is not yet fully understood.

Measurements of the increase in intracellular Ca^{2+} concentration, using arsenazo III (as in Fig. 7) indicate that the light-induced Ca^{2+}-increase does not coincide with the fast initial sodium ions influx of the light response. It may be that the delay between depolarization and intracellular Ca^{2+}-increase reflects the time needed for sodium to bring about the Ca^{2+} release into the cytoplasm.

In *Limulus* ventral nerve photoreceptor cell, a substantial part at least of the intracellular Ca^{2+}-increase following a light flash comes from extracellular sources (Maaz and Stieve, 1980, and Fig. 7). After lowering the extracellular calcium concentration to ca. 40 μmol/l, the light-induced arsenazo response becomes smaller than the limits of accuracy of the measurement; however this decrease is delayed by more than 10 min. This delay may mean that some time is needed to deplete the extracellular space close to the cell membrane sufficiently of calcium.

The recovery of the arsenazo response after return of the photoreceptor to a normal Ca^{2+}-environment takes even longer: more than 30 min. Fig. 7 also shows that the rate of

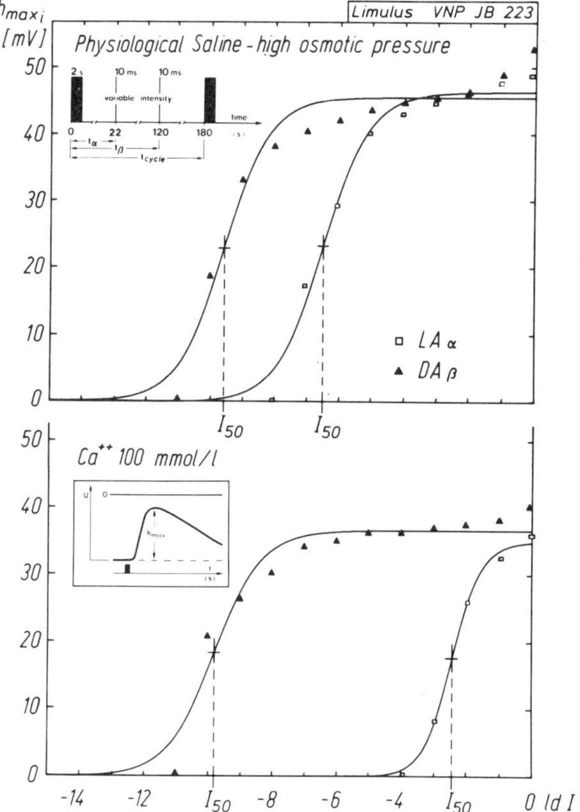

Figure 8 Response height *vs* stimulus intensity curves at 2 different states of adaptation of *Limulus* ventral nerve photoreceptor superfused by salines containing 10 mmol/l or 100 mmol/l Ca^{2+}. The inset in the upper curve describes the stimulus program which was repeated every 3 min. A strong constant light-adapting 2 s illumination (I_{LA} ca. 2×10^{16} 550 nm photons $cm^{-2} s^{-1}$) is followed by two 10 ms test stimuli of variable intensity in order to obtain two stimulus-response curves. The first test stimulus is to record the relatively light-adapted α curve, the second test stimulus for the dark-adapted β curve.

The response height h_{max} of the receptor potential (*inset lower curve*) is plotted *vs* the logarithm to base 2 (ld) of the intensity of the white light stimulus; I_o ca. 8×10^{16} 550 nm photons $cm^{-2} s^{-1}$. Upper curves in physiological saline containing 10 mmol/l Ca^{2+} and 270 mmol/l sucrose to adjust the osmotic pressure to be identical with that of the test saline. *Lower curves*: the ventral nerve is superfused by a saline containing 100 mmol/l Ca^{2+}; all the other ion concentrations identical to the reference saline (*upper curve*). The stimulus program (intensity and timing) is unchanged relative to upper curves. The drawn curves through the measured points are calculated by a computer program according to the equation of Naka and Rushton (1966) modified by Pak *et al.* (1973) (15°C).

repolarization of the receptor potential recovers much sooner than the arsenazo-response. This may indicate that the recorded arsenazo-response (a measure of intracellular Ca^{2+}-increase) is not responsible for the acceleration of the repolarization rate of the electrical light response.

Sodium could cause an increase in intracellular Ca^{2+} by causing a Ca^{2+}-release from intracellular sources such as vesicles, cisternae, mitochondria, pigment granules or calcium-binding proteins. In the visual cell of the crayfish *Astacus*, there are pigment granules acting as Ca-stores (Schröder *et al.*, 1980). In *Limulus* ventral nerve photoreceptor, however, no large intracellular Ca-stores could be found (Schröder, unpublished). Walz (1979) demonstrated that the endoplasmic reticulum of the photoreceptor of the leech can accumulate calcium while utilizing metabolic energy (ATP).

It seems conceivable (and would explain several experimental findings) that the rise in intracellular calcium may be due to a Ca^{2+}/Na^{+}-antiport across the cell membrane in which calcium is taken into the cell, in simultaneous exchange for extruded sodium; the energy for such a (possibly neutral) transport can be supplied from the ion gradients. Such a Ca^{2+}/Na^{+}-antiport was demonstrated—although in the opposite direction—in the squid axon membrane by Baker and Glitsch (1975). Calcium could also enter the cell during excitation via calcium permeable ion channels mentioned above.

Does calcium enter the photoreceptor cell only during the electrical light response, or is there a considerable exchange between extracellular and intracellular calcium in the dark when the external calcium concentration is varied? We have carried out a number of experiments which may cast light on this question.

Illumination causes a transient decrease in sensitivity (light adaptation) i.e. a constant light stimulus evokes a smaller light response. In *Limulus* ventral nerve photoreceptor we measured two response height *vs* stimulus intensity curves at two different delay times following a 2 s light-adapting illumination, each curve at a defined level of adaptation (Figs. 8 and 9): α in a (relatively) light-adapted state and β in a dark-adapted state.

Sensitivity can be characterized by the intensity I_{50} of the light stimulus evoking half saturation of the height of the intracellularly-measured receptor potential. I_{50} was determined for the α and β curves, while the photoreceptor was superfused either by reference saline, containing physiological ion concentrations including 10 mmol/l Ca^{2+}, or by test salines in which the Ca^{2+}-concentration was varied between 40 μmol/l and 100 mmol/l. Also, the Na^{+}-concentration was varied (Figs. 8 and 9, Table 2).

The sensitivity of the dark-adapted state does not depend significantly on the extracellular calcium concentration. However the extent of the sensitivity shift due to light adaptation measured as the difference between the β and the α-value of I_{50} is strongly reduced when the external Ca^{2+}-concentration is low and enlarged in raised external Ca^{2+}-concentration.

These results are consistent with the assumption that extracellular calcium enters the visual cell mainly during the electrical light response, causing a transient increase of the intracellular Ca^{2+}-concentration; this in turn is responsible for the measured transient decrease of sensitivity in light adaptation.

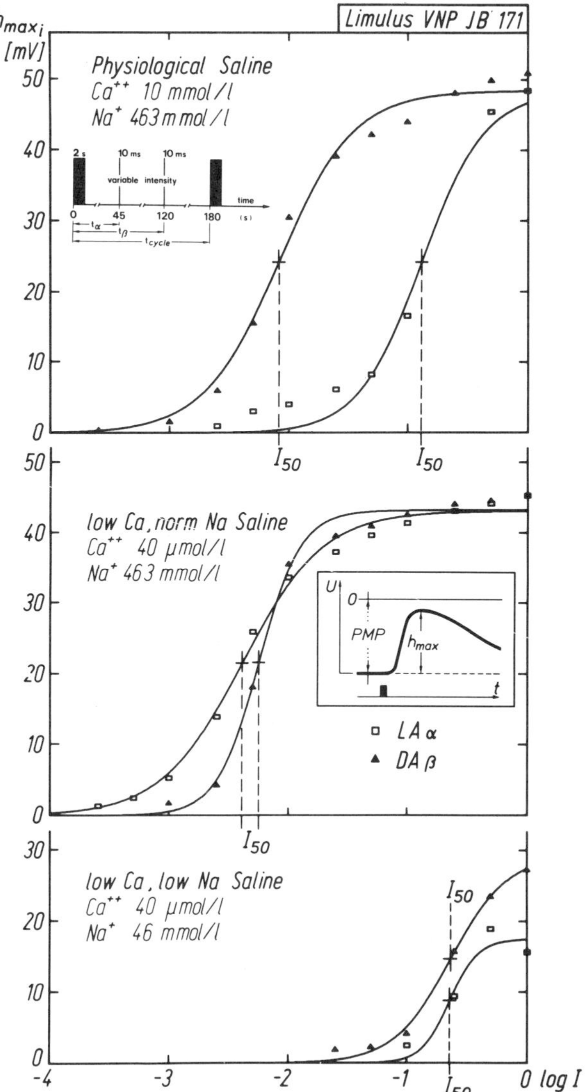

Figure 9 Response height *vs* stimulus intensity curves at 2 different states of adaptation of *Limulus* ventral nerve photoreceptors superfused by salines containing physiological (10 mmol/l) and low (ca. 40 μmol/l) calcium, and normal or low (10% of normal) sodium concentration. *Abscissa*: log (base 10) of light stimulus intensity (I_o ca. 10^{17} 550 nm photons $cm^{-2}\,s^{-1}$). *Upper curves*: reference curves recorded from the photoreceptor in physiological saline. After that the superfusion was switched to a low (40 μmol/l) Ca^{2+} saline (all the other ion concentrations unchanged) (*middle curves*) and then to a saline low in Ca^{2+} (40 μmol/l) and in Na^+ (10% of normal) (*lower curves*). Intensity of 2 s light-adapting illumination I_{LA} about 10^{17} 550 nm photons $cm^{-2}\,s^{-1}$. Remainder as in Fig. 8.

Table 2 Sensitivity of light- and dark-adapted *Limulus* ventral nerve photoreceptor superfused by salines containing various Ca^{2+} and Na^+ concentrations. Sensitivity determined as the stimulus intensity I_{50} evoking half saturation of receptor potential amplitude. Mean ± S.E., 15°C. I_0 ca. 8×10^{16} 550 nm photons $cm^{-2}\,s^{-1}$. In parentheses: number *n* of experiments. Whereas the sensitivity of the relatively dark-adapted photoreceptor does not depend significantly on external Ca^{2+} concentration, the sensitivity shift due to light adaptation is augmented in raised, and diminished in lowered, external Ca^{2+} concentration. Lowering Na^+ concentration decreases both the sensitivity of light- and of dark-adapted photoreceptor independent of Ca^{2+} concentration. The stimulus program is outlined in Figs. 8 and 9; the α values correspond to a relatively light-adapted, the β values to a fairly dark-adapted state of the photoreceptor (see Figs. 8 and 9).

$[Ca^{2+}]$	40 μmol/l	10 mmol/l	40 mmol/l	100 mmol/l	10 mmol/l	40 μmol/l
$[Na^+]$	463 mmol/l	485 mmol/l	485 mmol/l	440 mmol/l	48 mmol/l	46 mmol/l
$\alpha \frac{I_{50}}{I_0} \log I$	−2.3 ± 0.3	−1.5 ± 0.1	−1.3 ± 0.2	−0.5 ± 0.1	−0.5 ± 0.1	−1.1 ± 0.4
light-adapted	(*n* = 4)	(15)	(5)	(2)	(3)	(3)
$\beta \frac{I_{50}}{I_0} \log I$	−2.4 ± 0.2	−2.4 ± 0.1	−2.4 ± 0.2	−2.6 ± 0.1	−1.4 ± 0.1	−1.3 ± 0.4
dark-adapted	(4)	(15)	(5)	(2)	(3)	(3)

Lowering of external Na^+ concentration to 50 mmol/l causes an equal diminution both of the sensitivity of the dark-adapted and the light-adapted H–I-curve. This decrease in sensitivity induced by reduced sodium concentration occurs both in normal and in low external calcium concentration (Table 2). This desensitization caused by reduction in extracellular sodium is therefore different from that caused by raised extracellular calcium and there is no real Ca^{2+}/Na^+ antagonism in adaptation.

The observed effects are partially influenced by the fact that the time course of recovery of sensitivity (dark adaptation) depends upon the external calcium and sodium concentration. We have found in the crayfish retina (Stieve and Hanani, 1976) and in *Limulus* ventral nerve photoreceptor (Stieve and Bruns, unpublished) that dark adaptation following a light-adapting illumination is accelerated in salines low in calcium. Wulff *et al.* (1975) reported that dark adaptation in retinular cell of the *Limulus* lateral eye is slowed down considerably by superfusion with a saline which contains 10% of the normal sodium concentration. Fein and Charlton (1978) found that lowering the external sodium concentration to ca. 50 mmol/l (10%) greatly prolongs the time needed for the recovery of sensitivity (dark adaptation) of the *Limulus* ventral nerve photoreceptor, independent of whether lithium or choline was used as sodium substitute. Additional reduction of the external calcium concentration from 10 to 1 mmol/l reversed the effect of lowering sodium on dark adaptation.

It is a widely accepted hypothesis, first formulated by Dodge, Knight and Toyoda (1968) and called the "adapting bump model", that the electrical light response of the invertebrate photoreceptor is the sum of elementary excitatory events, called "bumps", which vary in size according to the state of adaptation. Bumps display a distribution in size (Fig.

11). Light adaptation causes a diminution of average bump size (Figs. 10 and 11). We have tested the calcium dependence of the bump light adaptation (Stieve and Bruns, 1980). If the external Ca^{2+}-concentration is raised, the bump size is increased in the dark-adapted state, but the bump diminution due to light adaptation by identical flashes is augmented (Fig. 11).

(d) *Quantum efficiency*

Additionally it is seen that the number of bumps evoked by the identical light stimuli is increased equally well by a moderate light adaptation as by

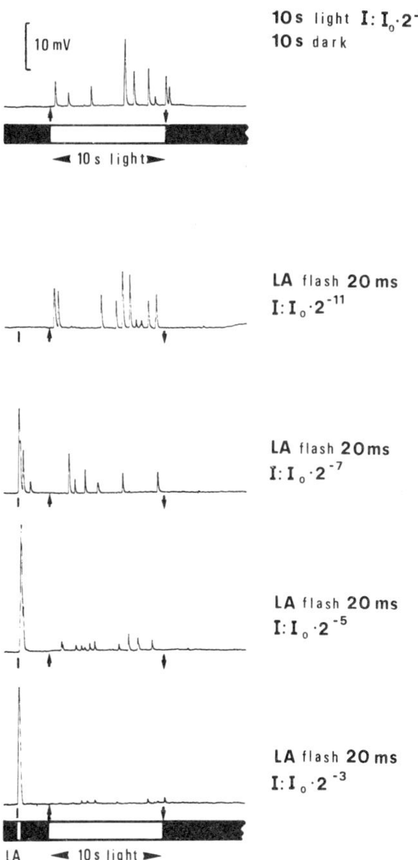

Figure 10 Bump registrations at different levels of light adaptation of a *Limulus* ventral nerve photoreceptor (pen trace of membrane voltage). The 10 s bump evoking stimulus is identical in all records whereas the intensity I_p of the preadapting flash varies from line to line as indicated. *Upper trace*: no preadapting flash. $I_0 = 3 \times 10^{13}$ 550 nm photons $cm^{-2} s^{-1}$. The ventral nerve was superfused by physiological saline at 15°C containing 10 mmol/l Ca^{2+}

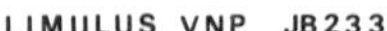

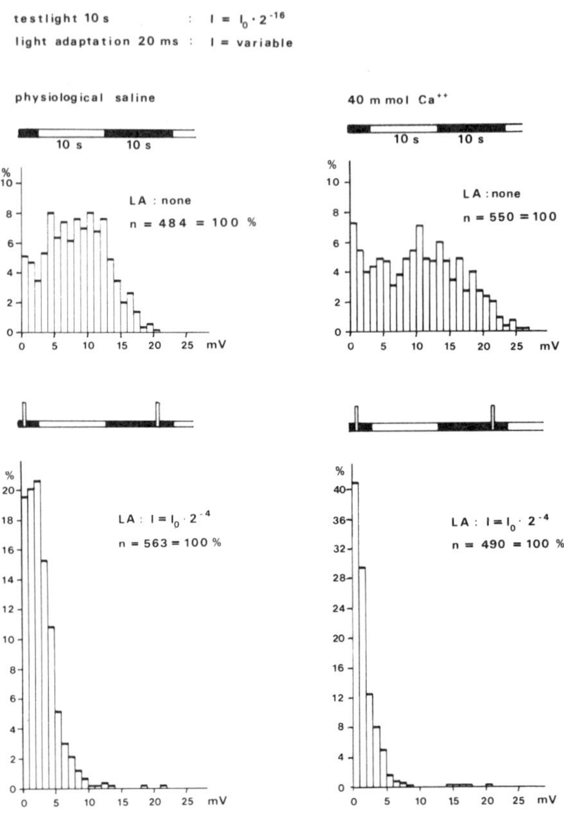

Figure 11 Frequency distribution of the amplitudes of the bumps recorded during illumination by the 10 s bump evoking stimuli at 2 different levels of adaptation and at 2 different external calcium concentrations (10 and 40 mmol/l), 15°C. In a saline with calcium concentration raised from 10 to 40 mmol/l, the average bump size in the dark-adapted state becomes larger and the diminution in bump size due to light adaptation by the same preadapting flash becomes more pronounced. Only the amplitudes of single (or first) bumps are plotted. About 15 % were multiple bumps (riding on top of others). Remainder as in Fig. 10.

raised extracellular Ca^{2+}-concentration (Table 3). This means that the quantum efficiency can be raised by light adaptation or by raised external Ca^{2+}-concentration. This may be the basis of facilitation, a phenomenon observed by Hanani and Hillman (1976), Fein and Charlton (1977*a*), and Stieve and Pflaum (1978*a*) where a weak conditioning illumination can raise the sensitivity of the *Limulus* or barnacle photoreceptor for a succeeding stimulus.

As can be seen in Fig. 12, bumps can be generated with a long delay following the light flash. They have latencies between 10 ms and more

Table 3 Bump frequencies at different levels of light adaptation and at two different external Ca^{2+} concentrations. Each bump frequency listed as mean ± S.E. per 20 s cycle recorded in 50 repetitions. Each cycle consists of a 10 s bump-evoking stimulus of constant light intensity $I_e = I_o \times 2^{-16}$; $I_o = 3 \times 10^{13}$ 550 nm photons $cm^{-2}\,s^{-1}$, followed by a 10 s dark period. The preadapting light flash, if applied, is provided 2 s before the bump which evokes illumination (i.e. at the start of the 19th second). I_p: intensity of preadapting flash. The corresponding number of bumps is listed in parentheses. Light bumps: bumps recorded during the 10 s of the bump evoking illumination. Dark bumps: bumps recorded in the dark during the 13th and 17th second of the cycle (i.e. over 5 s) 15°C, (see Fig. 10); from Stieve and Bruns, 1980).

preadapting light flash (I_p)	*bumps in*	*bump frequency* $(n + n_m)\,s^{-1}$ 10 mmol Ca^{2+}/l	40 mmol Ca^{2+}/l
—	light	1.05 ± 0.04 ($n + n_m = 527$)	1.33 ± 0.03 (666)
	dark	0.16 ± 0.03 (40)	0.40 ± 0.03 (99)
$I_o \times 2^{-12}$	light	1.41 ± 0.05 (700)	1.39 ± 0.04 (690)
	dark	0.15 ± 0.02 (37)	0.37 ± 0.03 (92)
$I_o \times 2^{-8}$	light	1.39 ± 0.04 (694)	1.36 ± 0.03 (681)
	dark	0.16 ± 0.03 (39)	0.34 ± 0.03 (85)
$I_o \times 2^{-4}$	light	1.34 ± 0.04 (668)	1.13 + 0.04 (565)
	dark	0.20 ± 0.02 (50)	0.44 ± 0.04 (111)

than 300 ms. The light-induced reaction converting rhodopsin to metarhodopsin is comparatively short (in *Limulus* ca. 5 ms, Fein and Cone, 1973; Lisman and Sheline, 1976). In the time between this light-induced rhodopsin reaction and the increase of the membrane conductance, unknown reactions, which finally cause the membrane conductance change, take place. Fig. 13 shows a hypothetical flow chart for the bump generation with the help of which the actions of calcium, described above, can be summarized:

(1) There seems to be no influence of calcium on the rhodopsin reactions (Wilms and Stieve, unpublished). The quantum efficiency of this reaction is assumed to be about 0.65–0.7, which is, according to Dartnall (1972), the value for vertebrate rhodopsin.

(2) The coupling factor *c*, coupling the rhodopsin reactions with the light-induced increase in membrane conductance is calcium-

dependent; *c* which may vary between 1 and smaller values is raised, probably by an increase in the intracellular Ca^{2+}-concentration.

(3) The delay responsible for the latency period is shortened by increased intracellular calcium concentration but probably in an indirect way.

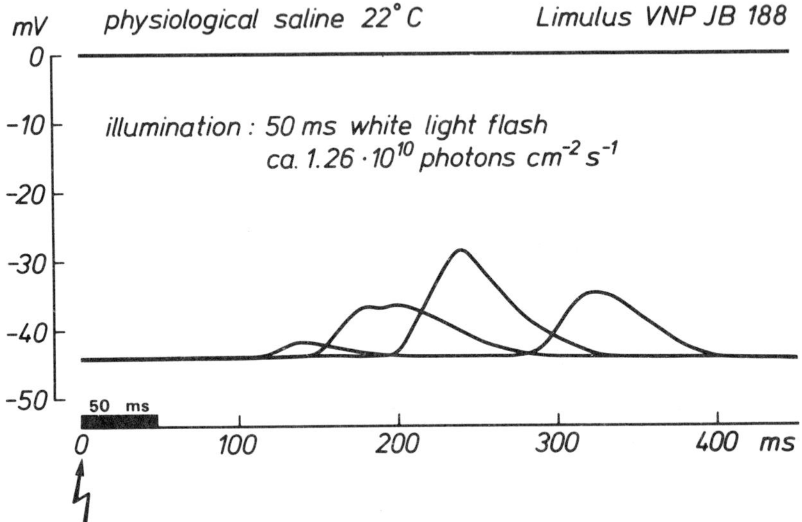

Figure 12 Light-induced bumps (slow potential fluctuations). *Limulus* ventral nerve photoreceptor.

(4) Dark-light adaptation is most probably brought about via the control of the amplification factor *a* by the intracellular Ca^{2+}-concentration. This amplification characterized by *a* causes—in the dark adapted state—many light-activated channels to be opened per bump, i.e. following a single successful photon absorption. The amplification factor *a* can be estimated, using the data of Brown and Coles (1979) and Wong (1978), to be ca. 10^3–10^4 light channels per bump in the dark-adapted state, and according to Wong (1978), about 1 light channel per bump in the strongly light-adapted state.

Although a major role of calcium in the adaptation mechanism of invertebrate photoreceptors has been well established, it is not yet clear whether in these photoreceptors calcium is the only agent controlling desensitization in light adaptation.

(5) The opening and closing of light-activated channels depends on an antagonistic action of Ca^{2+} and Na^+, via a Ca^{2+}/Na^+ binding competition to sites probably located at the extracellular surface of the cell membrane.

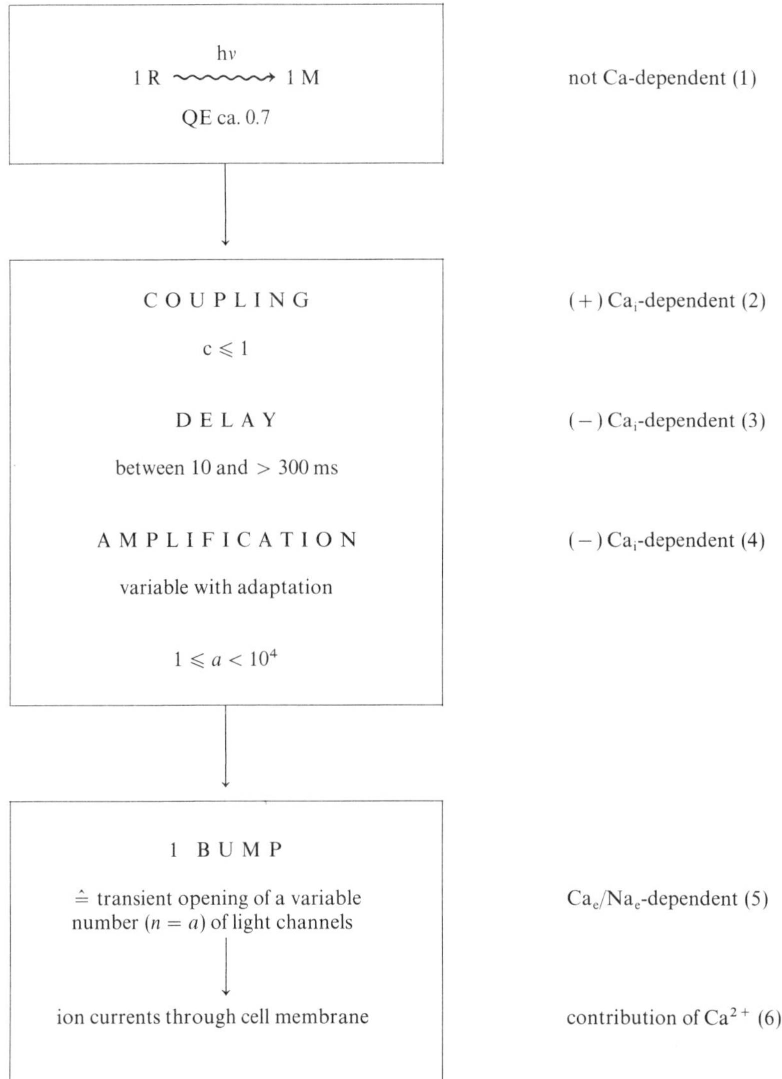

Figure 13 Flow chart of causal chain of events in visual excitation in invertebrates (see text). R—rhodopsin; M—metarhodopsin; Q.E.—quantum efficiency.

(6) Calcium ions can participate in membrane current, carrying positive charge into the cell.

Bumps occur also after the *Limulus* ventral nerve photoreceptor has been in the dark for a prolonged period (more than 1 hour). Several authors believe that these bumps are generated spontaneously, i.e. not evoked by photon absorption with an extremely long delay. If this is true, it may provide a clue to the understanding of vertebrate vision (Kramer and Widmann, 1977).

Acknowledgements

I wish to thank I. Claßen-Linke for critical reading and valuable suggestions, T. Malinowska for the reference list, and M. Bruns, A. Eckert and C. Nieveler for considerable technical help with the manuscript. This study was supported by the DFG (SFB 160).

REFERENCES

Baker, P. F. and Glitsch, H. G. (1975) Voltage-dependent changes in the permeability of nerve membranes to calcium and other divalent cations *Phil. Trans. R. Soc. Lond. B.*, **270** (908), 389–409.

Brown, H. M. (1976) Intracellular Na^+, K^+ and Cl^- activities in *Balanus* photoreceptors *J. Gen. Physiol.*, **68**, 281–296.

Brown, H. M., Hagiwara, S., Koike, H. and Meech, R. W. (1970) Membrane properties of a barnacle photoreceptor examined by the voltage-clamp technique *J. Physiol.*, **208**, 385–413.

Brown, H. M. and Ottoson, D. (1976) Dual role for potassium in *Balanus* photoreceptor: antagonist of calcium and suppression of light-induced current *J. Physiol.*, **257**, 355–378.

Brown, J. E. and Blinks, J. R. (1974) Changes in intracellular free calcium concentration during illumination of invertebrate photoreceptors *J. Gen. Physiol.*, **64**, 643–665.

Brown, J. E., Brown, P. K. and Pinto, L. H. (1977) Detection of light-induced changes of intracellular ionized calcium concentration in *Limulus* ventral photoreceptors using arsenazo III *J. Physiol.*, **267**, 299–320.

Brown, J. E. and Coles, J. A. (1979) Saturation of the response of light in *Limulus* ventral photoreceptor *J. Physiol.*, **296**, 373–392.

Clark, R. B. and Duncan, G. (1978) Two components of extracellularly recorded photoreceptor potentials in the cephalopod retina: differential effects of Na^+, K^+ and Ca^{2+} *Biophys. Struct. Mechanism*, **4**, 263–300.

Dodge, F. A., Knight, B. W. and Toyoda, J. (1968) Voltage noise in *Limulus* visual cells *Science*, **160**, 88–90.

Duncan, G. and Pynsent, P. B. (1979) An analysis of the wave forms of photoreceptor potentials in the retina of the cephalopod *Sepiola atlantica J. Physiol.*, **288**, 171–188.

Fein, A. and Charlton, J. S. (1977*a*) Enhancement and phototransduction in the ventral eye of *Limulus J. Gen. Physiol.*, **69**, 553–569.

Fein, A. and Charlton, J. S. (1977*b*) A quantitative comparison of the effects of intracellular calcium injection and light adaptation on the photoresponse of *Limulus* ventral photoreceptors *J. Gen. Physiol.*, **70**, 601–620.

Fein, A. and Charlton, J. S. (1978) A quantitative comparison of the time-course of sensitivity changes produced by Ca injection and light adaptation in *Limulus* ventral photoreceptors *Biophys. J.*, **22**, 105–113.

Fein, A. and Cone, R. A. (1973) *Limulus* rhodopsin: rapid return of transient intermediates to the thermally stable state *Science*, **182**, 495–497.

Fein, A. and Lisman, J. (1975) Localized desensitization of *Limulus* photoreceptors produced by light or intracellular calcium ion injection *Science*, **187**, 1094–1096.

Fioravanti, R. and Fuortes, M. G. F. (1972) Analysis of responses in visual cells of the leech *J. Physiol.*, **227**, 173–194.

Hagins, W. A., Zonana, H. V. and Adams, R. G. (1962) Local membrane current in the outer segments of squid photoreceptors *Nature*, **194**, 844–846.

Hamdorf, K. (1970) Korrelation zwischen Sehfarbstoffgehalt und Empfindlichkeit bei Photorezeptoren *Verh. Dtsch. Zool. Ges.*, 148–157.

Hamdorf, K. and Kirschfeld, K. (1980) Prebumps: evidence for double-hits at functional subunits in a rhabdomeric photoreceptor *Z. Naturforsch.*, **C 35**, 173–174.

Hanani, M. and Hillman, P. (1976) Adaptation and facilitation in the barnacle photoreceptor *J. Gen. Physiol.*, **67**, 235–250.

Hanani, M. and Shaw, C. (1977) A potassium contribution to the response of the barnacle photoreceptor *J. Physiol.*, **270**, 151–163.

Kramer, L. (1975) Interpretation of invertebrate photoreceptor potential in terms of a quantitative model *Biophys. Struct. Mechanism*, **1**, 239–257.

Kramer, L. and Widmann, T. (1977) Quantitative model for the electrical response of invertebrate and vertebrate photoreceptors *Biophys. Struct. Mechanism*, **2**, 333–336.

Lisman, J. E. and Brown, J. E. (1972) The effects of intracellular iontophoretic injection of calcium and sodium ions on the light response of *Limulus* ventral photoreceptors *J. Gen. Physiol.*, **59**, 701–719.

Lisman, J. E. and Sheline, Y. (1976) Analysis of the rhodopsin cycle in *Limulus* ventral photoreceptors using the early receptor potential *J. Gen. Physiol.*, **68**, 487–501.

Maaz, G. and Stieve, H. (1980) The correlation of the receptor potential with the light induced transient increase in intracellular calcium concentration measured by absorption change of Arsenazo III injected into *Limulus* ventral nerve photoreceptor cell *Biophys. Struct. Mechanism*, **6** (in press).

Meech, R. W. (1978) Calcium-dependent potassium activation in nervous tissues *Ann. Rev. Biophys. Bioenerg.*, **7**, 1–18.

Pepose, J. S. and Lisman, J. E. (1978) Voltage sensitive potassium channels in *Limulus* ventral photoreceptors *J. Gen. Physiol.*, **71**, 101–120.

Stieve, H. (1965) Interpretation of the generator potential in terms of ionic processes *Cold Spring Harbor Symp. Quant. Biol.*, XXX, 451–456.

Stieve, H. (1974) "On the ionic mechanisms responsible for the generation of the electrical response of light sensitive cells" in *Biochemistry of sensory functions* (ed. Jaenicke, L.) Springer-Verlag, Berlin-Heidelberg-New York, 79–105.

Stieve, H. and Bruns, M. (1978) Extracellular calcium, magnesium and sodium ion competition in the conductance control of the photosensory membrane of *Limulus* ventral nerve photoreceptor *Z. Naturforsch.*, **33c**, 574–579.

Stieve, H. and Bruns, M. (1980) Dependence of bump rate and bump size in *Limulus* ventral nerve photoreceptor on light adaptation and calcium concentration *Biophys. Struct. Mechanism*, **6** (in press).

Stieve, H. and Claßen-Linke, I. (1980) The effect of changed extracellular calcium and sodium concentration on the electroretinogram of the crayfish retina *Z. Naturforsch.*, **35c**, 308–318.

Stieve, H. and Hanani, M. (1976) Light and dark adaptation of crayfish visual cells depending on extracellular calcium concentration *Z. Naturforsch.*, **31c**, 324–327.

Stieve, H. and Pflaüm, M. (1978*a*) The response height versus stimulus intensity curve of the ventral nerve photoreceptor of *Limulus* depending on adaptation and external calcium concentration *Vision Res.*, **18**, 747–749.

Stieve, H. and Pflaum, M. (1978*b*) Lowering the ratio of extracellular calcium to sodium mimics the effect of light on the photosensory membrane of *Limulus* ventral nerve photoreceptor *Vision Res.*, **18**, 883–885.

Walz, B. (1979) Subcellular calcium localization and ATP-dependent Ca^{2+}-uptake by smooth endoplasmic reticulum in an invertebrate photoreceptor cell—ultrastructural, cytochemical and X-ray microanalytical study *Eur. J. Cell Biol.*, **20**, 83–91.

Weeks, F. I. and Duncan, G. (1974) Photoreception by a cephalopod retina: Response Dynamics *Exp. Eye Res.*, **19**, 493–509.

Wong, F. (1978) Nature of light induced conductance changes in ventral photoreceptors of *Limulus Nature*, **276**, 76–79.

Wulff, V. J., Stieve, H. and Fahy, J. L. (1975) Dark adaptation and sodium pump activity in *Limulus* lateral eye retinular cells *Vision Res.*, **15**, 759–765.

See additional references, page 216.

CHAPTER ELEVEN
MECHANISMS OF STIMULUS TRANSDUCTION IN CHEMORECEPTORS

C. J. DEN OTTER

Introduction

The transducer mechanisms underlying olfactory and gustatory reception are still poorly understood. The solution of the problem is hampered by the enormous variability in molecular structure of the chemical stimulants and an apparent large variability in the morphology of the receptors. Several theories have been proposed to explain how interactions between stimulant molecules and the organs of smell and taste may lead to generation of receptor potentials and, consequently, to action potential generation.

Morphology

The olfactory and gustatory cells in invertebrates and the olfactory cells in vertebrates are primary sensory cells with a distal dendrite and a proximal unmyelinated axon. Vertebrate taste cells, however, are secondary sensory cells, without axon, but with synaptic contacts with gustatory nerve fibres.

On close examination it appears that the basic scheme of organization of epithelial receptor cells is remarkably similar throughout the animal kingdom (Thurm, 1974). Independent of stimulus modality the receptor cells all possess a distal receptive segment connected to a proximal segment. The former usually contains neurotubules, often associated with ciliary structures, the latter characteristically has many mitochondria and vesicles. Between the proximal and distal segment, the cell forms a tight junctional complex with adjacent cells. This separates the intercellular fluid surrounding the proximal segment from the external medium bathing the distal segment. This may result in different ionic gradients across the proximal and distal membrane areas, and may also lead to a transjunction voltage gradient. A similar organization is found in the organs of smell and taste (Fig. 1, p. 196).

The initial chemosensory process includes selective filtering of ions and molecules from the environment. Before coming into contact with the olfactory or taste cell membranes, the substances must be adsorbed and then transported through structures shielding the receptor endings from the environment. The stimulus adsorbing and transporting structures may act as chemical filters restricting the set of stimuli and concentration ranges to which the receptors can respond. In insects, the lipophilic material covering the exo-skeleton and filling the pores in the olfactory hairs favours the adsorption and diffusion of lipophilic molecules (Hawke and Farley, 1970; Altner *et al.*, 1977). In contrast, the passage of these molecules will be hampered in the aqueous "receptor lymph" and "viscous substance" of insect chemosensory sensilla, and in the mucus separating the vertebrate olfactory and taste cells from the environment.

The chemical composition of the liquids bathing the receptive parts of vertebrate and invertebrate chemoreceptors is still poorly known. Mucopolysaccharides appear to be a common feature of these fluids (Scalzi, 1967; Moulins and Noirot, 1972; Bannister, 1974; Bernays *et al.*, 1975; Kaissling and Thorson, 1980). Polyanionic mucopolysaccharides have been reported in vertebrate and invertebrate olfactory receptors and in the "viscous substance" of insect taste hairs. These polyanions may be capable of binding molecules with polar groups. In addition they may provide an important store of inorganic cations usable in the electrical events associated with sensory transduction (Bannister, 1974). Finally, various enzymes have been demonstrated histochemically on the surface of olfactory and taste receptors, and these are thought to play a part in the receptor mechanism or to be involved in elimination of the stimulus molecules (Ottoson, 1963, 1971; Murray, 1971; Kasang and Kaissling, 1972; Bannister, 1974; Hansen, 1978).

It is unlikely however that the high specificity of olfactory and taste cells can be completely accounted for by the processes of adsorption and transportation (Beets, 1974). It has, for example, been found that the adsorption of odour molecules on the surface of insect olfactory hairs is a rather unspecific process (Kasang and Kaissling, 1972). Also, studies on binding of radioactive olfactory and gustatory stimulus molecules to membrane fractions from receptor-containing tissues support the role of the plasma membrane as the major location for selective filtering in olfaction and gustation (Cagan, 1977).

Electrophysiology

Generally, the primary effect of an appropriate stimulus on a receptor cell is a transient change in ion permeability (conductivity) of part of the apical sensory membrane. This leads to an ionic "receptor current", which evokes a "receptor potential", either by a local depolarization or hyperpolarization of the membrane.

The receptor potential is generally believed to spread electrotonically to more proximal parts of the receptor cell membrane. A depolarizing receptor potential ("generator potential") may lead to discharge of self-propagating action potentials provided the depolarization reaches a critical threshold level. Hyperpolarization, however, inhibits the production of nerve impulses and results in a decrease of the spontaneous impulse activity often present in unstimulated receptor cells. In primary sensory cells, receptor and action potential generation take place in the same cell, the latter process occurring in or near the cell body. In secondary sensory cells, the action potentials are initiated in the nerve cell that is in synaptic contact with the receptor cell. This may occur either directly in an electrical way, or by the release of a synaptic transmitter substance by the basal part of the receptor cells.

In this discussion, only the initial step transforming the external stimulus into the local receptor current is considered. This is based on a "changing permeability" model of the chemoreceptor membrane. For an understanding of the effects chemicals may have on a membrane, some knowledge of the latter's structure and composition is essential.

The plasma membrane

The frame of a plasma membrane is a bimolecular layer of phospholipids in which the molecules are perpendicular to the plane of the membrane. In many membranes cholesterol also occurs in the bilayer. Intercalated into the bilayer are integral (intrinsic) proteins, which may span its full width and thus be exposed on both sides of the membrane. These proteins cannot be removed without disrupting the structure. In addition, peripheral (extrinsic) proteins are found, which are bound at one or the other surface of the membrane. They can be dissociated from the membrane relatively easily. Finally, carbohydrates are invariably present on the outer surface of most cells.

The bilayer of biological membranes can be thought of as a two-dimensional viscous fluid at normal physiological temperatures (Singer and Nicolson, 1972). Lateral diffusion of molecules is possible in this fluid (Edidin, 1974). The molecular mobility in the membrane is lower when the lipid molecules are longer and more saturated, and also decreases at low temperatures and when higher proportions of cholesterol are present; these latter molecules obstruct the movements of neighbouring hydrocarbon chains by their large size and inertia (Booij and Bungenberg De Jong, 1956; Vandenheuvel, 1963; O'Brien, 1967). Moreover, interactions between the hydrophilic groups at the surface of the bilayer may affect the mobility of the molecules. The bilayer has a surplus of negative sites on its surface, which is not necessarily uniformly distributed, but may show local variations in density. At physiological pH, the phospholipid hydrophilic groups may either have a small (e.g., phosphatidyl ethanolamines) or a large (e.g., phosphatidic acids) net negative charge, or they may have electrostatically balanced, zwitterionic endgroups (e.g., lecithins and sphingomyelins) (Dawson, 1968). Dipole-dipole interactions between the zwitterions and the hydroxyl groups of sugar residues, and interactions between ions from the environment and the polar endgroups of the phospholipids may lead to a decrease in the mobility of the membrane molecules (Booij and Bungenberg De Jong, 1956).

Functionally, the lipid bilayer is commonly believed to be the major permeability barrier of the membrane to hydrophilic solutes. According to Booij (1963), however, the membrane lipid layer need not be completely impermeable to hydrophilic substances. Because of the thermal motion of the lipid hydrocarbon chains, the distance between these chains will vary, resulting in the presence of a continuously changing pattern of a few large pores and a large number of small pores ("statistical pores"). Studies on artificial membranes have indeed demonstrated that hydrocarbon chain mobility is an important parameter in the passive diffusion of hydrophilic substances across lipid bilayers, and that pores are not essential to explain water and ion movements across the membrane (Bangham *et al.*, 1965; Bittman and Blau, 1972; Papahadjopoulos *et al.*, 1973; Oschman *et al.*, 1974).

The proteins are involved in many membrane functions. They may be enzymes, catalysing various metabolic activities of the cell, and may also function as carrier molecules or provide pores, mediating transport of specific ions and small molecules across the membrane. The protein and carbohydrate groups at the exterior may play a part in cell interaction, and may bear antigenic determinants or specific receptor sites for chemicals (Singer, 1971; Ginsburg and Kobata, 1971; Keynes, 1979; Stevens, 1979).

One can conceive of a metabolically highly active membrane containing a higher proportion of protein to lipid than membranes having a predominantly isolating function (O'Brien, 1967; Quinn, 1977). The plasma membrane therefore varies in structure between different types of cells. It may even vary from region to region around a given cell depending on the functions associated with these regions.

Receptor sites

In olfaction and gustation, there is little information available on the particular biochemical groups in the receptor cell membrane which interact with the stimulants and control ion permeabilities. It has been proposed that the specific differential activation of olfactory and taste cells relies on the presence of different types of "receptor sites" (Beidler, 1954) or "acceptors" (Kaissling, 1969) in the receptor cell membrane. These would select ions and molecules by their shape, charge or even vibrations. A single membrane may contain several different receptor sites; and different receptor cells may have different ratios of receptor site types in their membranes (Wolbarsht, 1965; Beidler and Gross, 1971). The first step in the stimulation of the chemoreceptor cell could be the formation of a reversible complex between the stimulus molecules and specific sites. Complex formation may then result in a conformational change in the receptor site molecules, which is supposed to incite changes in membrane permeability to ions.

The results of studies on the structure-activity relationships (SAR) in chemoreception are often used to determine the properties of receptor sites. The aim of SAR studies is to correlate the molecular properties of chemicals with their odour or taste, with the assumption that a direct relationship exists between these two. In this way, it has been possible to identify the molecular attributes of various substances which produce a similar sensation in man or a similar behavioural response in animals. It is reasonable to infer that these structural features govern receptor site interaction and, hence, the mechanism of transduction.

SAR studies in olfaction of man (Amoore, 1952, 1962*a*, 1962*b*, 1965; Amoore *et al.*, 1964) suggested that receptor sites are rather inflexible sockets on the surface of some macromolecule into which specific molecules fit like a key into a lock (stereochemical theory of olfaction). These highly specific sites should be found in a limited number in the membrane of chemoreceptors only. Each site should represent a distinct "primary odour".

Assuming that primary odours are recognized much more frequently than mixed odours, Amoore initially postulated that there were seven "primaries" from which every known odour might be made by mixing them in certain proportions, and was able to give a detailed description of profiles and dimensions of the seven corresponding receptor site types by comparing the molecular models of the primary odours. Later (1967, 1969, 1970, 1977) Amoore identified the number of primary odours by studying the occurrence of specific anosmias. Each specific anosmia is thought to be due to the absence or loss of a specific type of receptor site. These investigations have raised the number of site types to at least 32 (Amoore, 1977).

Beets (1974, 1978) proposed a "generalized concept" of the receptor site, where sites are normal to all membranes. In his view, the sites are more flexible, having structural features which are—or have the potential to be—in some way complementary to those of the stimulus molecules. They can accommodate the latter in a reversible complex. The binding properties of a site may vary depending upon the physicochemical properties of the groups surrounding it, and involve not only steric, but also polar interactions. SAR studies remain a potential means of increasing our knowledge of the nature of the stimulus-receptor site interactions (see, e.g., Benz, 1976).

Wright (1976, 1977*a*, 1977*b*; see also Wright and Burgess, 1970, 1975), studying olfaction in man and insects, proposes the olfactory specificity is associated with specific low-frequency vibrational patterns of molecules. The different sites should be selectively "tuned" to a narrow band of frequencies. For a number of odours, he was able to establish a statistically significant correlation between the sensation they produce and their patterns of vibratory frequency, as revealed by far infrared spectroscopy. The difference between so-called odour "generalists" and "specialists", which have been described in several insect species (Boeckh *et al.*, 1965), is explained by assuming that the membranes of the former contain sites which are all tuned to the same frequency, whereas the latter would have different types of sites, each type tuned to different frequencies. A specialist cell, which is responsive only to a small group of related compounds, would respond most strongly to molecules matching the complete set of frequencies its sites are tuned to. A generalist cell would respond to almost any of a large number of compounds matching the oscillation to which its sites are tuned. It is not however quite clear how this mechanism can account for the differential responses of a generalist cell to different compounds.

The recent discovery of neurotransmitter and hormonal receptor proteins (Lester, 1977; Nathanson and Greengard, 1977; Keynes, 1979; Stevens, 1979) has led to the assumption that the receptor sites are structural features of membrane proteins. In addition, the large discriminatory abilities of olfactory and taste cells—which would require a wide diversity of receptor site types—are considered to indicate that the majority of the receptor sites are proteinaceous. This has also been suggested by the hereditary characters of a specific anosmia (Whissel-Buechy and Amoore, 1973) and a taste blindness (Kalmus, 1971). Furthermore, there is some support from electron microscopical investigations. Studies on the olfactory mucosa of mouse (Kerjaschki and Hörandner, 1976; Kerjaschki, 1977), cow (Menco *et al.*, 1976), and rat (Menco, 1977) show larger numbers of intramembranous particles (IMPs) in the olfactory cilia and knob membranes by comparison to respiratory cilia membranes. These IMPs are regarded as fragments of integral membrane proteins (Pinto Da Silva and Branton, 1970; Elgsaeter and Branton, 1974). Masson *et al.* (1977) found a positive correlation between the IMP density in frog olfactory cilia and the amplitude of the electro-olfactogram. On the other hand, it has been proposed that the lipid components of the chemoreceptor membrane are also capable of providing receptor sites (Davies, 1970, 1971; Dodd, 1971, 1974; Den Otter, 1972*a*, *b*, *c*; Kurihara *et al.*, 1972; Kurihara, 1974).

There have been attempts to study the properties of the receptor site substances directly. Proteins which form weak complexes *in vitro* with bitter and sweet-tasting compounds were extracted from bovine (Dastoli and Price, 1966; Dastoli *et al.*, 1968*b*), porcine (Dastoli *et al.*, 1968*a*), and rat tongues (Hiji *et al.*, 1968, 1969; Hiji and Sato, 1972). However, subsequent studies have failed to support the original claim that these proteins are taste receptor molecules (Price and DeSimone, 1977; Cagan and Morris, 1979). Hansen (1969) found a positive correlation between the distribution of α-glucosidases and the numbers of taste hairs on the legs and proboscis of insects. This led him to propose that the primary process of sugar reception in insects is the formation of a sugar–glucosidase complex. The presence of α-glucosidases at the tip of blowfly taste hairs has been demonstrated by Kijima *et al.* (1973). It is not clear which of more than ten glucosidases which have been found to date might act *in vivo* as the receptor protein (Hansen, 1978). Whether splitting of α-glucosidic linkages by the receptor protein is needed to control the permeability of the receptor membrane is also still unsolved (Hansen, 1974; Kijima and Morita, 1977).

Rozental and Norris (1973) and Singer *et al.* (1975) isolated a sulphur-rich protein from the antennae of *Periplaneta americana* to which naphthoquinones, which inhibit feeding in this cockroach, were selectively bound. It was concluded that sulphydryl groups form the major reaction sites in this insect's olfactory and gustatory receptors, and that these are blocked by these inhibitory substances. Spectroscopic analyses of the inhibitory effects of a sulphydryl reagent on protein from antennae of tobacco budworm moths (*Heliothis virescens*) led to the same conclusion (Frazier and Heitz, 1975). Riddiford (1970) was able to remove proteins from the antennae of saturniid moths by elution for half an hour with Ringer's solution and found the animals with washed antennae no longer responded behaviourally to olfactory stimuli for three or more hours after the treatment. However, Kaissling (1971) found no significant decrease in the electrophysiological response (electroantennogram amplitudes) of these antennae even after washing them for up to 12 hours.

A number of authors have modified proteins in the olfactory and gustatory organs with chemical reagents, and studied the effects of this treatment on the behavioural or sensory responses of the organism. The results of these studies have lent support to the view that sulphydryl groups are involved in taste and olfaction in various insects (Koyama and Kurihara, 1971; Norris *et al.*, 1971; Shimada *et al.*, 1972; Norris and Chu, 1974; Villet, 1974; Frazier and Heitz, 1975; Ma, 1977; Norris, 1977), frog (Getchell and Gesteland, 1972), carp (Hidaka, 1970), rat (Beidler, 1975), and man (Henkin and Bradley, 1969). Several experiments, however, indicated that the SH-groups are not involved in the primary selective process in vertebrate taste cells. Administration of SH-group blocking agents in rat and carp inhibited stimulation by NaCl, sucrose, and HCl non-selectively, suggesting that the inactivation occurs at a secondary event which is common to the transduction of the responses for all three stimuli (Henkin and Bradley, 1969; Hidaka, 1970; Mooser, 1976; Mooser and Lambuth, 1977).

Spectroscopic studies on rabbit olfactory epithelium have indicated that interactions occur between linalool and related odorants and proteins, triggering changes in protein conformation (Ash, 1968, 1969). Similarly, Dodd (1971) has found evidence that butyric acid and some other odorants induce localized structural changes in lipids of rabbit olfactory cell membranes.

Models of chemoreceptive transduction

Conceptual models

One of the methods used to elucidate possible mechanisms of chemo-electrical transduction is to construct quantitative models of the interactions between stimulus and receptor sites. Here, the exact nature of the chemical structure of the sites is not considered in any detail.

Beidler (1954, 1971) has published a theory of salt stimulation based on classical enzyme-substrate kinetics, which was supported by his own quantitative data of the integrated response in the chorda tympani nerve of the rat. Quantitative models of the transductive process in insects have been developed by Kaissling (1969, 1971, 1974, 1975*a*, 1975*b*, 1976, 1977) and Morita (1969) for olfactory and taste receptors, respectively.

It is assumed that binding of the stimulus with the receptor site may lead to "activation" of the site, i.e., to a change in its conformation. This altered conformation may induce a local increase in membrane conductance and, hence, a generator potential. The size of the generator potential is supposed to be determined by (1) the affinity of the stimulus to the receptor molecules, according to the mass action law, (2) the ability to form an active stimulus-receptor site complex, (3) the increase of membrane conductance per activated complex, and (4) the velocity of the process of "inactivation" of the stimulus molecules (Kaissling, 1974).

These models all lead to a hyperbolic relationship between response amplitude and stimulus strength. Although some receptor cells show this relationship (e.g., salt, sucrose, and acid receptors in rats: Beidler, 1961, 1971; sex pheromone receptors in male *Bombyx mori* stimulated with some bombykol analogues: Kaissling, 1974, 1975*b*), others show a flatter curve (e.g., blowfly salt receptor cells: Den Otter, 1972*b*; sex pheromone receptors in male *Bombyx mori* stimulated with bombykol: Kaissling,

1974, 1975*b*; sex pheromone receptors in the summer fruit tortrix moth (*Adoxophyes orana*) stimulated with female sex pheromone components: Den Otter, 1977). Obviously, these kinetic models are still not completely adequate.

Molecular models

A second method of elucidating transduction mechanisms is to draw upon the properties of possible membrane constituents. Despite the volume of data accumulated to date only a few molecular models have emerged.

(*a*) *The carotenoid pigment model of olfaction*

Rosenberg *et al.* (1968) have investigated the effects of the adsorption of various odorous gases on the electrical properties of all-*trans*-*β*-carotene crystallites. This was intended to test the suggestion of Briggs and Duncan (1961, 1962) that carotenoids—which had been shown to be present in the olfactory region of cattle—are implicated in the primary mechanism of vertebrate olfactory transduction. It appeared that many vapours increased the semiconduction current of these crystals, the current increasing with concentration. Some vapours could increase the current by up to 10^7 times as much as an inert gas (argon, helium). The effects were completely reversible by dissipation of the odours. It was proposed that a weak-bond complex occurs, which would produce an increase in the number of charge carriers (Misra *et al.*, 1968). Strong odours evoked the largest current increase in *β*-carotene, with the exception of methyl and ethyl acetate. It turned out, however, that these esters elicited a large current increase in crystalline powder of vitamin A alcohol. The authors therefore concluded that different carotenoids function as different receptor site types. However, it is still not clearly demonstrated that the receptor cells contain the pigment and that carotenoids occur in the olfactory epithelium of all vertebrate groups (Moulton, 1962, 1971; Moulton and Beidler, 1967). In addition, some anomalous results still need clarification. For example, the weakly odorous short chain-length alcohols gave larger current increases than the longer-chain alcohols (Moulton, 1971).

(*b*) *The penetration and puncturing model of olfaction*

Davies (1970, 1971) proposed that stimulus molecules penetrate the membrane leaving punctures through which ions can pass. The increased ion fluxes should partially short-circuit the membrane resting potential, causing a generator potential.

Most odoriferous molecules are lipophilic and consequently, Davies suggested, these punctured the lipid part of the membrane. The hydrophilic substances having a strong odour, such as ammonia, hydrogen disulphide or sulphur dioxide, were supposed to interfere with the proteinaceous parts of the membrane, probably poisoning the sodium pumps, which would also have a membrane depolarizing effect.

Large, awkward-shaped and rather rigid odour molecules would be the most effective, a few molecules (or perhaps even one) being sufficient to disturb the structure of certain membranes. Smaller molecules would be less powerful odorants because they need to penetrate the membrane in larger numbers, side by side, before stimulation occurs. Differences in shape, size and rigidity could account for the large differences in sensitivity to molecules which are only slightly different in solubility and chemical properties. It is suggested (see discussion in Davies, 1970) that molecules which have passed through the membrane may return to the atmosphere when stimulus concentration decreases again. Obviously, this would again result in holes in the membrane through which ions may move. This may explain post-stimulation hyperpolarization or depolarization. The molecules, however, which have by then diffused into the cell interior may become complexed with proteins.

Davies (1970, 1971) proposed that odour quality is dependent on both the diffusion rate of the odour molecules through the membrane and the rate of "healing" of the lipid bilayer. Large, strongly adsorbed molecules will diffuse relatively slowly through the membrane. When the healing time is short, the membrane would heal as the odour molecules move through, i.e., the latter would not leave a channel through which ionic flow might occur. If, however, the rate of diffusion of molecules through the membrane is high relative to the latter's time of healing, a hole will remain open. The membrane's time of healing and its resistance to penetration by molecules will be dependent upon the fluidity of the lipid bilayer. The more fluid the membrane, the more easily it can be penetrated and the more rapidly a puncture will heal. As different olfactory membranes may have differing lipid compositions, identical molecules will stimulate some cells more strongly than others. Large molecules will hardly, or not, stimulate the cells with rapidly healing, fluid membranes, whereas small molecules are too weakly adsorbed to penetrate the large molecule-sensitive, slow-healing membranes. It is supposed that distinct groups of cells with identical membranes do not exist, but that there will be a more or less continuous distribution of membranes ranging from very fluid to semi-solid. Consequently, the different odour qualities would be a continuum, rather than being demarcated into "primaries".

Davies (1970, 1971) related the intensity of muskiness of different substances to the desorption rates of molecules (from a lipid monolayer-covered water surface into the air above) and found a parabolic relationship. He developed a theory predicting this parabolic relationship, and estimated the coefficients of the parabola with a curve-fitting procedure. It turned out, however, that this theory sometimes predicted muskiness for substances having non-musk odours. Therefore, desorption rate was expected to be a significant, but not exclusive factor in predicting intensity

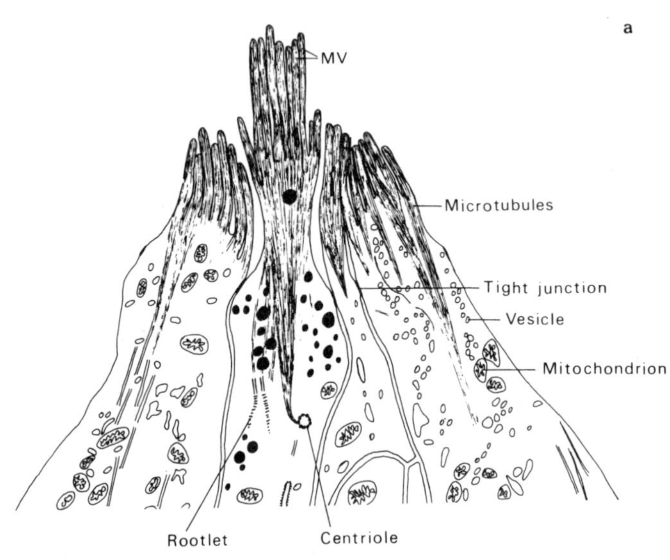

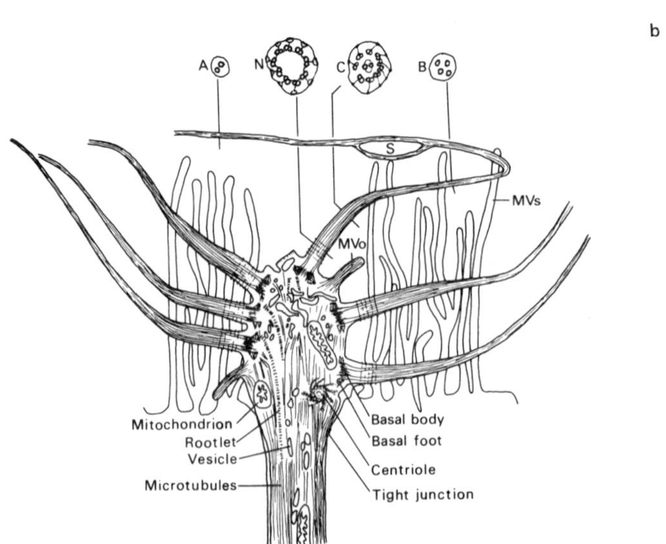

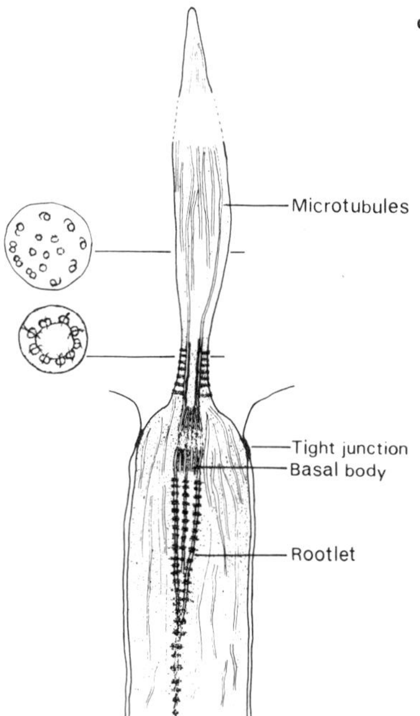

Figure 1 (a) Schematic drawing of apical cell portions of vertebrate taste cells (adapted and redrawn from Murray, 1973). A type of cell containing dark granules and having relatively long microvilli (MV) is flanked by cells whose cytoplasm is more vesicular. The microvilli and the neck region, which connects the microvilli with the proximal cell body, are filled with longitudinally orientated tubules, which are in relation to centrioles in the upper part of the cell.

Figure 1 (b) Schematic drawing of apical portion of a vertebrate olfactory cell surrounded by microvilli (MVs) of supporting cells (adapted and redrawn from Andres, 1969). The olfactory knob bears microvilli (MVo) and modified cilia. The proximal part of the cilia contains a $9 \times 2 + 2$ arrangement of microtubules (C). Just above the base a "necklace" of several rows of membrane particles is present on the ciliary shaft, which is related to linkage with the outer doublet structures (N) (Gilula and Satir, 1972). In the tapering distal ciliary segment the tubuli gradually diminish in number (B, A). The cilia have several spindle-shaped swellings (S).

Figure 1 (c) Schematic drawing of apical part of an insect chemoreceptor cell (adapted and redrawn from Gaffal and Bassemir, 1974). The thinner part connecting the proximal and distal dendrite segments contains a $9 \times 2 + 0$ arrangement of microtubules, which originate from basal bodies in the proximal segment. At the base of the distal segment, the B-tubules open and in the centre tubules appear which are not connected with basal bodies. The tapering distal segment passes up into a hair-shaped sensillum and may or may not be branched. The lumen of the hair is filled with an aqueous extracellular "receptor lymph". The wall of an olfactory hair is punctured by many minute pores filled with lipophilic material. A taste hair has only one or a few apical pores, in which an aqueous "viscous substance" is present (Stürckow, 1967; Steinbrecht, 1969).

of muskiness. This led Davies to introduce a second, geometrical facto., *viz.*, the size of the odorous molecule and the balance between its non-polar and polar portions. This factor is thought to cause a change in fluidity of the surrounding membrane into which the molecule has penetrated. Large molecules might reduce the fluidity by their size, inertia and shape; more flexible molecules might increase the membrane's fluidity. Taking the influence of the geometrical factor into account, Davies was able to construct an odour quality "map", i.e., a correlation of odour quality with cross-sectional areas of molecules (as a first approximation he neglected the ratio of non-polar to polar material in the molecule) and with free energies of desorption of the molecules from the lipid-water interface into the air. In the map various areas could be indicated which should uniquely denote the quality of the odour in physico-chemical terms.

(*c*) *The mechano-chemical model of taste stimulation*

Gross (see Beidler and Gross, 1971) has suggested that interactions take place between the stimulus molecules and macromolecular, proteinaceous sites spanning the full width of the membrane. Since a taste cell is excited by potassium salts at concentrations which would completely depolarize a nerve cell, Gross assumed that the part of the taste cell membrane outside the tight junctions with neighbouring cells (see Fig. 1) is impermeable to ions. Two types of sites, functionally and spatially separated, may be present:

(1) *receptors*, responding to chemicals in the environment, which are located mainly outside the junctions;

(2) *effectors*, which change ionic permeabilities, and which are located proximal to the junctions.

The primary reaction of the receptors to chemical changes in the environment is thought to be a general shrinkage of their molecular volumes, after diffusion of stimulating ions or molecules into the receptor matrix. The molecular residue density as well as the types of residues making up the receptor would determine which ions or molecules can diffuse into the matrix, and what kind of interaction between stimulus and receptor will result in an adequate shrinkage response. Hence, specificity of the receptor depends on its detailed structure.

Sugar molecules and bitter substances are assumed to affect the matrix of their receptors firstly by reducing the water activity, thereby causing the protein to lose water, which results in shrinkage of the matrix. Secondly, these compounds may form hydrogen bond cross-links between chain segments within the receptor, which also cause shrinkage of the protein. Salts and acids can modify the electrostatic field of the receptor structure as well as decrease its water content. Reduction of the repulsive field between fixed charges in the receptor will induce shrinkage of the protein.

Gross proposed that shrinkage of receptors may cause swelling or dilation of neighbouring membrane structures. A general shrinkage of receptors outside the tight junctions may allow the expansion of effectors proximal to the junctions. Coupling between these two sites may be accomplished by the membrane lipids. The expansion of effectors would permit ions to flow across the membrane causing a generator potential.

(*d*) *The ion antagonism model of salt stimulation*

Divalent cations and membrane permeability

Den Otter (1972*a*, *b*, *c*) has developed a theory based on studies of biocolloid systems, particularly on association colloids formed by amphipatic lipid molecules, i.e. lipid molecules consisting of a non-polar, hydrophobic part and a polar, hydrophilic end group (see Bungenberg De Jong, 1949; Booij and Bungenberg De Jong, 1956).

In an aqueous solution, the hydrophobic carbon chains of lipid molecules will tend to "flee" from the water. They will aggregate into micelles in which the charged groups are directed outwards, toward the aqueous phase. The shape of the micelles may vary considerably, from globular to large flat micelles having a bilayer "sandwich" structure. Globular micelles may change to sandwich micelles after adding ions which bind to the charged groups and diminish the repulsive forces between them. The membrane lipid bilayer is considered to be a phospholipid sandwich micelle, although gangliosides, containing sialic acid moieties, and cerebroside sulphate may occur to a lesser extent.

Investigations on many cell types have revealed that divalent cations, and particularly Ca^{2+}, are involved in regulating the permeability of plasma membranes. The calcium ions are supposed to hold the membrane molecules together by forming bridges between adjacent anionic sites, and by forming coordination complexes with several negative ligands (Danielli, 1958; Davson, 1962; Kavanau, 1965; Joos and Carr, 1967; Dawson, 1968). Den Otter (1972*b*) proposed that the calcium ions are bound to the membrane molecules according to the equilibrium

$$Ca^{2+} + A^{2-} \rightleftarrows CaA \tag{1}$$

On addition of calcium ions to the medium the number of anionic groups closely cross-linked by calcium will increase (equilibrium (1) shifts to the right). As a consequence, the compactness of the membrane will increase and its permeability decrease. Removing calcium ions frees more negative groups. These groups will be forced apart by electrostatic repulsion, which leads to a less compact packing of the molecules and to increased membrane permeability.

Differential effects of alkali and alkaline earth cations

Den Otter (1972*a*, *b*) stimulated taste hairs of blowflies (*Calliphora vicina*) with different alkali chlorides and found that the order of increasing stimulating effectiveness of the cations was irregular with respect to their atomic numbers. For so-called "salt cells" the order was $Li < Na \leqslant Cs < Rb < K$. This indicated that the stimulatory effect of the alkali cations cannot merely be a function of their atomic weight or ion volume and, hence, their ionic mobility, as was suggested from behavioural studies.

An irregular sequence of increasing stimulatory effect of alkali cations had also been found by Gillary (1966*a*, *c*) for taste hairs of the fly *Phormia regina* ($Li < Cs < Rb \leqslant Na < K$), and by Kusana and Yamashita (see Yamashita, 1963) for taste cells in the tongue of the frog *Rana nigromaculata* ($Li < Na < Cs < K$). Moreover, in *Phormia regina*, Rees and Hori (1968) found an irregular sequence of increasing hyperpolarizing effect of alkaline earth cations ($Ba < Mg < Sr < Ca$). A closer examination of the literature revealed that in many biological processes similar irregular sequences of alkali and alkaline earth cations occur (*cf.* Den Otter, 1972*a*).

Bungenberg De Jong (1949) determined the concentration (*Cn*) of various inorganic and organic cations which exactly neutralized the charge of different acidic biocolloids. It appeared that the "ion spectrum", i.e. the rank order of increasing *Cn* of the various ions, differed between the different biocolloids. For the alkali cations, the sequence $K < Na < Li$ of increasing *Cn* was found for carboxyl and sulphate colloids, whereas for phosphate colloids the reverse sequence $Li < Na < K$ was obtained. In addition, comparison of the neutralizing effects of all alkali cations (Li, Na, K, Rb, Cs) and the alkaline earth cations (Mg, Ca, Sr, Ba) yielded regular sequences of increasing *Cn* for carboxyl and sulphate colloids, whereas for phosphate colloids "transition sequences" were found, where the sequence of ions does not correspond to their atomic numbers. These transition series are thought to result because phosphate groups are more polarizable than water. The polarizability of ionized groups may also change depending on the nature of adjacent groups, and this can lead to different transition series for different phosphate colloids, depending on the latter's exact composition.

It was concluded (Den Otter, 1972*a*, *b*) that the irregular sequence of stimulatory effect of the alkali cations indicates binding of the cations to phosphate groups in the taste cell membrane. This was also supported by the fact that the responses of salt-sensitive cells in blowflies are not affected by pH over a range from about 3 to 10 (Evans and Mellon, 1962*b*; Gillary, 1966*a*, *b*), which excludes the relatively weakly acidic carboxyl groups of the membrane proteins (Bungenberg De Jong, 1942; Beidler, 1954).

The order of increasing stimulatory effect of the alkali cations is similar to that of the decreasing affinity of these ions to phosphate groups. It thus seems that the increase in taste cell membrane permeability is inversely correlated to the number of cations bound. The salt cells, however, respond more strongly when the salt concentration is increased. Direct binding of alkali cations to phosphate groups therefore cannot be the only process determining the changes in membrane permeability. Den Otter (1972*b*) concluded that antagonism between the calcium ions in the membrane and the stimulating salt ions may play an important part in the stimulation process.

Ion antagonism

For phosphate biocolloids, Bungenberg De Jong *et al.* (1936) determined *Cn* for $CaCl_2$ in the presence of NaCl. They found that more $CaCl_2$ is needed to discharge the colloids when NaCl is added; NaCl thus antagonizes the action of $CaCl_2$. On increasing the NaCl concentration, the *Cn* of $CaCl_2$ reaches a maximum, then decreases, and finally—when the NaCl concentration chosen equals the *Cn* of NaCl itself—becomes

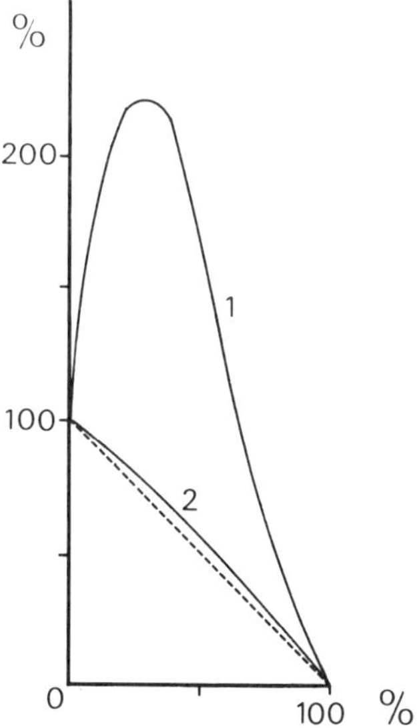

Figure 2 Neutralization of charge of alcohol soluble soya bean phosphatide with mixtures of $CaCl_2$ and NaCl (curve 1), and LiCl and NaCl (curve 2) (adapted and redrawn from Bungenberg De Jong *et al.*, 1936). Abscissa: NaCl concentrations in the salt mixture expressed as percentages of the concentration of neutralization of NaCl in the absence of another salt. Ordinate: Concentrations of $CaCl_2$ or LiCl in the salt mixture expressed as percentages of the concentrations of neutralization of these salts in the absence of NaCl. Only slight deviations from additivity (broken straight line) occur in the combination LiCl + NaCl.

zero. When, however, mixtures of LiCl and NaCl are chosen, only slight deviations from additivity are seen. Then, no antagonism proper occurs, for in the presence of NaCl the *Cn* for LiCl never exceeds the *Cn* value found when only LiCl is present. This is illustrated in Fig. 2, which shows the neutralization of alcohol soluble soya bean phosphatide with mixtures of $CaCl_2$ + NaCl and LiCl + NaCl.

The magnitude of the deviation from additivity depends on the relative positions of the cations in the ion spectrum. Antagonism of salts only occurs when the individual *Cn* values of the cations differ by at least a factor of 10. The phosphate colloids are the only biocolloids in which antagonism can be expected between alkali and alkaline earth salts.

Electrostatic interactions between anions and cations play an important part in antagonism. In solutions of $CaCl_2$ and NaCl, Cl^- ions will surround and thus screen Ca^{2+} ions, which will diminish the activity coefficient of the latter. The more NaCl is present, the more Cl^- ions will interfere with the Ca^{2+} ions, so that higher $CaCl_2$ concentrations are needed to bind the same amount of Ca^{2+} ions to the colloid. However, fixation of Na^+ ions to the polar groups of the colloid gradually becomes increasingly important, reducing the amount of Ca^{2+} ions needed to discharge the colloid. The antagonism curve ends at the *Cn* of NaCl.

The proposition is (Den Otter, 1972*b*) that on stimulation of taste cells with alkali chlorides, equilibrium (1) will shift to the left as a consequence of screening of calcium ions by added chlorine ions. This leads to opening of the membrane, which will partly be counteracted however, by binding of alkali cations to phosphate groups. The net result of this process will be an increase in membrane permeability. The higher the affinity of the alkali cations for the phosphate groups, the smaller the ultimate increase will be. Hence, the sequence of increasing stimulatory effect of the alkali cations is the same as their sequence of increasing *Cn* for phosphatides.

This theory can account for the effects of different concentrations of different alkali salts on an individual taste cell as well as for the responses of different taste cells to different concentrations of one and the same alkali salt (Fig. 3).

Responses to different alkali salts

In Fig. 3, the curves 1 to 5 illustrate the "opening" effect of different concentrations of the alkali salts 1 to 5 on a single cell membrane. Curve 1 shows the response to a potassium and curve 5 that to a lithium salt.

It appears that at lower concentrations the responses all follow the ascending branch of these curves. However, at higher concentrations the response will decline, and the higher the affinity of the cation for the phosphate group, the earlier the onset. Indeed, Gillary (1966*a*, *c*) found, when plotting response versus log molarity, that the onset of response

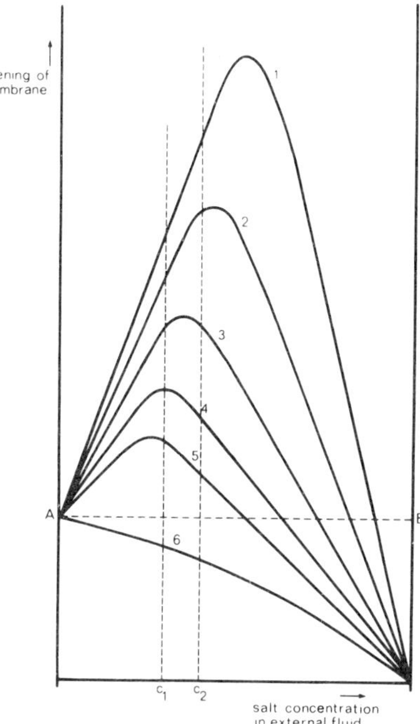

Figure 3 Opening of taste cell membranes (ordinate) as a function of the salt concentration in the external fluid (abscissa) (from Den Otter, 1972*b*). Point A represents the packing of membrane molecules in unstimulated cells. Above level AB, the membranes are less compact than in the unstimulated condition and, thus, more permeable. Below level AB, the compactness of the membranes will be increased, and their permeability decreased. The figure illustrates either (1) the opening of a membrane of an individual taste cell by different concentrations of different alkali salts (salts 1 to 5), or (2) the opening of different cell membranes (membranes 1 to 5) by different concentrations of one and the same alkali salt. Curve 6 illustrates the condensation of a membrane when treated with, e.g., alkaline earth salts or quinine hydrochloride.

decline agreed with the sequence of increasing stimulatory effect of alkali cations (Li < Cs < Rb ⩽ Na < K). A decrease in response at higher salt concentrations was also observed in salt cells of rat, cat, frog, and man (Tateda and Beidler, 1964; Pfaffmann, 1965; Borg *et al.*, 1970). Den Otter and Van Der Poel (1965) found that the stimulatory effect of ammonium salts was of about the same order of magnitude as that of potassium salts. As the ammonium cation resembles the potassium ion as regards its place in cation spectra for phosphate colloids, this is expected (Bungenberg De Jong *et al.*, 1940).

Salts with cations having *Cn* values not exceeding the *Cn* of calcium ions by more than tenfold will tighten the membrane over their entire concentration range (curve 6 in Fig. 3). This accounts for the hyper-polarizing effect of alkaline earth cations on blowfly taste cells (Rees and

Hori, 1968). Bungenberg De Jong (1949) has established that the (monovalent) cations of quinine hydrochloride have a far higher affinity for phosphate groups than the calcium ions. Hence, it is quite conceivable that quinine hydrochloride also hyperpolarizes taste cell membranes in blowflies (Morita, 1959, 1963; Morita and Yamashita, 1959), and produces a decrease in membrane conductance in taste cells of rat and frog (Ozeki, 1971; Akaike *et al.*, 1976; Akaike and Sato, 1976).

Responses of different cells

In Fig. 3 curves 1 to 5 can also be considered to illustrate the opening effect of one salt on five different cell membranes. *A* (Fig. 3) is the degree of opening of the membranes in unstimulated condition. Bungenberg De Jong *et al.* (1940) found that the antagonistic effect is smaller with phosphatides having a higher density of negative charge. Curves 1 and 5 may be considered as membranes having phospholipids with low and high density of negative charge, respectively; curves 2, 3, and 4 would be membranes with intermediate charge densities. When changing the alkali salt concentration from c_1 to c_2, the permeability of membranes 1 and 2 will increase, and that of membranes 4 and 5 decrease, whereas that of membrane 3 will remain unchanged.

Types of cells responding positively, negatively or not at all to an increase in alkali salt concentration have all been found in taste hairs of blowflies (Den Otter, 1971). The blowfly's classical "water cell", which is inhibited by inorganic salts as a direct function of the latter's concentration (Evans and Mellon, 1962*a*; Dethier, 1963), obviously has a high density of negative charge at the membrane surface (curves 4 and 5).

(e) The water/lipid distribution model of chemoreception

The investigations of Booij and Bungenberg De Jong (1956) have also revealed much of the possible effects of organic substances introduced into the aqueous environment on the lipid bilayer of plasma membranes. These effects were found to depend on the added substance's distribution in the water/lipid system, on its distribution within the bilayer, and on its size and shape. A substance may be found (see Fig. 4)

(*a*) in the aqueous medium (hydrophilic compounds, ions);
(*b*) at the bilayer's surface (ions fixed at polar groups);
(*c*) in the bilayer, parallel to its molecules (amphipatic molecules secured to the aqueous medium by their hydrophilic group);
(*d*) in between the monolayers (organic substances without or with a weakly hydrophilic group).

Substances at *a* will have no influence on the bilayer unless indirectly by interfering with ions bound to the head groups. The effects of the ions at *b*

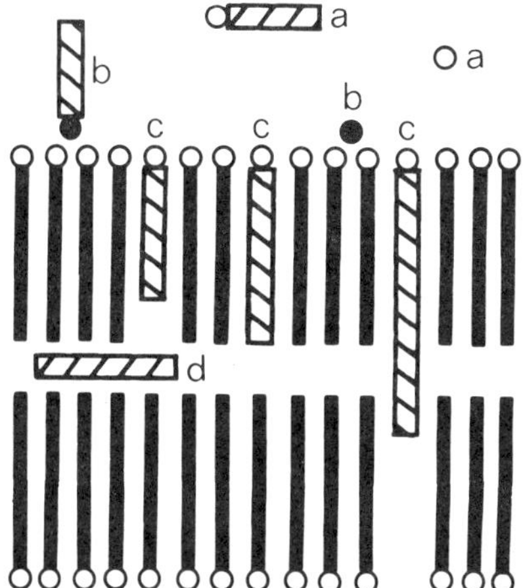

Figure 4 Possibilities as regards distribution of substances in the lipid bilayer/water system (from Den Otter, 1972*c*). The hydrophobic chains of lipid molecules are represented by shaded rods, those of added molecules by hatched rods. Open and shaded circles represent negative and positive groups or ions respectively.

have already been discussed. Molecules at position *d* will disturb the bilayer structure and will have an opening action. The effects of the molecules accumulating at *c* depend on both the hydrophobic and hydrophilic parts of the introduced molecules. The better the hydrophobic carbon chains fit into the bilayer, the less their disturbing effect will be on it. Shorter and longer carbon chains will cause a less compact packing of the molecules as they will disarrange the bilayer structure. This effect will, of course, be still larger when the introduced chains are branched or unsaturated. The hydrophilic head groups of the introduced molecules will generally have a condensing effect on the bilayer when they are positive or uncharged, because they will then locally reduce the repulsive negative forces.

This scheme of action of organic substances on the lipid bilayer can account for, for example, the inhibitory effects of normal alcohols on taste cells of the blowfly *Phormia regina* (Steinhardt *et al*., 1963, 1966; Dethier and Chadwick, 1947). The inhibition increases with increasing chain length of the alcohols, particularly beyond *n*-butanol. The alcohols enter the taste cell membrane, accumulating at position *c*, where they reduce the density of negative charge. The short alcohols, which are more water-soluble, have a relatively small effect, but when the alkyl group contains more than four carbons the condensing action increases considerably (Den Otter, 1972*c*).

Steinhardt *et al*. (1966) found one exception to the depressing effect of alcohols, occurring during salt inhibition of the classical "water cell".

Addition of depressing alcohol concentrations to a NaCl concentration which inhibits the water cell response produces a higher response of this cell than NaCl alone. This effect can be understood from Booij's results (1952; quoted in Booij and Bungenberg De Jong, 1956), which demonstrated that the condensing action of alcohols on lipid bilayers changes into an opening action when the bilayer has been condensed beforehand with cations. In olfaction, responsiveness increases with increasing chain length of the alcohols (Ottoson, 1958). This may indicate that the membranes of olfactory cells are more strongly condensed than those of insect taste cells.

(*f*) *Phospholipid membrane models*

The possibility that phospholipids may be involved in salt reception is supported by studies on phospholipid model taste cell membranes, initiated by Kamo *et al.* (1974*a*, *b*). The model consists of a Millipore filter impregnated with phospholipids extracted from bovine tongue epithelium. Kamo *et al.* (1974*a*) showed that the transmembrane potentials in this model closely paralleled receptor potentials recorded intracellularly from vertebrate taste cells during stimulation with salts, acids, and water. In addition, the model also demonstrated pH independence of salt stimulation between pH 3 and 12. Kamo *et al.* (1974*b*) concluded that the potential differences across the model membrane originated mainly from differences in the phase boundary potentials at both surfaces of membrane and solution. Diffusion potentials are considered to be of minor importance in the model, but may play a more prominent role in natural membranes.

Using different model membranes containing either single phospholipids or total lipid extract from bovine tongue epithelium led to the conclusion that variations in phospholipid composition may be responsible for the variations in responses observed between individual taste cells (Miyake *et al.*, 1975). The phase boundary potential is a function of both the charge density at the membrane surface and the ionic strength in the solution. The phase boundary potential of a negatively charged membrane will increase with increasing salt concentration, but that of a positively charged membrane decreases.

The differential effect of $CaCl_2$ on taste cell membranes (e.g., depolarization in frog taste cells (Akaike *et al.*, 1976), hyperpolarization in flies (Rees and Hori, 1968)) is explained by the strong affinity of Ca^{2+} for the negative phospholipid head groups. $CaCl_2$ will depolarize a membrane containing a surplus of zwitterionic phospholipids, because Ca^{2+} will bind to the negative groups, making the membrane surface charge positive. The phase boundary potential of this membrane will therefore decrease with increasing $CaCl_2$ concentration. In membranes retaining a net negative charge, the phase boundary potential will steadily increase on increasing the $CaCl_2$ concentration. Thus a membrane consisting of phosphatidyl ethanolamine (which has a slightly negative surface charge) will depolarize at lower, and hyperpolarize at higher $CaCl_2$ concentrations (Miyake *et al.*, 1975).

This theory could also account for the suppressive effect of salts on the sugar response in frog, and the inhibitory action of anions on cation response in rat (Miyake *et al.*, 1976*b*; Aiuchi *et al.*, 1976). The molecular mechanism of sugar reception is not as yet known. According to Miyake *et al.* (1976*b*) non-electrolytic stimuli may cause a conformational change in membrane structure, which causes the surface charge to become more positive locally. Increase of salt concentration will then cause the phase boundary potential to decrease. Anions would induce similar changes of conformation in the membrane (Aiuchi *et al.*, 1976).

Miyake *et al.* (1975, 1976*a*) also interpreted the response of taste cells to water, suggesting that when water was applied to a membrane adapted to a salt solution, ions dissolved in or adsorbed to the membrane surface will diffuse out into the bulk water phase. The water response would be attributable to the diffusion potential produced. This potential depends on the difference in the anionic and cationic transference numbers in the adapting solution. If the transference number of the anions exceeds that of the cations, the membrane surface would become positive with respect to the bulk phase. Therefore, the latter will become more negative to an electrode in the reference bath on the other side of the membrane, i.e., the taste cell interior. This theory allows the water response of frog taste cells to be explained quantitatively (Miyake *et al.*, 1976*a*).

Conclusion

All the models surveyed have a common goal in that they attempt to explain how receptor potentials are caused by chemical stimulation. Each has its particular point of emphasis, which ranges from changes in semiconductance, membrane conformational changes to phase boundary potentials. There is as yet no clear evidence favouring one of these hypotheses over any other, although the current tendency seems to give more weight to the role of the lipid part of the membrane. In fact, it seems likely that chemo-electrical transduction will eventually be shown to incorporate several of the processes suggested.

At this point, the next exciting question is how the electrical signal is transmitted through the cell to the action potential generator. Work has already begun on this problem and suggests three possible pathways. The extant hypothesis is that of electrotonic transmission of the receptor potential. Recently, however, Atema (1973, 1975) and Maes (1977) have suggested that the potential change evoked by the stimulus might lead to conformational changes in the microtubules, which are chemically transmitted to the proximal part of the cell. Finally, it is also conceivable that transmission occurs along the plane of the membrane. It is possible that local transient changes in membrane conformation produce "pressure waves" along the lipid bilayer of successive compressions and decompressions (Singer, 1971). The "fluid mosaic model" of plasma membrane (Singer and Nicolson, 1972) could indeed favour this idea.

It could therefore pay to take these latter hypotheses into consideration when considering transduction across the membrane, as it is possible that this process is intimately related to transmission through the cell.

Acknowledgements

I am very grateful to Dr G. Thomas for his helpful suggestions and corrections of the English text. Thanks are also due to Dr P. L. Cuperus for help in preparing some figures.

REFERENCES

Aiuchi, T., Kamo, N., Kurihara, K. and Kobatake, Y. (1976) Physicochemical Studies of Taste Reception. VI. Interpretation of Anion Influences on Taste Response *Chem. Senses Flavor*, **2**, 107–119.

Akaike, N., Noma, A. and Sato, M. (1976) Electrical Responses of Frog Taste Cells to Chemical Stimuli *J. Physiol.*, **254**, 87–107.

Akaike, N. and Sato, M. (1976) Mechanism of Action of Some Bitter-Tasting Compounds on Frog Taste Cells *Jap. J. Physiol.*, **26**, 29–40.

Altner, H., Sass, H. and Altner, I. (1977) Relationship between Structure and Function of Antennal Chemo-, Hygro-, and Thermoreceptive Sensilla in *Periplaneta americana Cell Tiss. Res.*, **176**, 389–405.

Amoore, J. E. (1952) The Stereochemical Specificities of Human Olfactory Receptors *Perf. and Ess. Oil Rec.*, **43**, 321–330.

Amoore, J. E. (1962*a*) The Stereochemical Theory of Olfaction. 1. Identification of the Seven Primary Odors *Proc. Sci. Sect. Toilet Goods Assoc., Special Suppl. to No. 37*, 1–12.

Amoore, J. E. (1962*b*) The Stereochemical Theory of Olfaction. 2. Elucidation of the Stereochemical Properties of the Olfactory Receptor Sites *Proc. Sci. Sect. Toilet Goods Assoc., Special Suppl. to No. 37*, 13–23.

Amoore, J. E. (1965) Psychophysics of Odor *Cold Spr. Harb. Symp. quant. Biol.*, **30**, 623–637.

Amoore, J. E. (1967) Specific Anosmia: A Clue to the Olfactory Code *Nature, Lond.*, **214**, 1095–1098.

Amoore, J. E. (1969) "A Plan to Identify Most of the Primary Odors" in *Olfaction and Taste III* (ed. Pfaffmann, C.) Rockefeller University Press, New York, 158–171.

Amoore, J. E. (1970) "Computer Correlation of Molecular Shape with Odour: A Model for Structure-Activity Relationships" in *Taste and Smell in Vertebrates* (eds. Wolstenholme, G. E. W., Knight, J.) J. & A. Churchill, London, 293–312.

Amoore, J. E. (1977) Specific Anosmia and the Concept of Primary Odors *Chem. Senses Flavor*, **2**, 267–281.

Amoore, J. E., Johnston, J. W. and Rubin, M. (1964) The Stereochemical Theory of Odor *Scient. Amer.*, **210**, 42–49.

Andres, K. H. (1969) Der Olfaktorische Saum der Katze *Z. Zellforsch.*, **96**, 250–274.

Ash, K. O. (1968) Chemical Sensing: An Approach to Biological Molecular Mechanisms Using Difference Spectroscopy *Science*, **162**, 452–454.

Ash, K. O. (1969) Ascorbic Acid: Cofactor in Rabbit Olfactory Preparations *Science*, **165**, 901–902.

Atema, J. (1973) Microtubule Theory of Sensory Transduction *J. theor. Biol.*, **38**, 181–190.

Atema, J. (1975) "Stimulus Transmission along Microtubules in Sensory Cells: An Hypothesis" in *Microtubules and Microtubule Inhibitors* (eds. Borgers, M., De Brabander, M.) North-Holland Publishing Co., Amsterdam, 247–257.

Bangham, A. D., Standish, M. M. and Watkins, J. C. (1965) Diffusion of Univalent Ions across the Lamellae of Swollen Phospholipids *J. Molec. Biol.*, **13**, 238–252.

Bannister, L. H. (1974) "Possible Functions of Mucus at Gustatory and Olfactory Surfaces" in *Transduction Mechanisms in Chemoreception* (ed. Poynder, T. M.) Information Retrieval Ltd, London, 39–48.

Beets, M. G. J. (1974) "Stimulant Structure, Information and Discrimination" in *Transduction Mechanisms in Chemoreception* (ed. Poynder, T. M.) Information Retrieval Ltd, London, 129–148.

Beets, M. G. J. (1978) *Structure-Activity Relationships in Human Chemoreception* Applied Science Publishers Ltd, Barking.

Beidler, L. M. (1954) A Theory of Taste Stimulation *J. gen. Physiol.*, **38**, 133–139.

Beidler, L. M. (1961) Taste Receptor Stimulation *Prog. Biophys. biophys. Chem.*, **12**, 107–151.

Beidler, L. M. (1971) "Taste Receptor Stimulation with Salts and Acids" in *Handbook of Sensory Physiology, Vol. IV: Chemical Senses, Part 2: Taste* (ed. Beidler, L. M.) Springer-Verlag, Berlin, 200–220.

Beidler, L. M. (1975) "Transductive Coupling in the Gustatory System" in *Functional Linkage in Biomolecular Systems* (eds. Schmitt, F. O., Schneider, D. M., Crothers, D. M.) Raven Press, New York, 255–262.

Beidler, L. M. and Gross, G. W. (1971) "The Nature of Taste Receptor Sites" in *Contributions to Sensory Physiology, Vol. 5* Academic Press, New York, 97–127.

Benz, G. (1976) *Structure-Activity Relationships in Chemoreception* Information Retrieval Ltd, London.

Bernays, E. A., Blaney, W. M. and Chapman, R. F. (1975) "The Problems of Perception of Leaf-Surface Chemicals by Locust Contact Chemoreceptors" in *Olfaction and Taste V* (eds. Denton, D. A., Coghlan, J. P.) Academic Press, New York, 227–229.

Bittman, R. and Blau, L. (1972) The Phospholipid-Cholesterol Interaction. Kinetics of Water Permeability in Liposomes *Biochem.*, **11**, 4831–4839.

Boeckh, J., Kaissling, K.-E. and Schneider, D. (1965) Insect Olfactory Receptors *Cold Spr. Harb. Symp. quant. Biol.*, **30**, 263–280.

Booij, H. L. (1963) "Colloid Chemistry of Living Membranes" in *Permeability. Lectures Held at the Conference on Permeability, Wageningen, May 1–4, 1962* N.V. Uitgevers-Maatschappij W. E. J. Tjeenk Willink, Zwolle, The Netherlands, 5–35.

Booij, H. L. and Bungenberg De Jong, H. G. (1956) "Biocolloids and their Interactions, with Special Reference to Coacervates and Related Systems" in *Protoplasmatologia. Handbuch der Protoplasmaforschung* (eds. Heilbrunn, L. V., Weber, F.) Springer-Verlag, Vienna, 1–162.

Borg, G., Diamant, H. and Zotterman, Y. (1970) "Neural and Perceptual Responses to Taste Stimuli" in *Taste and Smell in Vertebrates* (eds. Wolstenholme, G. E. W., Knight, J.) J. & A. Churchill, London, 99–113.

Briggs, M. H. and Duncan, R. B. (1961) Odour Receptors *Nature*, **191**, 1310–1311.

Briggs, M. H. and Duncan, R. B. (1962) Pigment and the Olfactory Mechanism *Nature*, **195**, 1313–1314.

Bungenberg De Jong, H. G. (1942) "Kolloidsystemen als Variabele Systemen. II. Complexe Systemen en hun Regulatie door pH en Electrolyten" in *Leerboek der Algemene Plantkunde. II. Physiologie en Erfelijkheid* (ed. Koningsberger, V. J.) Scheltema en Holkema's Boekhandel en Uitgeversmaatschappij, Amsterdam, 96–121.

Bungenberg De Jong, H. G. (1949) "Reversal of Charge Phenomena, Equivalent Weight and Specific Properties of the Ionised Groups" in *Colloid Science, Vol. 2* (ed. Kruijt, H. R.) Elsevier, Amsterdam, 259–334.

Bungenberg De Jong, H. G., Booij, H. L. and Wakkie, J. G. (1936) Zur Kenntnis der Lyophilen Kolloide. Zum Mechanismus des in Gemischen von Neutralsalzen Auftretenden Antagonismus hinsichtlich der Umladung von Phosphatiden *Kolloid-Beihefte*, **44**, 254–284.

Bungenberg, De Jong, H. G., Teunissen-Van Zijp, L. and Teunissen, P. H. (1940) Biokolloide als Hochmolekulare Elektrolyte. III a) Sphingomyelin. b) Stellung des Rubidiums und Cäsiums in der Wirkungsreihe der Alkalikationen *Kolloid-Z.*, **91**, 311–315.

Cagan, R. H. (1977) "Recognition of Gustatory and Olfactory Stimulus Molecules at Receptor Sites" in *Food Intake and Chemical Senses* (eds. Katsuki, Y., Sato, M., Takagi, S. F., Oomura, Y.) University of Tokyo Press, 131–138.

Cagan, R. H. and Morris, R. W. (1979) Biochemical Studies of Taste Sensation: Binding to Taste Tissue of ^{3}H-Labeled Monellin, a Sweet-Tasting Protein *Proc. Nat. Acad. Sci. U.S.A.*, **76**, 1692–1696.

Danielli, J. F. (1958) "Surface Chemistry and Cell Membranes" in *Surface Phenomena in Chemistry and Biology* (eds. Danielli, J. F., Pankhurst, K. G. A., Riddiford, A. C.) Pergamon Press, London, 246–265.

Dastoli, F. R., Lopiekes, D. V. and Doig, A. R. (1968*a*) Bitter-Sensitive Protein from Porcine Taste Buds *Nature*, **218**, 884–885.

Dastoli, F. R., Lopiekes, D. V. and Price, S. (1968*b*) A Sweet-Sensitive Protein from Bovine Taste Buds. Purification and Partial Characterization *Biochem.*, **7**, 1160–1164.

Dastoli, F. R. and Price, S. (1966) Sweet-Sensitive Protein from Bovine Taste Buds: Isolation and Assay *Science*, **154**, 905–907.

Davies, J. T. (1970) "Recent Developments in the 'Penetration and Puncturing' Theory of Odour" in *Taste and Smell in Vertebrates* (eds. Wolstenholme, G. E. W., Knight, J.) J. & A. Churchill, London, 265–291.

Davies, J. T. (1971) "Olfactory Theories" in *Handbook of Sensory Physiology, Vol. IV: Chemical Senses, Part 1: Olfaction* (ed. Beidler, L. M.) Springer-Verlag, Berlin, 322–350.

Davson, H. (1962) Growth of the Concept of the Paucimolecular Membrane *Circulation*, **26**, 1022–1037.

Dawson, R. M. C. (1968) "The Nature of the Interaction between Protein and Lipid during the Formation of Lipoprotein Membranes" in *Biological Membranes. Physical Fact and Function* (ed. Chapman, D.) Academic Press, London, 203–232.

Den Otter, C. J. (1971) Tarsal and Labellar Taste Hairs of *Calliphora vicina* Robineau-Desvoidy: Location, Sensitivity to NaCl *Neth. J. Zool.*, **21**, 464–484.

Den Otter, C. J. (1972*a*) Differential Sensitivity of Insect Chemoreceptors to Alkali Cations *J. Insect Physiol.*, **18**, 109–131.

Den Otter, C. J. (1972*b*) Interactions between Ions and Receptor Membrane in Insect Taste Cells *J. Insect Physiol.*, **18**, 389–402.

Den Otter, C. J. (1972*c*) Mechanism of Stimulation of Insect Taste Cells by Organic Substances *J. Insect Physiol.*, **18**, 615–625.

Den Otter, C. J. (1977) Single Sensillum Responses in the Male Moth *Adoxophyes orana* (F.v.R.) to Female Sex Pheromone Components and Their Geometrical Isomers *J. comp. Physiol.*, **121**, 205–222.

Den Otter, C. J. and Van Der Poel, A. M. (1965) Stimulation of Three Receptors in Labellar Chemosensory Hairs of *Calliphora erythrocephala* Mg. by Monovalent Salts *Nature*, **206**, 31–32.

Dethier, V. G. (1963) *The Physiology of Insect Senses* Methuen, London.

Dethier, V. G. and Chadwick, L. E. (1947) Rejection Thresholds of the Blowfly for a Series of Aliphatic Alcohols *J. gen. Physiol.*, **30**, 247–253.

Dodd, G. H. (1971) Studies on Olfactory Receptor Mechanisms *Biochem. J.*, **123**, 31*P*–32*P*.

Dodd, G. H. (1974) "Structure and Function of Chemoreceptor Membranes" in *Transduction Mechanisms in Chemoreception* (ed. Poynder, T. M.) Information Retrieval Ltd, London, 103–113.

Edidin, M. (1974) "Two-Dimensional Diffusion in Membranes" in *Transport at the Cellular Level. Symposium XXVIII of the Society for Experimental Biology* (eds. Sleigh, M. A., Jennings, D. H.) Cambridge University Press, 1–14.

Elgsaeter, A. and Branton, D. (1974) Intramembrane Particle Aggregation in Erythrocyte Ghosts. I. The Effects of Protein Removal *J. Cell Biol.*, **63**, 1018–1036.

Evans, D. R. and Mellon, D. (1962*a*) Electrophysiological Studies of a Water Receptor Associated with the Taste Sensilla of the Blowfly *J. gen. Physiol.*, **45**, 487–500.

Evans, D. R. and Mellon, D. (1962*b*) Stimulation of a Primary Taste Receptor by Salts *J. gen. Physiol.*, **45**, 651–661.

Frazier, J. L. and Heitz, J. R. (1975) Inhibition of Olfaction in the Moth *Heliothis virescens* by the Sulfhydryl Reagent Fluorescein Mercuric Acetate *Chem. Senses Flavor*, **1**, 271–281.

Gaffal, K.-P. and Bassemir, U. (1974) Vergleichende Untersuchung Modifizierter Cilienstrukturen in den Dendriten Mechano- und Chemosensitiver Rezeptorzellen der Baumwollwanze *Dysdercus* und der Libelle *Agrion Protoplasma*, **82**, 177–202.

Getchell, M. L. and Gesteland, R. C. (1972) The Chemistry of Olfactory Reception: Stimulus-Specific Protection from Sulfhydryl Reagent Inhibition *Proc. Nat. Acad. Sci. U.S.A.*, **69**, 1494–1498.

Gillary, H. L. (1966*a*) *Quantitative Electrophysiological Studies on the Mechanisms of Stimulation of the Salt Receptor of the Blowfly* Doct. Diss. Johns Hopkins University, Baltimore, Maryland.

Gillary, H. L. (1966*b*) Stimulation of the Salt Receptor of the Blowfly. I. NaCl *J. gen. Physiol.*, **50**, 337–350.

Gillary, H. L. (1966*c*) Stimulation of the Salt Receptor of the Blowfly. III. The Alkali Halides *J. gen. Physiol.*, **50**, 359–368.

Gilula, N. B. and Satir, P. (1972) The Ciliary Necklace. A Ciliary Membrane Specialization *J. Cell Biol.*, **53**, 494–509.

Ginsburg, V. and Kobata, A. (1971) "Structure and Function of Surface Components of Mammalian Cells" in *Structure and Function of Biological Membranes* (ed. Rothfield, L. I.) Academic Press, New York, 439–459.

Hansen, K. (1969) "The Mechanism of Insect Sugar Reception, a Biochemical Investigation" in *Olfaction and Taste III* (ed. Pfaffmann, C.) Rockefeller University Press, New York, 382–391.

Hansen, K. (1974) "α-Glucosidases as Sugar Receptor Proteins in Flies" in *Biochemistry of Sensory Functions* (ed. Jaenicke, L.) Springer-Verlag, Berlin, 207–233.

Hansen, K. (1978) "Insect Chemoreception" in *Taxis and Behavior* (*Receptors and Recognition, Series B, Vol. 5*) (ed. Hazelbauer, G. L.) Chapman and Hall, London, 231–292.

Hawke, S. D. and Farley, R. D. (1970) Chemical Filtering at Pores in the Antennal Chemoreceptors of the Desert Burrowing Cockroach, *Arenivaga* sp. *Amer. Zool.*, **10**, 521.

Henkin, R. I. and Bradley, D. F. (1969) Regulation of Taste Acuity by Thiols and Metal Ions *Proc. Nat. Acad. Sci. U.S.A.*, **62**, 30–37.

Hidaka, I. (1970) The Effects of Transition Metals on the Palatal Chemoreceptors of the Carp *Jap. J. Physiol.*, **20**, 599–609.

Hiji, Y., Kobayashi, N. and Sato, M. (1968) A Sweet-Sensitive Protein from the Tongue of the Rat *Kumamoto med. J.*, **21**, 137–139.

Hiji, Y., Kobayashi, N. and Sato, M. (1969) Binding Capacities of Sugars with the "Sweet-Sensitive Protein" from the Rat Tongue *Kumamoto med. J.*, **22**, 104–107.

Hiji, Y. and Sato, M. (1972) "Properties of Sweet-Sensitive Protein Extracted from the Rat Tongue" in *Olfaction and Taste IV* (ed. Schneider, D.) Wissenschaftliche Verlagsgesellschaft, Stuttgart, 221–225.

Joos, R. W. and Carr, C. W. (1967) The Binding of Calcium in Mixtures of Phospholipids *Proc. Soc. Exper. Biol. Med.*, **124**, 1268–1272.

Kaissling, K.-E. (1969) "Kinetics of Olfactory Receptor Potentials" in *Olfaction and Taste III* (ed. Pfaffmann, C.) Rockefeller University Press, New York, 52–70.

Kaissling, K.-E. (1971) "Insect Olfaction" in *Handbook of Sensory Physiology, Vol. IV: Chemical Senses, Part 1: Olfaction* (ed. Beidler, L. M.) Springer-Verlag, Berlin, 351–431.

Kaissling, K.-E. (1974) "Sensory Transduction in Insect Olfactory Receptors" in *Biochemistry of Sensory Functions* (ed. Jaenicke, L.) Springer-Verlag, Berlin, 243–273.

Kaissling, K.-E. (1975*a*) "Transduction in the Olfactory System" in *Functional Linkage in Biomolecular Systems* (eds. Schmitt, F. O., Schneider, D. M., Crothers, D. M.) Raven Press, New York, 262–271.

Kaissling, K.-E. (1975*b*) Sensorische Transduktion bei Riechzellen von Insekten *Verh. Dtsch. Zool. Ges.*, **67**, 1–11.

Kaissling, K.-E. (1976) "The Problem of Specificity in Olfactory Cells" in *Structure-Activity Relationships in Chemoreception* (ed. Benz, G.) Information Retrieval Ltd, London, 137–148.

Kaissling, K.-E. (1977) "Structure of Odour Molecules and Multiple Activities of Receptor

Cells" in *Olfaction and Taste VI* (ed. Le Magnen, J., MacLeod, P.) Information Retrieval Ltd, London, 9–16.

Kaissling, K.-E. and Thorson, J. (1980) "Insect Olfactory Sensilla: Structural, Chemical and Electrical Aspects of the Functional Organization" in *Receptors for Neurotransmitters, Hormones, and Pheromones* (eds. Hall, L. M., Hildebrand, J. G., Satelle, D. B.) Elsevier, Amsterdam, 261–282.

Kalmus, H. (1971) "Genetics of Taste" in *Handbook of Sensory Physiology, Vol. IV: Chemical Senses, Part 2: Taste* (ed. Beidler, L. M.) Springer-Verlag, Berlin, 165–179.

Kamo, N., Miyake, M., Kurihara, K. and Kobatake, Y. (1974*a*) Physicochemical Studies of Taste Reception. I. Model Membrane Simulating Taste Receptor Potential in Response to Stimuli of Salts, Acids and Distilled Water *Biochim. Biophys. Acta*, **367**, 1–10.

Kamo, N., Miyake, M., Kurihara, K. and Kobatake, Y. (1974*b*) Physicochemical Studies of Taste Reception. II. Possible Mechanism of Generation of Taste Receptor Potential Induced by Salt Stimuli *Biochim. Biophys. Acta*, **367**, 11–23.

Kasang, G. and Kaissling, K.-E. (1972) "Specificity of Primary and Secondary Olfactory Processes in *Bombyx* Antennae" in *Olfaction and Taste IV* (ed. Schneider, D.) Wissenschaftliche Verlagsgesellschaft, Stuttgart, 200–206.

Kavanau, J. L. (1965) *Structure and Function in Biological Membranes. Vol. I and II* Holden-Day, Inc., San Francisco.

Kerjaschki, D. (1977) "Some Freeze-Etching Data on the Olfactory Epithelium" in *Olfaction and Taste VI* (eds. Le Magnen, J., MacLeod, P.), Information Retrieval Ltd, London, 75–85.

Kerjaschki, D. and Hörandner, H. (1976) The Development of Mouse Olfactory Vesicles and Their Cell Contacts: A Freeze-Etching Study *J. Ultrastruct. Res.*, **54**, 420–444.

Keynes, R. D. (1979) Ion Channels in the Nerve-Cell Membrane *Scient. Amer.*, **240**, 98–107.

Kijima, H., Koizumi, O. and Morita, H. (1973) α-Glucosidase at the Tip of the Contact Chemosensory Seta of the Blowfly, *Phormia regina J. Insect Physiol.*, **19**, 1351–1362.

Kijima, H. and Morita, H. (1977) "Receptor Site Properties and the 'α-Glucosidase Hypothesis' in Regard to the Sugar Receptor Molecule of Flies" in *Food Intake and Chemical Senses* (eds. Katsuki, Y., Sato, M., Takagi, S. F., Oomura, Y.) University of Tokyo Press, 139–148.

Koyama, N. and Kurihara, K. (1971) Modification by Chemical Reagents of Proteins in the Gustatory and Olfactory Organs of the Fleshfly and Cockroach *J. Insect Physiol.*, **17**, 2435–2440.

Kurihara, K. (1974) "Physico-Chemical Aspects of Chemoreceptor Mechanism: Stimuli Receptor Interaction and Receptor Potential in Taste Stimulation" in *Transduction Mechanisms in Chemoreception* (ed. Poynder, T. M.) Information Retrieval Ltd, London, 163–176.

Kurihara, K., Koyana, N. and Kurihara, Y. (1972) "Chemical Architecture and Model System of Gustatory and Olfactory Receptor Membrane" in *Olfaction and Taste IV* (ed. Schneider, D.) Wissenschaftliche Verlagsgesellschaft, Stuttgart, 234–240.

Lester, H. A. (1977) The Response to Acetylcholine *Scient. Amer.*, **236**, 106–118.

Ma, W.-C. (1977) Alterations of Chemoreceptor Function in Armyworm Larvae (*Spodoptera exempta*) by a Plant-Derived Sesquiterpenoid and by Sulfhydryl Reagents *Physiol. Entom.*, **2**, 199–207.

Maes, F. W. (1977) Simultaneous Chemical and Electrical Stimulation of Labellar Taste Hairs of the Blowfly *Calliphora vicina J. Insect Physiol.*, **23**, 453–460.

Masson, C., Kouprach, S., Giachetti, I. and MacLeod, P. (1977) "Relation between Intramembranous Particle Density of Frog Olfactory Cilia and EOG Response" in *Olfaction and Taste VI* (eds. Le Magnen, J., MacLeod, P.) Information Retrieval Ltd, London, 195.

Menco, B. P. M. (1977) "Freeze-Etch Morphology of Olfactory and Respiratory Cilia in Rat, Cow and Frog" in *Olfaction and Taste VI* (ed. Le Magnen, J., MacLeod, P.) Information Retrieval Ltd, London, 199.

Menco, B. P. M., Dodd, G. H., Davey, M. and Bannister, L. H. (1976) Presence of Membrane Particles in Freeze-Etched Bovine Olfactory Cilia *Nature*, **263**, 597–599.

Misra, T. N., Rosenberg, B., Switzer, R. (1968) The Effect of Adsorption of Gases on the Semiconductive Properties of All-*Trans-β*-Carotene *J. chem. Phys.*, **48**, 2096–2102.

Miyake, M., Kamo, N., Kurihara, K. and Kobatake, Y. (1975) Physico-Chemical Studies of Taste Reception. IV. Response of Individual Phospholipid Membrane to a Variety of Chemical Stimuli *J. Membrane Biol.*, **22**, 197–209.

Miyake, M., Kamo, N., Kurihara, K. and Kobatake, Y. (1976*a*) Physicochemical Studies of Taste Reception. III. Interpretation of the Water Response in Taste Reception *Biochim. Biophys. Acta*, **436**, 843–855.

Miyake, M., Kamo, N., Kurihara, K. and Kobatake, Y. (1976*b*) Physicochemical Studies of Taste Reception. V. Suppressive Effect of Salts on Sugar Response of the Frog *Biochim. Biophys. Acta*, **436**, 856–862.

Mooser, G. (1976) N-Substituted Maleimide Inactivation of the Response to Taste Cell Stimulation *J. Neurobiol.*, **7**, 457–468.

Mooser, G. and Lambuth, N. (1977) Inactivation of Taste Receptor Cell Function by Two Cationic Protein Modification Reagents *J. Neurobiol.*, **8**, 193–206.

Morita, H. (1959) Initiation of Spike Potentials in Contact Chemosensory Hairs of Insects. III. D.C. Stimulation and Generator Potential of Labellar Chemoreceptor of *Calliphora* *J. cell. comp. Physiol.*, **54**, 189–204.

Morita, H. (1963) Generator Potential of Insect Chemoreceptors *Proc. XVI Internat. Congr. Zool.*, **3**, 105–106.

Morita, H. (1969) "Electrical Signs of Taste Receptor Activity" in *Olfaction and Taste III* (ed. Pfaffmann, C.) 370–381.

Morita, H. and Yamashita, S. (1959) Generator Potential of Insect Chemoreceptor *Science*, **130**, 922.

Moulins, M. and Noirot, Ch. (1972) "Morphological Features Bearing on Transduction and Peripheral Integration in Insect Gustatory Organs" in *Olfaction and Taste IV* (ed. Schneider, D.) Wissenschaftliche Verlagsgesellschaft, Stuttgart, 49–55.

Moulton, D. G. (1962) Pigment and the Olfactory Mechanism *Nature*, **195**, 1312–1313.

Moulton, D. G. (1971) "The Olfactory Pigment" in *Handbook of Sensory Physiology, Vol. IV: Chemical Senses, Part 1: Olfaction* (ed. Beidler, L. M.) Springer-Verlag, Berlin, 59–74.

Moulton, D. G. and Beidler, L. M. (1967) Structure and Function in the Peripheral Olfactory System *Physiol. Rev.*, **47**, 1–52.

Murray, R. G. (1971) "Ultrastructure of Taste Receptors" in *Handbook of Sensory Physiology, Vol. IV: Chemical Senses, Part 2: Taste* (ed. Beidler, L. M.) Springer-Verlag, Berlin, 31–50.

Murray, R. G. (1973) "The Ultrastructure of Taste Buds" in *The Ultrastructure of Sensory Organs* (ed. Friedmann, I.) North-Holland Publishing Company, Amsterdam, 1–81.

Nathanson, J. A. and Greengard, P. (1977) "Second Messengers" in the Brain *Scient. Amer.*, **237**, 108–119.

Norris, D. M. (1977) "A Molecular and Submolecular Mechanism of Insect Perception of Certain Chemical Information in their Environment" in *Colloques Internationaux du C.N.R.S. No. 265*, 81–102.

Norris, D. M. and Chu, H.-M. (1974) Chemosensory Mechanism in *Periplaneta americana*: Electroantennogram Comparisons of Certain Quinone Feeding Inhibitors *J. Insect Physiol.*, **20**, 1687–1696.

Norris, D. M., Ferkovich, S. M., Baker, J. E., Rozental, J. M. and Borg, T. K. (1971) Energy Transduction in Quinone Inhibition of Insect Feeding *J. Insect Physiol.*, **17**, 85–97.

O'Brien, J. S. (1967) Cell Membranes-Composition: Structure: Function *J. theor. Biol.*, **15**, 307–324.

Oschman, J. L., Wall, B. J. and Gupta, B. L. (1974) "Cellular Basis of Water Transport" in *Transport at the Cellular Level. Symposium XXVIII of the Society for Experimental Biology* (eds. Sleigh, M. A., Jennings, D. H.) The University Press, Cambridge, 305–350.

Ottoson, D. (1958) Studies on the Relationship between Olfactory Stimulating Effectiveness and Physico-Chemical Properties of Odorous Compounds *Acta physiol. scand.*, **43**, 167–181.

Ottoson, D. (1963) Some Aspects of the Function of the Olfactory System *Pharmacol. Rev.*, **15**, 1–42.

Ottoson, D. (1971) "The Electro-Olfactogram. A Review of Studies on the Receptor Potential of the Olfactory Organ" in *Handbook of Sensory Physiology, Vol. IV: Chemical Senses, Part 1: Olfaction* (ed. Beidler, L. M.) Springer-Verlag, Berlin, 95–131.

Ozeki, M. (1971) Conductance Change Associated with Receptor Potentials of Gustatory Cells in Rat *J. gen. Physiol.*, **58**, 688–699.

Papahadjopoulos, D., Jacobson, K., Nir, S. and Isac, T. (1973) Phase Transitions in Phospholipid Vesicles. Fluorescence Polarization and Permeability Measurements Concerning the Effect of Temperature and Cholesterol *Biochim. Biophys. Acta*, **311**, 330–348.

Pfaffmann, C. (1965) "The Sense of Taste" in *Handbook of Physiology. Section 1: Neurophysiology, Vol. 1* (eds. Field, J., Magoun, H. W., Hall, V. E.) American Physiological Society, Washington, 507–533.

Pinto Da Silva, P. and Branton, D. (1970) Membrane Splitting in Freeze-Etching. Covalently Bound Ferritin as a Membrane Marker *J. Cell Biol.*, **45**, 598–605.

Price, S. and DeSimone, J. A. (1977) Models of Taste Receptor Cell Stimulation *Chem. Senses Flavor*, **2**, 427–456.

Quinn, P. J. (1977) *The Molecular Biology of Cell Membranes*, 2nd ed. Macmillan, London.

Rees, C. J. C. and Hori, N. (1968) The Effect of Electrolytes of the General Formula XCl_2 on the Response of the Type 1 Labellar Chemoreceptor of the Blowfly *Phormia J. Insect. Physiol.*, **14**, 1499–1513.

Riddiford, L. M. (1970) Antennal Proteins of Saturniid Moths: Their Possible Role in Olfaction *J. Insect Physiol.*, **16**, 653–660.

Rosenberg, B., Misra, T. N. and Switzer, R. (1968) Mechanism of Olfactory Transduction *Nature*, **217**, 423–427.

Rozental, J. M. and Norris, D. M. (1973) Chemosensory Mechanism in American Cockroach Olfaction and Gustation *Nature*, **244**, 370–371.

Scalzi, H. A. (1967) The Cytoarchitecture of Gustatory Receptors from the Rabbit Foliate Papillae *Z. Zellforsch. mikrosk. Anat.*, **80**, 413–435.

Shimada, I., Shiraishi, A., Kijima, H. and Morita, H. (1972) Effects of Sulphydryl Reagents on the Labellar Sugar Receptor of the Fleshfly *J. Insect Physiol.*, **18**, 1845–1855.

Singer, S. J. (1971) "The Molecular Organization of Biological Membranes" in *Structure and Function of Biological Membranes* (ed. Rothfield, L. I.) Academic Press, New York, 145–222.

Singer, S. J. and Nicolson, G. L. (1972) The Fluid Mosaic Model of the Structure of Cell Membranes *Science*, **175**, 720–731.

Singer, G., Rozental, J. M. and Norris, D. M. (1975) Sulphydryl Groups and the Quinone Receptor in Insect Olfaction and Gustation *Nature*, **256**, 222–223.

Steinbrecht, R. A. (1969) "Comparative Morphology of Olfactory Receptors" in *Olfaction and Taste III* (ed. Pfaffmann, C.) Rockefeller University Press, New York, 3–21.

Steinhardt, R. A., Morita, H. and Hodgson, E. S. (1963) Electrophysiological Analysis of Inhibition and Specificity in Labellar Chemoreceptors of the Blowfly *Proc. XVI Internat. Congr. Zool.*, **3**, 99–101.

Steinhardt, R. A., Morita, H. and Hodgson, E. S. (1966) Mode of Action of Straight Chain Hydrocarbons on Primary Chemoreceptors of the Blowfly, *Phormia regina J. cell Physiol.*, **67**, 53–62.

Stevens, C. F. (1979) The Neuron *Scient. Amer.*, **241**, 49–59.

Stürckow, B. (1967) "Occurrence of a Viscous Substance at the Tip of the Labellar Taste Hair of the Blowfly" in *Olfaction and Taste II* (ed. Hayashi, T.) Pergamon Press, Oxford, 707–720.

Tateda, H. and Beidler, L. M. (1964) The Receptor Potential of the Taste Cell of the Rat *J. gen. Physiol.*, **47**, 479–486.

Thurm, U. (1974) "Mechanisms of Electrical Membrane Responses in Sensory Receptors, Illustrated by Mechanoreceptors" in *Biochemistry of Sensory Functions* (ed. Jaenicke, L.) Springer-Verlag, Berlin, 367–390.

Vandenheuvel, F. A. (1963) Study of Biological Structure at the Molecular Level with Stereomodel Projections. I. The Lipids in the Myelin Sheath of Nerve *J. Am. Oil Chem. Soc.*, **40**, 455–471.

Villet, R. H. (1974) Involvement of Amino and Sulphydryl Groups in Olfactory Transduction in Silk Moths *Nature*, **248**, 707–709.

Whissell-Buechy, D. and Amoore, J. E. (1973) Odour-Blindness to Musk: Simple Recessive Inheritance *Nature*, **242**, 271–273.

Wolbarsht, M. L. (1965) Receptor Sites in Insect Chemoreceptors *Cold Spr. Harb. Symp. quant. Biol.*, **30**, 281–288.

Wright, R. H. (1976) Odour and Molecular Vibration: A Possible Membrane Interaction Mechanism *Chem. Senses Flavor*, **2**, 203–206.

Wright, R. H. (1977*a*) The Olfactory Transmission of Information *Colloques Internationaux du C.N.R.S. No. 265*, 61–71.

Wright, R. H. (1977*b*) Odor and Molecular Vibration: Neural Coding of Olfactory Information *J. theor. Biol.*, **64**, 473–502.

Wright, R. H. and Burgess, R. E. (1970) "Specific Physicochemical Mechanisms of Olfactory Stimulation" in *Taste and Smell in Vertebrates* (eds. Wolstenholme, G. E. W., Knight, J.) J. & A. Churchill, London, 325–342.

Wright, R. H. and Burgess, R. E. (1975) Molecular Coding of Olfactory Specificity *Can. J. Zool.*, **53**, 1247–1253.

Yamashita, S. (1963) Stimulating Effectiveness of Cations and Anions on Chemoreceptors in the Frog Tongue *Jap. J. Physiol.*, **13**, 54–63.

ADDITIONAL REFERENCES TO CHAPTER 10

Brown, J. E. (1977) Calcium ion, a putative intracellular messenger for light adaptation in *Limulus* ventral photoreceptors *Biophys. Struct. Mechanism*, **3**, 141–143.

Dartnall, H. J. A. (1972) "Photosensitivity" in *Handbook of Sensory Physiology*, Vol. VII/1, Springer-Verlag, Berlin, 122–145.

Fein, A. and Charlton, J. S. (1977*c*) Increased intracellular sodium mimics some but not all aspects of photoreceptor adaptation in the ventral eye of *Limulus J. Gen. Physiol.*, **70**; 601–620.

Lisman, J. E. and Brown, J. E. (1975*a*) Light induced changes of sensitivity in *Limulus* ventral photoreceptors *J. Gen. Physiol.*, **66**, 473–488.

Lisman, J. E. and Brown, J. E. (1975*b*) Effects of intracellular injection of calcium buffers on light adaptation in *Limulus* ventral photoreceptors *J. Gen. Physiol.*, **66**, 489–506.

Naka, K. J. and Rushton, W. A. H. (1966) S-potentials from colour units in the retina of fish (Cyprinidae) *J. Physiol.* (*Lond.*), **185**, 536–555.

Pak, W. L., Grabowski, S. R. and Pinto, L. H. (1973) "Adaptation and receptor interactions: some results of intracellular recordings (preliminary note)" in *Biochemistry and Physiology of Visual Pigments* (ed. Langer, H.) Springer-Verlag, Berlin, Heidelberg, New York, 225–228.

Schröder, W., Frings, D. and Stieve, H. (1980) Measuring Ca-uptake and release by invertebrate photoreceptor cells by a laser microprobe mass spectroscopy *Scanning Electron Microsc.*, 647–654.

Stieve, H. (1977) On the mechanism of conductance control of the arthropod visual cell membrane *Biophys. Struct. Mechanism*, **3**, 145–151.

Stieve, H. (1979) "Charge separation by rhodopsin containing photosensory membranes" in *Light Induced Charge Separation in Biology and Chemistry*, Dahlem Konferenz, Verlag Chemie, Weinheim, 503–523.

Part 2

ORGANIZATION OF SENSORY SYSTEMS

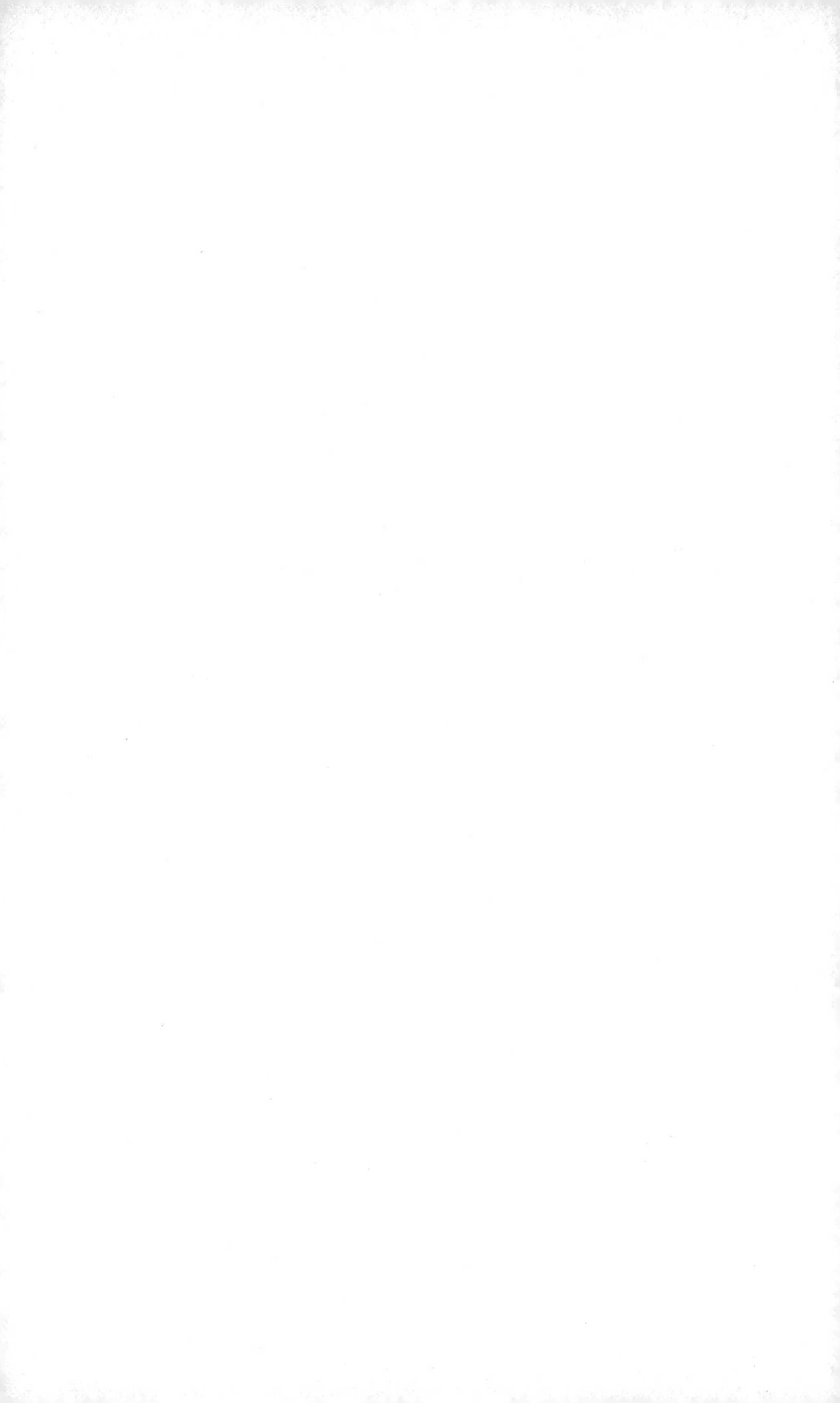

CHAPTER TWELVE
INTRODUCTION

O. LOWENSTEIN

Part 2 is devoted to the functional analysis of sensory systems. We may ask in what way our approach to the analysis of sensory function in the second part of this book differs from what has been examined in Part 1, and this in turn may lead us to redefine sensory systems more closely.

A system may be defined as a compound entity composed of a number of associated components organized into a functional "organic" whole. Purely formally, such components may be ideas or concepts making up a specific doctrine e.g. in religion, philosophy or science. Alternatively, we may deal descriptively or analytically with a complex of related objects such as galaxies of stars or organs within a living organism. In the latter context, a sensory system may comprise the sum total of all sensory inputs in a particular animal with special reference to their combined role in the control of the animal's behaviour. Alternatively, we may deal with the receptors representing a single sensory modality in order to analyse the co-ordinated functional integration of their component structures or tissue elements. Thus, one might view a retinal bipolar cell as an element, a bipolar amacrine–ganglion network as a circuit and an entire retina as a subsystem.

The critical distinction between circuit and subsystem is to be viewed in terms of a "bounded domain" characterized by observable input and output "terminals". Within such a domain there may be one or more circuits with profuse interactions (interconnections) which make cause and effect obscure. Outside the domain the signal flow is discernible. The bounded domain may be treated as a "black box". Viewed from the outside such a domain is a subsystem, seen from the inside it is a circuit (Harmon, 1970).

The subject of the first chapter in Part 2—the hair cell serving as a common mechanosensitive transducer in the diverse receptor endings of the vestibular and cochlear organs of the vertebrate inner ear as well as of the lateral line of aquatic vertebrates—is a good example of such a system component. Its functional characteristics *per se* have already been discussed in Part 1. Here our attention will be directed to the special aspects connected with its functional adaptation to the conditions of aquatic life.

A fascinating aspect of the study of the hair cell is the complexity of the deployment of this tissue element in the various end organs of the acoustico-lateralis system serving in the control of posture movement and orientating behaviour. The hair cell's directional sensitivity finds its expression in its assembly within given sensory epithelia in patterns of fixed topographic distribution and alignment of axes of greatest sensitivity to mechanical displacement. Furthermore, a number of ultrastructurally distinct types of hair cells differing, for instance, in relative length of hair processes and other dimensional characteristics, in their mode of innervation, and their association with the overlying auxiliary structures such as cupulae and otolith or otoconial membranes are found organized into patterned assemblies within given end organs.

The wider aspects of spatial orientation are introduced in chapter 15, in which the role of so-called proprioceptors is discussed with reference to the total complex of sensory-motor subsystems serving in the control of posture and movement of organisms in a wide variety of environments. The degree of complexity of integration between the component orientation systems varies widely within the animal kingdom and is naturally closely related to environmental factors and behavioural characteristics.

Yet another mechano-receptor system is covered in chapter 17, which deals with the sensory function of the vertebrate skin. This incorporates complex arrays of inputs organized into coordinated systems of receptors for stimuli of touch, pressure and heat. It is interesting to see how much our insight into the "systems" aspect in this field of sensory science has advanced in recent years.

The structural and functional complexity of the retina of the camera eye furnishes us with another example of a compound receptor system. Here we shall find the co-ordination between two or more types of primary receptor cells associated with subsystems of neuronal elements representing an outpost of the central nervous processor. When discussing the relationship between the peripheral visual organ and the brain itself, we are confronted by systems on a still higher level of complexity, characterized by hierarchically organized patterns of input–output interactions. The study of such complex assemblies calls for the application of various methods of mathematical systems analysis, biocybernetics or biological control science.

The electric sense and the sensitivity of organisms to magnetic fields differ in the way in which they enter into our consideration here. The first has long passed from the realm of speculation into the sphere of accurate measurement and quantitative analysis, thanks to the fact that the adequate and quantifiable stimulus originates in the animal itself and that the relevant receptor structures are well known. The second has for some time been a matter of postulate and conjecture, but has now gained a more tangible status in behavioural research through the discoveries of its importance in the orientation of the honey bee to parameters of the earth-magnetic field.

A final contribution under the heading of "Unusual Senses" deals with the sensory role of the effects of "pervasive" electromagnetic fields on organisms. The question is how much nearer we are to forming an idea concerning the relevant receptor structures and mechanisms. This would be the prerequisite for accepting this "modality" into the framework of a sensory system.

The systems concept has so far been defined in terms of association, combination and organization of elements into "functional organic wholes". There is an immanent suggestion of "design" in such an integration of parts for an overall functional effect. Present-day biological theory deals with this by asserting that the apparent purposiveness of such functional systems is explicable as a *pro tempore* final result of the selective process in phylogenetic evolution of organisms and their adaptation to environmental circumstances. Environmental constraints are themselves considered as modifiable by the activities of organisms in a mutual interplay of "formative" influences. This blurs the boundaries between organism and environment, establishing an effective "continuum" of material reality. Observed after the evolutionary process, functional systems appear to be designed for a specific end, but before their assembly the final effect of their association into systems will be seen as "certainly compatible with first principles, but not deducible from those principles and therefore essentially unpredictable" (Monod, 1972).

In Part 2, therefore, we shall be interested in the configurations and mode of functioning of our systems, and in the relationship between their component elements, i.e. units, circuits and subsystems. In the unravelling of these complex relationships we shall hope to gain some better understanding of the fundamental significance of the "structural and functional" features of the unit elements examined in the first part of the book.

REFERENCES

Harmon, D. L. (1970) "Neural Subsystems: An interpretive summary" in *The Neurosciences, Second Study Program* (ed. Schmitt, F. O.) Rockefeller University Press, New York, 486–494.

Monod, J. (1972) *Chance and Necessity* Collins, London.

CHAPTER THIRTEEN

THE ACOUSTICO LATERALIS SYSTEM OF AQUATIC VERTEBRATES

A. D. HAWKINS AND K. HORNER

Introduction

The acoustico lateralis system is a collection of homologous sense organs found in the primitively aquatic vertebrates, the cyclostomes, fishes and amphibians. It consists of a series of superficial receptor organs on the head and body, the lateral-line system, and a pair of auditory organs, the ears, embedded deep inside the head. In present-day aquatic vertebrates the acoustico lateralis system is highly evolved and serves a multiplicity of functions. Various end organs are sensitive to local movements of the surrounding medium, small electrical currents, linear and angular accelerations of the head, gravitational forces and propagated sound waves. Because of this functional diversity, the term octavo lateralis has been applied to the system by some authors to avoid any implication that it is exclusively auditory (see Bullock, this volume).

The idea that this range of different sense organs forms a common system, and that the most highly developed of them—the ear—is derived from the simpler superficial forms, is based on the morphological and developmental similarities between them. The evolutionary origin of the acoustico lateralis system is obscure. It is present in a developed state in all fossil fishes but is absent from vertebrate precursors. In the Cephalaspids, the jawless earliest fish, the ear has only two semicircular canals and the lateral line is only fragmentary, but this condition is paralleled in modern day cyclostomes and is not necessarily primitive. In the Acanthodians, the oldest jawed fishes, the ear is complete with a full set of three semicircular canals and three small otoliths while the lateral line is also well developed (Watson, 1938). Some fossil fish show a development of the acoustico lateralis system which is not present in modern forms. This pore canal system, found in both Agnathan and

Gnathostome fishes, is a series of interconnected ampullae beneath the surface of the head, connected to the surface by small pores (Thompson, 1977). Its function is unknown.

Thus, the aquatic vertebrates possess a unique, highly developed and diversified system of sense organs which, though of unknown origin, has clearly played a highly significant part in the rise of this successful group.

The hair cell

The unity of the acoustico lateralis system is largely based on a common sensory cell, found in all the mechanoreceptive parts of the system, including the auditory and vestibular parts of the ear and the unspecialized lateral line organs. This is the hair cell, an elongate epithelial cell with a bundle of fine hairs or cilia projecting from its apical end into some form of tectorial structure. Details of the arrangements and structure of hair cells are given by Russell (this volume) for those of the ear. The ultrastructure of the hair cell has principally been investigated by Flock (1965, 1971).

There is some variation in hair cell type, based mainly on differences in the ciliary bundle. Each bundle normally consists of a single kinocilium, and a group of up to 150 stereocilia, arranged in a staircase leading up to the kinocilium. Each stereocilium is composed of an external triple layered membrane surrounding a fibrillar core, which at its base continues as an axial filament piercing an apical cuticular region of the cell (Flock, 1965). The kinocilium, like many motile cilia, is composed of a bundle of nine peripheral double filaments surrounding a central pair of simple filaments and emerges from a basal body or centriole outside the area of the cuticular plate. In the lateral line of the dogfish there are two forms of sensory cell (Roberts and Ryan, 1971). In one type, the stereocilia are of similar length, adjacent to a single rather longer kinocilium. In the other, there are many long microvilli surrounding a single cilium. As a general rule, however, stereocilia are found in all the mechanoreceptors of the acoustico lateralis system.

Among the more specialized and non-mechanoreceptive end organs of the lateral line system like the ampullae of Lorenzini of marine elasmobranchs and the microampullae of freshwater elasmobranchs, the sensory cells are hair cells (Szabo, 1972), but the sensory cells of other specialized neuromasts, like the ampullary organs of teleosts, bear only microvilli at their apical surfaces. Bennett (1971) suggested that the specialized lateral line organs developed from ordinary lateral line organs, in which case the sensory cells of the ampullary and tuberous organs may represent modified hair cells. A further aspect in which these cells differ from the more typical hair cells is that they lack efferent innervation (Szabo, 1974).

Little is known about the nature of the supporting or sustentacular cells which surround the more typical hair cells of the acoustico lateralis system. The supporting cells are normally longer than the hair cells and bear only a few microvilli at their apical surface. They extend to the basement membrane of the end organ, unlike the hair cells. Jande (1966), however, has reported that some of the supporting cells in the labyrinth of the frog tadpole do not contact the basement membrane. Furthermore, in the labyrinth of the thornback ray *Raja clavata* (Lowenstein *et al.*, 1964), the goldfish, *Carassius auratus* and loach, *Cobitus* (Saito, 1973), and of other species of teleost (Popper, 1977) the supporting cells have one long microvillus located centrally among the shorter microvilli. This central microvillus has a fibrillar structure similar to that of the typical kinocilium. Lewis and Li (1975) for the bullfrog, *Rana catesbeiana*, distinguished between a range of different hair cell types, based on the morphology of the ciliary bundles. In the cod, *Gadus morhua*, Dale (1976) has reported that the first indication of the development of a ciliary bundle is the appearance of the stereocilia among the microvilli, and that this is followed later by the development of the kinocilium. It is not clear whether there is any interstitial development or replacement of hair cells in the sensory epithelia, or whether the supporting cells might play a part in this.

It is evident that the principal function of the typical hair cell is mechanoreceptive. Mechanical deflection of the cilia by applied shearing forces eventually activates the synapse with the afferent nerve fibre. The hair cells of the lateral line canal have quite small time constants and are capable of conducting signals in the kHz range without attenuation, though these hair cells are situated in an organ which is restricted by its mechanical coupling to the water to have a natural resonance frequency of only about 100 Hz (Flock *et al.*, 1973).

The possible modes of ciliary movement in the hair cells have been considered by Flock *et al.* (1977). It is clear that the displacements involved are very small; Hudspeth and Corey (1977) have estimated the threshold sensitivity of hair cells in the amphibian sacculus to be about 5 Å ($1\ \text{Å} = 1 \times 10^{-10}$ m).

Quite apart from its acute sensitivity it is also clear that the hair cell is fundamentally directional in its mechanical response. The morphological asymmetry, with the kinocilium placed eccentrically with respect to the stereocilia, is correlated with a degree of functional polarization. The hair cell depolarizes (and firing of the afferent fibre is stimulated) when the hair cell bundle is displaced towards the kinocilium, and the cell hyperpolarizes (with firing of the afferent fibre inhibited) when the bundle is displaced away from the kinocilium (Lowenstein and Wersall, 1959; Flock, 1964). Thus the axis of sensitivity of the hair cell can be defined by an arrow bisecting the top of the cell, with its head towards the kinocilium (Fig. 1).

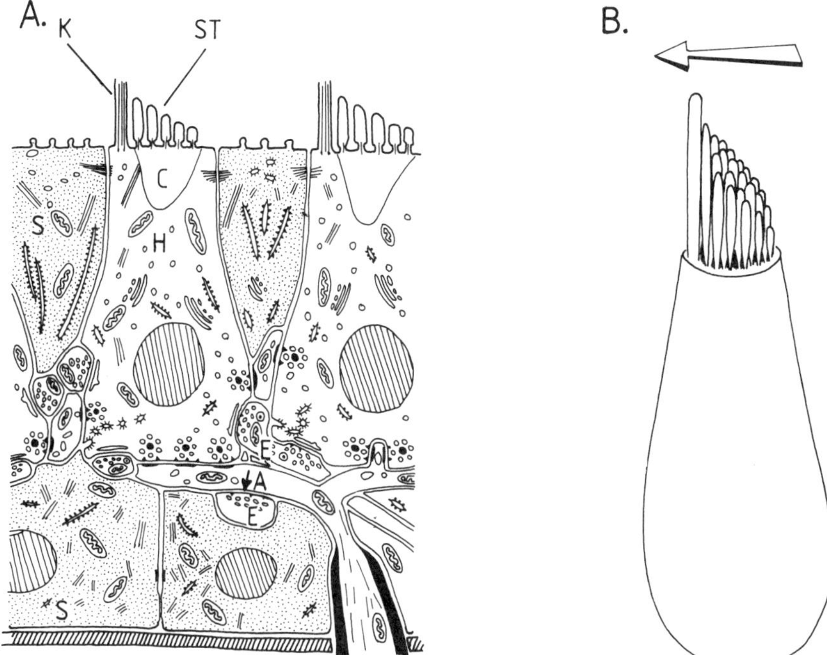

Figure 1 (A) Schematic diagram of the sensory epithelium of the goldfish saccular macula. The arrow marks a synapse between an efferent and an afferent nerve fibre. A, afferent nerve endings. E, efferent nerve endings. H, hair cell. S, sustentacular cell. C, cuticular plate. K, kinocilium. ST, stereocilia. (Modified from Nakajima and Wang, 1974.)
(B) Showing direction of functional polarization of hair cell.

The lateral line system

The lateral line system is a collection of essentially epidermal sense organs on the head and trunk. Dijkgraaf (1963) has distinguished between two types of organ, the ordinary or unspecialized lateral line organs, and the ampullary or specialized organs. Both comprise groups of sensory cells, or neuromasts, which are scattered about the skin or arranged in well defined lines. The former may also be rolled up into canals.

The ordinary lateral line organs

The best known part of the lateral line system is the lateral line itself, an extended array of neuromasts aligned along the trunk of many fishes and often prominently marked. However, the lateral line system is more highly developed on the head of most fish (Fig. 2), and is also present, though less conspicuously, on the body and head of aquatic amphibians. Each lateral line organ consists of a group of hair cells and their supporting

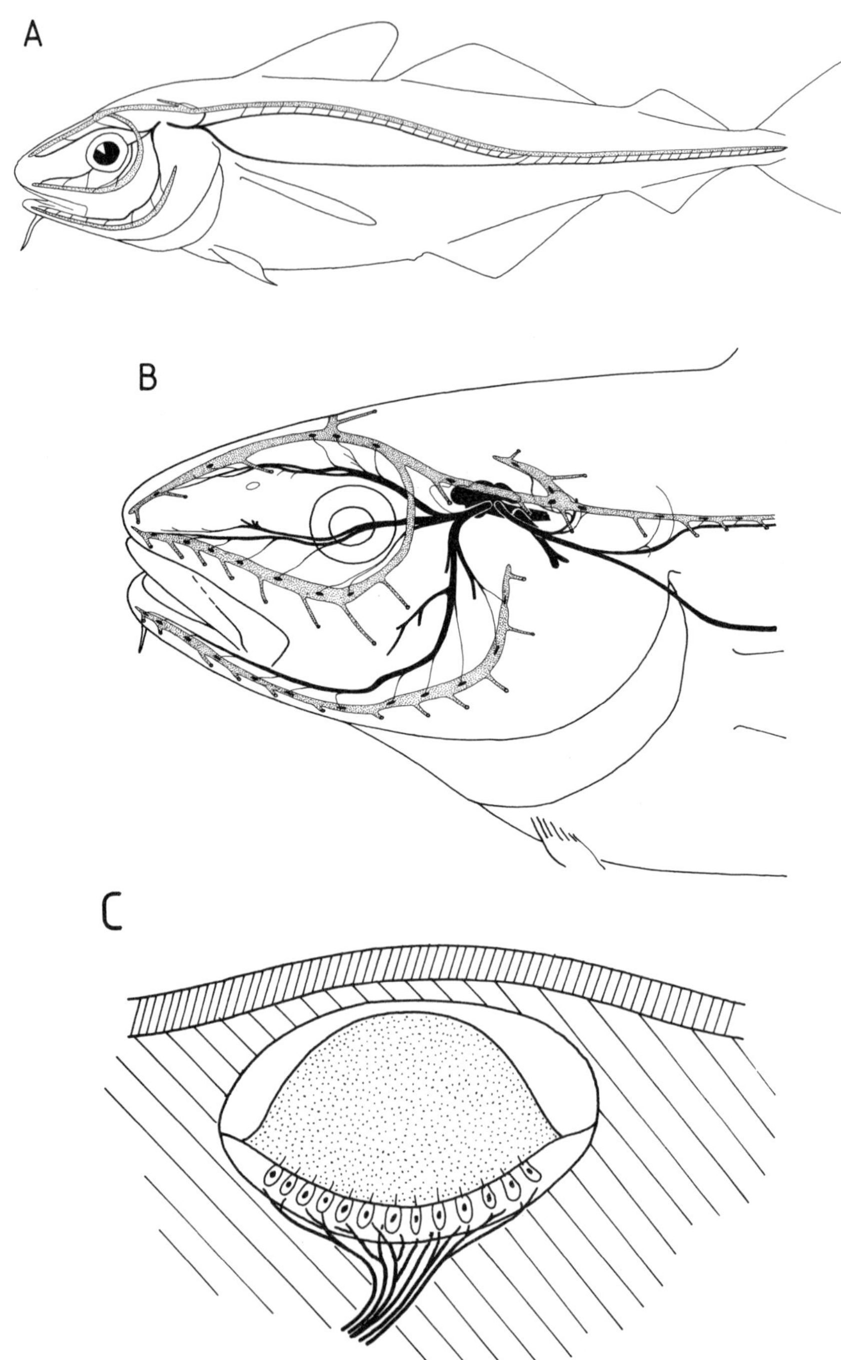
A
B
C

cells, forming a sensory epithelium, resting on a network of blood capillaries and the dendritic branches of the afferent nerve fibres. The hair bundles from the hair cells project into a jelly-like cupula resting upon the sensory epithelium.

The free standing neuromasts may occur singly at the bottom of pits or on raised eminences, the cupula projecting into the surrounding medium. In some cases the neuromasts are arranged in groups. For example, in the adult toad, *Xenopus laevis*, groups of three to twelve neuromasts are arranged more or less in a line on a slightly elevated ridge called a stitch (Murray, 1955; Gorner, 1963; Harris and Milne, 1966; Pabst, 1977). Many stitches run parallel to the long axis of the body, while others are orientated transversely to this axis (Fig. 3). The cupula is a flat rectangle in shape, rising 100 μm above the surface of the sensory membrane. The distal end is flaccid, and bends easily along its flat face, but the structure is relatively stiff along its long axis, which corresponds to the main axis of orientation of the polarized hair cells.

Canal neuromasts are usually completely surrounded by a constriction in the wall of the canal containing them and thus do not project into the surrounding medium. However, the canals themselves may open to the exterior by a system of pores, the neuromasts often lying midway between adjacent pores. The pores themselves may be multiple, or funnel shaped, but in some species of fish the canals are open only at the extreme ends, or are effectively closed off altogether with contact to the exterior only via a thin membrane. The surrounding fluid can then be substantially different in composition to the surrounding medium. In the burbot, *Lota lota*, it has a high potassium and low sodium content like the endolymph of the ear (Flock, 1965). In other fish the canal fluid resembles either seawater or an ultrafiltrate of the blood. The cupula of a canal organ is often dome-shaped as in the burbot where the cupula almost fills the canal. In most fish, despite the great variability in the development of the lateral line system the various canals or lines of organs follow a common pattern of a line on the flank, one over the eye, one beneath the eye and one running along the lower jaw.

One of the most striking electrophysiological features of the intact lateral line system is that the afferent fibres from the neuromasts show a high level of activity even in the absence of overt stimulation. Hoagland (1933) first described this so-called "spontaneous" discharge, while Sand (1937) pointed to the value of such a discharge in providing the sense

Figure 2 (A) Lateral line sensory canals on the head and flank of the cod (stippled) with the course of the lateralis nerves shown.
(B) Sensory canals of the head of the cod, showing the main neuromasts, and their innervation (modified from Cole, 1898).
(C) Schematic cross section of a neuromast from the trunk lateral line of the cod. Note the cupula almost filling the canal, and sitting upon the sensory hair cells.

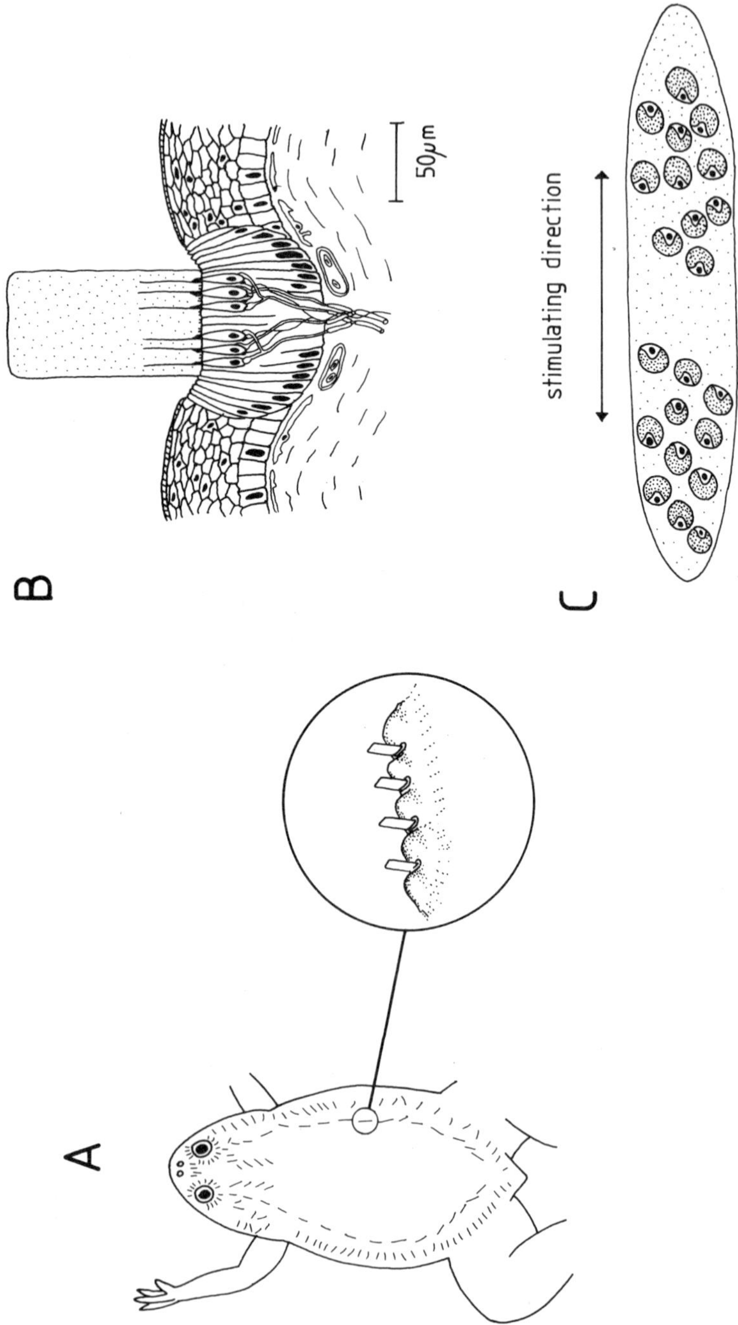
A
B
50μm
C
stimulating direction

organ with a mechanism for two-way modulation of its response. Indeed, Sand (loc. cit.) demonstrated that for a particular lateral line sense organ deflection of the cupula in one direction stimulated the activity of the afferent fibres, while deflection in the opposite direction inhibited the spontaneous rate of discharge. The spontaneous activity is irregular and is believed to be due to the spontaneous release of chemical transmitter at the afferent synapse of the hair cell (Harris and Flock, 1967). Recently, Pabst (1977) has shown for *Xenopus laevis* that each neuromast has its own impulse generation site and that the afferent activity of each stitch is thus the result of the combined activity of a number of spike generators on the same afferent fibre. It is clear, however, that all hair cells in one stitch having the same orientation are innervated by the same branching afferent fibre, while a second fibre innervates the hair cells of opposing orientation (Kroese *et al.*, 1978). Thus the inherent bidirectionality of the organ is preserved.

The functions of the ordinary lateral line system

Schulze (1870), who erroneously thought that water flowed through the sensory canals, regarded the lateral line system as detecting mass movement of the water but also thought it might be an accessory auditory organ. He was followed in this latter view by Mayser (1882). This early confusion of the function of the lateral line system with that of the auditory organs has persisted until the present day.

The view which has predominated is that the lateral line organs are not sound detectors but the water flow detectors of the integument. This idea was first proclaimed by Hofer (1908) and has since been strongly supported by the behavioural studies of Dijkgraaf (1934, 1947, 1956, 1963, 1967). Dijkgraaf has shown that the lateral line organs are sensitive to the movements of water acting locally upon the animal's body and produced by what he called "damming" phenomena in front of moving objects. He has stressed the role of the system in enabling the animal to orientate towards such sources of stimulation. Many of these water disturbances are generated by the animal's own activities (Dijkgraaf, 1963; Roberts, 1972). Gertychowa (1970) has shown that the blind catfish, *Anoptichthys jordani*, can locate nearby objects by detecting self-generated water displacements.

Figure 3 (A) In the clawed toad, *Xenopus*, groups of free standing neuromasts are lined up in rows (after Flock, 1967).
(B) The sensory epithelium is composed of hair cells and their supporting cells. Water motion displaces the cupula, which through the sensory hairs activates the receptor mechanism. Course of nerve fibres is conjectural.
(C) Adjacent hair cells are orientated with their kinocilia pointing in opposite directions. The kinocilium is indicated as a black dot on the periphery of each hair cell.

The function of the lateral line system in enabling fish to orientate to local hydrodynamic disturbances is also well established for aquatic amphibians. Görner (1963) has described how the lateral line organs of the clawed toad, *Xenopus*, respond differently to water displacements from different directions.

The lateral line system performs a more specialized function in some surface-dwelling fish, like the topminnow *Fundulus notatus*. The neuromasts serve in the detection of waves and ripples generated at the air–water interface (Schwartz, 1965, 1971; Schwartz and Hasler, 1966). The stimulus is essentially a low frequency transverse wave, whose propagation velocity depends on the frequency. When a floundering fly on the water surface generates such waves, the fish can orientate with respect to it, and thereby attack it. The orientation is abolished if parts of the lateral line system are removed. Different groups of lateral line organs are especially sensitive to surface waves approaching the fish from specific directions (Fig. 4), though the perceptual fields overlap one another, and this degree of overlap may be important in conveying an ability to respond precisely. Removal of the sense organs from one side of the head results in a disorientated response, and evidently the detection of direction depends on the collaboration of symmetrically located organs (Schwartz, 1967).

Though the lateral line system detects moving water there is no evidence that the organ has a proprioceptive function or that it is involved in the control of normal swimming (Dijkgraaf, 1963). Indeed, it is now

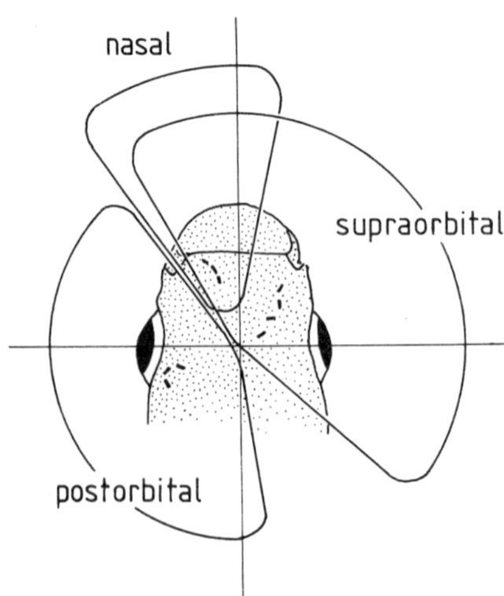

Figure 4 Receptive field of the nasal supraorbital and postorbital groups of sense organs in *Aplocheilus lineatus*. The symmetrically located fields and organs are not illustrated (after Schwartz, 1967).

clear from the work of Russell and Roberts (1972) on the dogfish *Scyliorhinus*, of Russell (1971) on *Xenopus*, and of Russell (1974) on the goldfish *Carassius*, that vigorous movement of the body results in activation of the efferent fibres innervating the lateral line sense organs. This efferent activity has an inhibitory effect upon spontaneous activity of the afferent fibres of the lateral line, a result which suggests that rather than the lateral line playing a part in locomotion its sensitivity is actually reduced during active movement. These neurophysiological findings are supported by the behavioural observation that when surface-feeding fish and toads are swimming they are less responsive to surface waves (Schwartz, 1967; Shelton, 1971). Russell (1974) has also reported an inhibition of second order lateral line neurones in the goldfish during active movement and has proposed that the role of the inhibitory pathways is to ensure that at the end of a period of vigorous movement the primary and second order sensory neurones are non-adapted, with their sensitivities fully preserved.

Kuiper (1967) has suggested that the lateral line system may not be disturbed by currents generated during normal swimming, by virtue of the so-called "boundary layer" of water carried along with the fish. Burying the lateral line organs in canals might also be expected to isolate them from the direct effects of many of the animal's own movements. That the lateral line system does not detect massive water currents which displace the whole fish, was stressed by Dijkgraaf (1963). Evidently the system does not inform a fish that it is being carried along in an ocean current at constant velocity. The cupulae, or the pores of the canals, must be stimulated by a local jet or wave of water movement.

Kuiper (1967) drew attention to the similarity between the lateral line system, and a differential Pitot system of instruments for measuring pressure gradients and hence water velocities, along a surface. The positioning of lateral line organs in canals, as well as affording the organs some protection against overstimulation during swimming, might also serve to define the axis of directionality of each individual organ. An organ placed in a canal between two openings will have its axis of maximal sensitivity defined by the line drawn between the two pores. Kuiper (1967) considered that the presence of the array of directional sense organs probably allowed quite sophisticated detection and spatial localization of moving objects.

This analysis of directional information by the lateral line system, whether the stimulus is a propagated surface wave, a moving turbulent eddy, or a linear jet of moving water, is of great interest but has hardly been touched upon. Schwartz (1967) performed a series of behavioural trials with a surface wave-detecting fish, and concluded that the curvature of the wave was a decisive factor in enabling the fish to locate the source. Kuroki (1967) treated the lateral line system (as opposed to the individual organ) as a time difference or phase difference detector determining the direction of a source by measuring differences in the time of receipt of the signals at the different organs. Harris (1967), questioned this approach, pointing out that the time differences were too small to be useful, and suggested that instead the system detected intensity gradients of water velocity. Recent electrophysiological studies have certainly confirmed that the individual neuromasts are detectors of water velocity. Kroese *et al.* (1978) and Strelioff and Honrubia (1978) have shown that the lateral line stitches of *Xenopus* show their response not to sustained deflection of the cupula but to the velocity of cupular movement. This supports the earlier suggestion by Harris and Milne (1966) that because of the elliptical shape of the cupula in *Xenopus*, the movement of the cupula would be proportional to fluid drag and therefore to velocity. The way signals of differing intensity received by the array of sense organs are integrated by the central nervous system deserves closer study.

The function of the lateral line in detecting local water movements has not always been apparent to all workers. Lowenstein (1967) has described some of the alternative functions that have been suggested for the system. They include sensitivity to chemicals, tactile stimuli, water velocity, hydrostatic pressure, and changes in temperature. The system has also been attributed with an equilibrium function, and has been implicated in the detection of sounds.

The lateral line as an auditory organ

The idea that the lateral line might constitute an accessory hearing organ has proved extraordinarily persistent since it was originally mooted by Schulze (1870) and Mayser (1882). After a particularly careful series of behavioural experiments with fish, Parker (1904) concluded that though the lateral line organs were *not* stimulated by sound, they were sensitive to water vibrations of low frequency. Parker described the effective stimulus as intermediate in character between that effective for the skin and the ear. In addition, studies by Suckling and Suckling (1951) have shown that small vibratory movements of the water can cause firing of the afferent fibres from the lateral line. However, perhaps the most influential work in rehabilitating the idea that the lateral line serves as an auditory organ has been that of Harris and van Bergeijk (1962), who showed that the lateral line organ responded electrophysiologically to the near field particle displacements generated in the water close to a sound source. These results led van Bergeijk (1967*a*, *b*) to postulate that the lateral line system, operating in the near field, provided the fish with its ability to localize a sound source. Furthermore, it led a number of workers to suggest that the low frequency auditory threshold curves obtained from fish through psychophysical experiments represented the response of the lateral line system rather than that of the inner ear (see, for example, Wodinsky and Tavolga, 1964, and Cahn, Siler and Wodinsky, 1969).

To consider more fully the implications of Harris and van Bergeijk's experiments we must consider the properties of sound in water.

Sound is a propagated mechanical disturbance generated by the movement of a source within any elastic medium. The speed of propagation (the velocity of sound) depends on the density of the medium and its elastic constants, and is some 4–5 times faster in water than in air. The travelling wave consists of a back and forth motion of the component particles of the medium (designated either the particle velocity, u, or the particle displacement d). However this motion of the medium is also accompanied by local changes in pressure (the sound pressure, p) above or below the prevailing hydrostatic pressure. The ratio of pressure to velocity is dependent upon the acoustic properties of the particular medium. Distant from a sound source, and in the absence of any discontinuities or perturbations in the sound field, the plane wave equation applies:

$$p = u\rho c$$

where ρc is the acoustic impedance of the medium.

Detection of a sound wave requires that energy from the travelling sound wave be transformed into some other form of energy, such as the movement of cilia relative to the sensory cell. This transformation operates only if the receptor has rather different acoustic properties to the medium in which it is placed. That is, there must be a change in mechanical impedance to generate relative motion between the receptor and the medium through which the sound is propagating.

From simple *a priori* considerations it would seem that the lateral line system does not constitute an ideal sound receptor. Unlike the inner ear, where the tectorial structure is loaded with a dense calcareous material of very different acoustic properties to the surrounding fluid, both the cupula and the tissue surrounding it are effectively transparent to underwater sound (Pumphrey, 1950). This inability of the lateral line neuromasts to detect sound waves has been confirmed by the experiments of Cahn, Siler and Fujiya (1973), who showed that the lateral line was not stimulated in the pressure null of a standing wave, despite the very large particle motions that are characteristic of such a sound field. Evidently the whole fish is moved back and forth along with the particle oscillations and the non-mass-loaded neuromasts fail to register this motion (Schuijf and Buwalda, personal communication). To stimulate the lateral line neuromasts, local water movements must impinge directly upon the cupula, as they do when the organs are stimulated by local hydrodynamic disturbances. The inner ear, on the other hand, is protected from direct stimulation, being totally enclosed within the head. The mass-loaded hair cells are stimulated by sound waves travelling through the tissues. A very good response is obtained from the otolith organs in the pressure null of a standing wave (Hawkins and MacLennan, 1976) in contrast to the result obtained from the lateral line. Harris and van Bergeijk (1962) nevertheless showed that in some circumstances the unloaded neuromasts of the lateral line could be stimulated by sound. These authors pointed out that close to a sound source there is a zone, which they called the near field, characterized by very high particle motions. The near field effect is associated with the fact that sound sources whose linear dimensions are small compared with one wavelength, produce diverging or spherical waves, in which the acoustic energy spreads over an increasingly greater area as the wave progresses. General equations describing this three-dimensional acoustic wave are derived in most textbooks of acoustics (e.g., Camp, 1970). In a spherical wave, the relationship between sound pressure and particle velocity or displacement is much more complicated than in the plane wave equation described earlier. Particle velocity is no longer in phase with sound pressure, but lags by up to 90°. Furthermore, the particle velocity is no longer related to sound pressure by a simple ratio but is dependent upon the distance from the sound source. Close to the source, increasingly higher particle velocities (and particle displacements, $d = u/2\pi f$ where f is the frequency) are associated with a given sound pressure.

Fig. 5 illustrates the near field effect for a simple sound source. In this figure the particle displacements for a standard sound pressure of 1 μbar ($0.1\ \mathrm{N\,m^{-2}}$) are given at different distances from a source. Data are provided for several frequencies. It can be seen that not only do relatively large particle displacements accompany a given sound pressure close to the source, an effect which is more pronounced at low frequencies, but that there is an extremely strong displacement gradient with distance. We shall return to this point later. More distant from the source, in the far field, where the plane wave equation applies, particle displacement is dependent only upon the sound pressure.

Harris and van Bergeijk (1962) demonstrated that for the killifish, *Fundulus heteroclitus*, microphonic potentials could be recorded from the lateral line neuromasts when the fish was placed in the near field of a sound source operating at 100 Hz. Harris and van Bergeijk concluded that since the cupula is in a mucus-filled canal in the killifish, the motion of the cupula is probably proportional to the particle displacement rather than to the particle velocity.

This finding is at first rather surprising and appears to contradict the later observation of Cahn, Siler and Fujiya (1973) that the neuromasts are not stimulated in the pressure null of a standing wave where particle motion is also very large. The difference lies in the gradient of particle motion in the two experimental situations. In the pressure null of a low

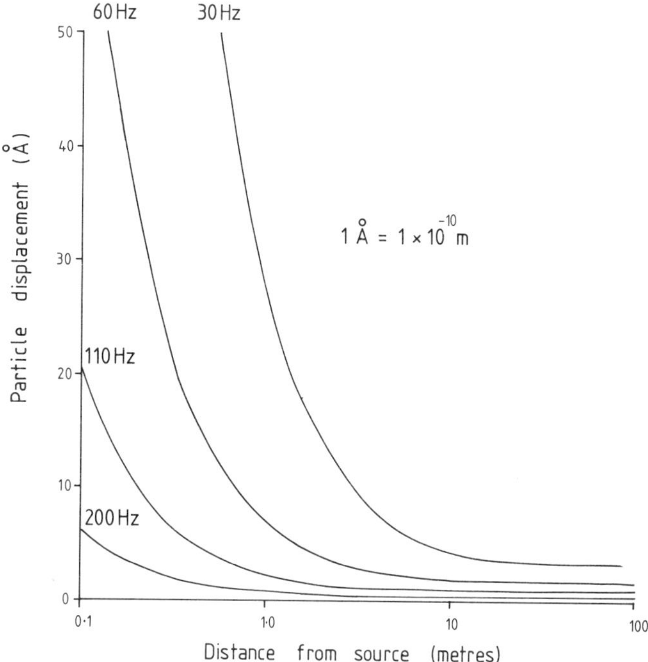

Figure 5 The "near field" effect, showing the steep decline in the amplitude of displacement with distance from a monopole sound source. All values are for a sound pressure of 1 μbar (0.1 N m^{-2}).

frequency standing wave the magnitude of particle displacement is large but does not vary greatly with distance. In the near field of a sound source, however, there is a very steep gradient in displacement. It would seem that for the fish, and perhaps even the individual neuromast, to detect particle motion there must be a steep intensity gradient along the body or between adjacent pores of the lateral line.

One might expect the lateral line neuromasts, and other lightly loaded end organs, to be sensitive to sound waves under other circumstances where there is a steep particle motion gradient, for example, near an air/water interface, where a pressure release effect results in the generation of large local particle motions. It should therefore be noted that in Clupeid fish some of the sense organs of the cranial part of the lateral line are in close proximity to a gas filled bulla (Denton and Blaxter, 1976), and may therefore be stimulated in a sound field.

Despite these examples of possible sound detection by the lateral line we must accept Dijkgraaf's (1963) conclusion that the lateral line does not have sound reception as its principal function. The system clearly has other behaviour-related functions in the majority of fish and amphibians.

Nor is it the only, or even the most sensitive sound receptor. Kuiper (1967) has measured the sensitivity of the lateral line neuromasts of the fish *Acerina cernua* to displacement and gives a figure of about 25 Å at 75 Hz, with the response dropping off steeply above this frequency. This compares with about 0.5 Å for the estimated displacement sensitivity in the saccular otolith organ of the cod, *Gadus morhua* (Chapman and Hawkins, 1973), at the same frequency, this more sensitive response extending to even higher frequencies.

The specialized lateral line organs

The main lateral line organs are to be viewed principally as mechanoreceptors, though their precise functions may sometimes be debated. In many fish there is also present in the integument an array of sense organs also innervated by the lateralis nerve, and clearly forming part of the lateral line system, but having other more specialized non-mechanoreceptive functions.

The ampullae of Lorenzini are receptors found in the skin of sharks and rays (Fig. 6B). Other types of ampullae are also found in elasmobranchs, and also in certain teleost groups, notably the Siluridae, Gymnotidae, Mormyridae, Gymnarchidae, Brachiopterygii and Dipnoi. Though the ampullae of elasmobranchs correspond to a basic structural pattern, those of the teleosts show great variation and apparent specialization and may have a range of different names applied to them by different authors. In contrast to the ordinary lateral line organs, amongst the more specialized lateral line organs, only the ampullae of Lorenzini of marine elasmobranchs and the microampullae of freshwater elasmobranchs are provided with hair cells. The sensory cells of the ampullary organs of teleosts generally bear only microvilli at their apical surfaces (Szabo, 1972, 1974, and Fig. 6C).

In the ampullary organs of teleosts and elasmobranchs the apical surfaces of the sensory cells lining each ampulla are in contact with a jelly-filled canal which travels to the epidermal surface (Fig. 6A). Marine fish generally have long canals and freshwater fish short ones. In the skin of the teleost families Mormyridae, Gymnotidae and Gymnarchidae is what appears to be a functionally distinct type of specialized lateral line organ, the so-called tuberous organ or *Knollenorgane* (Fig. 6D). These differ from the ampullary organs in that the sensory cells do not communicate with a cavity leading to the surface but the greater part of them are covered by specialized epidermal cells, while only a small basal part attaches to the supporting cell hillock.

Bullock (1974) has recounted the fascinating story of the discovery of those various specialized sensory receptors of the lateral line, and the gradual assignment to them of an electroreceptive function. A detailed

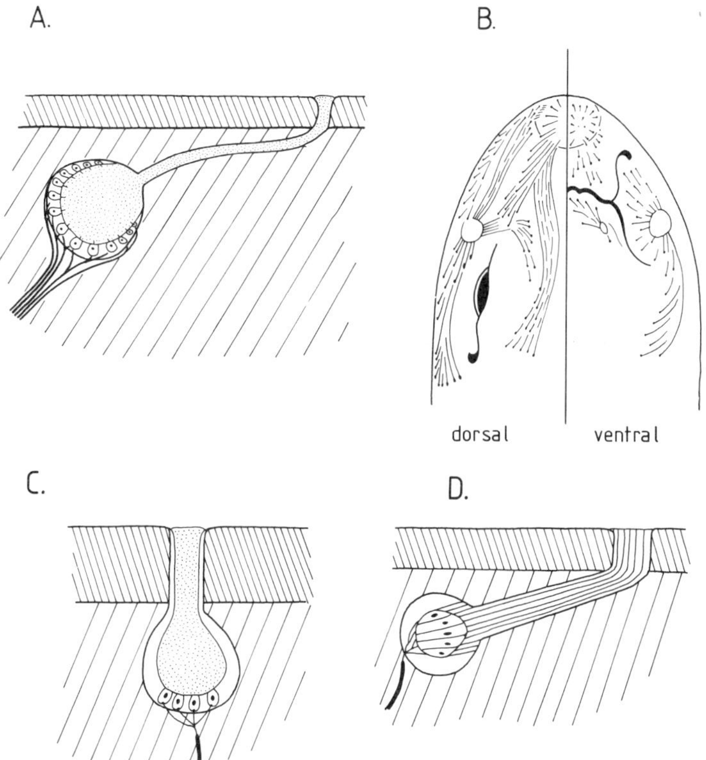

Figure 6 (A) Schematic diagram of an ampullary lateral line organ, leading to the surface by a jelly-filled canal (after Dijkgraaf, 1963).
(B) Dorsal and ventral views of the ampullae of Lorenzini in the dogfish, *Scyliorhinus canicula*.
(C) Ampullary lateral line organ of a Gymnotid fish (after Szabo, 1974).
(D) Tuberous organ of a Gymnotid fish (after Szabo, 1974).

consideration of the electroreceptive function of the various specialized lateral line organs is given by Szabo and by Bullock (this volume). It would seem that passive reception by low-frequency electroreceptors has evolved independently several times in the vertebrates (Bullock, 1974), and that the specialized lateral line organs have developed from ordinary lateral line organs (Lissman and Mullinger, 1968; Bennett, 1970).

The ear

The fish ear

The fully developed fish ear may vary greatly from species to species in its general shape and in the relative proportion of its different parts. In the

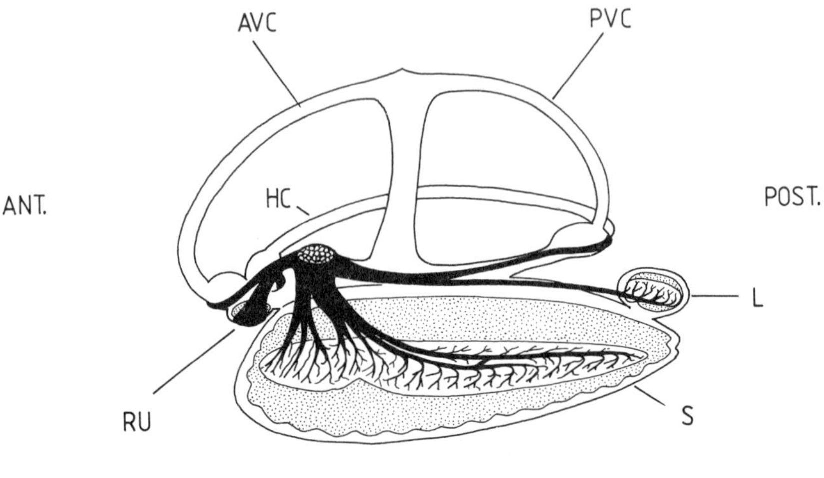

Figure 7 Medio-lateral view of the right ear of the cod, showing the three semicircular canals, and the three otolith organs. The various nerve rami are shown in black. AVC, anterior vertical canal. HC, horizontal canal. PVC, posterior vertical canal. L, lagena. RU, recessus utriculi. S. sacculus. Note that in this fish the endolymphatic duct is absent.

majority of fish, and in amphibia, the semicircular canals come to lie in three closely orthogonal planes (i.e., at mutual right angles), each canal having an expansion at one end, the ampulla (Fig. 7). Each ampulla contains a receptor organ, the crista, consisting of a group of sensory hair cells and an overlying cupula. Two of the canals lie predominantly in the vertical plane—the anterior and posterior vertical canals. They are joined medially by the crus communis which fuses ventrally with a caudal extension of the utriculus—the utricular canal. The ampulla of the anterior vertical canal joins with the rostral end of the main part of the utriculus—the utricular recess. The ampulla of the posterior canal generally joins with the utricular canal, posterior to the crus communis. However, in the shark *Carcharhinus* (Tester *et al.*, 1972) the posterior canal duct joins directly to the sacculus of the pars inferior (see Fig. 10). The remaining semicircular canal lies in the horizontal plane, with its ampulla adjacent to that of the anterior vertical canal entering the utricular recess. Essentially, in teleosts and amphibia all three canals join at the utriculus, which provides fluid continuity between them. Even in those sharks where the posterior canal duct joins with the sacculus there is still fluid continuity via the utriculo-saccular duct or canal.

In the cyclostomes, or lampreys, a horizontal canal is absent, leaving

A.

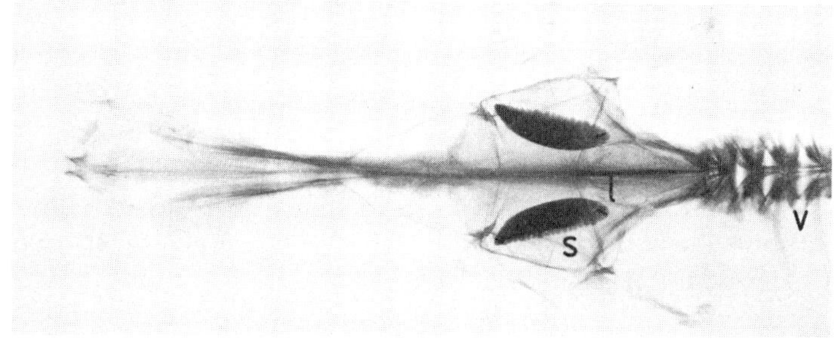

B.

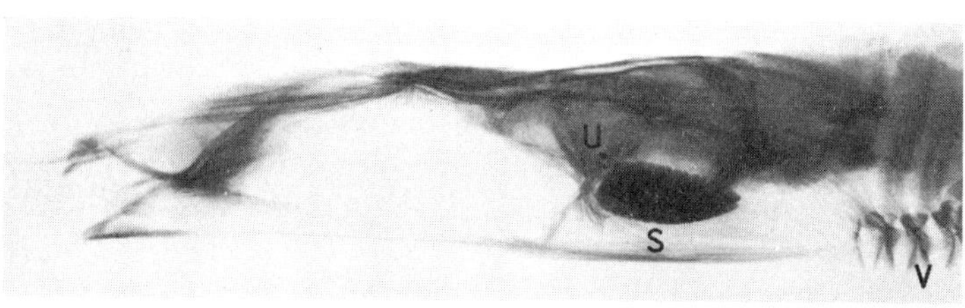

Figure 8 Radiographs of the cranium of the cod, showing the locations of the three principal otoliths.
(A) Dorsal view, showing the large paired saccular otoliths and the small lagenar otoliths (l) at the caudal end. The vertebral column is indicated (v).
(B) Lateral view. The utricular otoliths can be seen at the rostral end of the ear (u).

only two vertical canals (Lowenstein *et al.*, 1968), while the hagfish, *Myxine*, has a single canal, though with two canal receptors or cristae (van Bergeijk, 1967; Lowenstein and Thornhill, 1970).

In most elasmobranchs the endolymphatic duct remains open to the exterior via a small pore, thereby connecting the sacculus to the surrounding medium. In many teleosts the duct ends blindly, and may be much reduced in size.

Beneath the utriculus of the pars superior, and in fluid continuity with it, lie the sacculus and lagena of the pars inferior. Each of these, together with the utriculus, contains a sensory membrane or macula composed of hair cells and their supporting cells. Each macula is surmounted by a dense layer of crystalline calcium carbonate, which in the elasmobranchs and amphibia consists of a mass of separate crystals, the otoconia, bound together by a web-like membrane. In most teleosts, the separate crystals are replaced by a solid "stone" or otolith of calcium carbonate.

The structural organization of the maculae in fish has been examined by Lowenstein *et al.* (1964, 1968); Lowenstein and Thornhill (1970); Nakajima and Wang (1974); Dale (1976); Jorgensen (1976); Enger

(1967); Popper (1977, 1978); Jenkins (1979) and others. The otoliths or otoconia are separated from the hair cells of the macular surface by an intervening otolithic membrane, divisible into several layers. The apical surface of each sensory cell shows a ciliary bundle projecting into the subcupular part of the membrane, consisting of the typical arrangement of a single kinocilium and a large number of shorter stereocilia. There is some differentiation into different hair cell types across the macula, the more peripheral hair cells generally having longer kinocilia. In the central part of the macula the hair bundles project into cavities in the reticular, subcupular part of the membrane. On the periphery, the taller processes of the hair cells may attach to the membrane. The calcareous otolith does not contact the hair cells directly.

The different maculae within the ear have quite different orientations. The utricular macula lies mainly in the horizontal plane, with the otolith sitting upon it. The saccular and lagenar maculae and their respective otoliths lie predominantly in vertical planes (Figs. 7 and 8). A striking feature of the maculae in all the aquatic vertebrates is the high degree of directional organization of the hair cells within them. Whereas in the

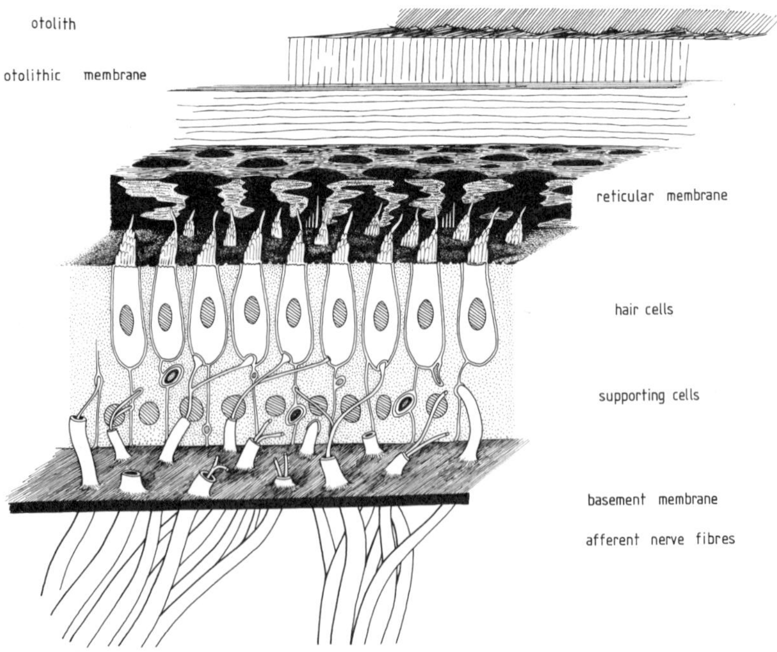

Figure 9 Schematic section through the saccular macula of the cod. Note the common orientation of the sensory hair cells. The hairs do not contact the calcareous otolith but are separated from it by several membranes. In the living animal the basement membrane lies in the vertical plane, with the otolith in a lateral position.

cristae of the semicircular canals the morphologically polarized hair cells are orientated in one direction only, in the maculae they may be segregated into several zones, the cells of each zone having a characteristic orientation, often differing from that of adjacent zones. In general, where there are hair cells orientated in a particular direction there will be another zone in which the hair cells have an opposing orientation. It would seem that this directional pattern is preserved in the afferent nerve fibres which synapse with the hair cells (Furukawa and Ishii, 1967; Hawkins and Horner, 1980), many of the afferent fibres giving a spike discharge on movement of the otolith in one direction only. However, in the goldfish saccular macula there are some fibres which are linked to hair cells of opposing orientation, and these discharge spikes on both phases of the sound stimulus (Furukawa, 1978). Perhaps the simplest pattern of hair cell orientation is found in the sacculus of the Ostariophysan fish, and in the lagena of a great range of species where there are simply two zones of hair cells with opposing or complementary orientations. In the utriculus, and in the sacculus of many non-Ostariophysans the pattern of hair cell orientation may be much more complex.

In most elasmobranchs, and in some teleosts, a macula is found which is not loaded by an otolithic structure. This is the macula neglecta, a sensory membrane with its own nerve ramus situated in the utricular canal, or in the posterior canal duct, depending on the species (Tester *et al.*, 1972). In elasmobranchs, the part of the canal duct containing the macula neglecta may be placed close to a membrane-covered fenestra in the chondrocranium, leading to the endolymphatic fossa, a depressed part of the cranium containing gelatinous connective tissue (Fig. 10). In the more active pelagic sharks the macula neglecta consists of two strips of membrane containing sensory hair cells inside a tubular structure which

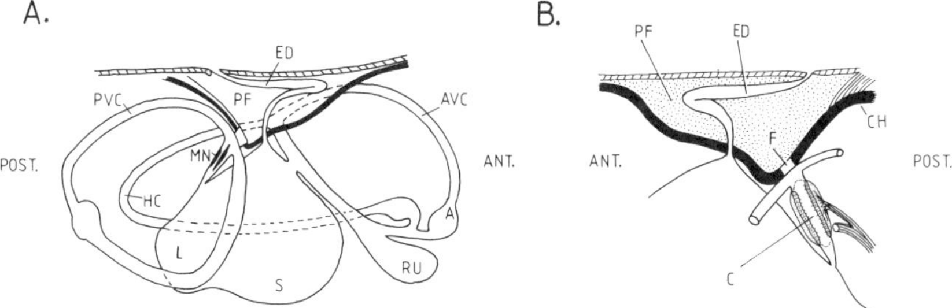

Figure 10 (A) Schematic diagram of the left ear of *Carcharhinus menisorrah* showing the relationship of the posterior canal duct to the fenestra, parietal fossa, and endolymphatic duct.
(B) Schematic section through the right ear. AVC, anterior vertical canal. PVC, posterior vertical canal. HC, horizontal canal. A, ampulla. C, cupula of macula neglecta. CH, chondrocranium. ED, endolymphatic duct. F, fenestra. MN, macula neglecta. PF, parietal fossa.

houses a single sausage-shaped cupula (Fay *et al.*, 1974). Corwin (1977) describes the cupula as having a light collagenous structure, and reports that the two sensory membranes each contain very large populations of hair cells. In orientation, the hairs of one patch oppose the hairs of the other, along the length of the tube. In the less active sharks, and in the bottom-dwelling rays, the macula consists of a single epithelial patch containing few hair cells, with a rather disordered orientation (Lowenstein *et al.*, 1964; Corwin, 1980).

It is clear that lightly loaded maculae are also found in the utriculus of the Clupeid fishes (Wohlfahrt, 1936; O'Connell, 1955; van Bergeijk, 1967; Gray and Denton, 1979). The pattern of hair cell orientation shown by the utriculus of the herring, *Clupea*, appears to be unique (Popper and Platt, 1979). In the Clupeidae, and in a number of other teleost groups, there is a close association between particular parts of the ear and gas-filled spaces. Thus, in the herring, *Clupea harengus*, there are two gas-filled bullae, one on either side of the head, each mechanically linked with the utriculus, and with lateral line neuromasts in adjacent head canals. These bullae are connected by exceedingly fine gas-filled tubes to the swimbladder, and with change of depth the volumes of the gas-filled parts of the bullae are maintained constant by exchanges of gas with the swimbladder. A change in pressure in the gas-filled part of the bulla causes a displacement of a membrane, which is transferred as a movement of liquid through a fenestra by means of a thin membrane acting as a release window to the exterior. The motion which is set up stimulates the maculae of the utriculus and also several lateral line sense organs adjacent to the release window (Denton and Blaxter, 1976).

In the Ostariophysi there is a link between the gas-filled swimbladder and the sacculus. A separate anterior chamber of the swimbladder is mechanically connected by a chain of small bones, the Weberian ossicles, to a perilymphatic space, the sinus impar, which in turn is connected with a transverse canal filled with endolymph, running into the sacculus (von Frisch, 1938; Alexander, 1962). The saccular otolith has a wing-like projection extending into the endolymph, adjacent to the opening of the transverse canal. Van Bergeijk (1967) suggested that fluid displacements from the transverse canal rock the otolith on its long axis, and Jenkins (1979) suggests that the pivotal axis of the otolith is established by its attachment to the perimacular epithelium. The fluid motion within the sacculus is possible because there is a flexible region, or pressure release window, in the saccular wall.

Many other teleost fish also have a connection between a gas sac and the ear. In the Mormyridae, two gas-filled vesicles lie alongside the sacculi, the boundary between the structures being filled by a fine membrane. A gas-secretory rete mirabile is found in each vesicle and presumably maintains the volume of gas in the vesicle in the absence of any connection to the swimbladder (Stipetic, 1939). In the Moridae or deep sea cod, an anterior extension from the gas-filled swimbladder contacts the endolymph of the sacculus through a membrane stretched across a foramen in the basi-occipital bone.

The ear of aquatic amphibians

The pars superior of the amphibian ear, like that of most vertebrates, follows the typical pattern of three semicircular canals, and an otolith-filled sac, the utriculus. The pars inferior, however, has undergone further development in comparison with that of teleosts. There is usually a greatly expanded endolymphatic duct, ending blindly in a capacious sac, which fills the intracranial space. In addition, two additional maculae develop in many amphibia, the basilar papilla, and the amphibian papilla. The latter is found in the salamanders, frogs and toads, but is absent from some primitive perennibranchiate amphibians. It is the basilar papilla which in reptiles, birds and mammals develops into a more prominent appendage to the ear, the cochlea. The amphibian papilla, on the other hand, is found in all amphibia, but is lacking in the amniotes (Witschi, 1949). Each of these auditory papillae has its own set of hair cells and a separate gelatinous tectorial membrane.

The basilar papilla develops in a tubular exvagination of the wall of the sacculus, adjacent to the lagena. In the adult bullfrog, *Rana catesbeiana*, the papilla contains about 95 hair cells innervated by 300–500 nerve fibres (Capranica, 1978). The hair bundles of the sensory cells project into recesses within the overlying tectorial membrane. Fluid motions set up in the extensive perilymphatic spaces of the head are coupled to the endolymph by way of a thin membrane, producing movement of the tectorial membrane and hence exciting the hair cells.

The amphibian papilla is a protuberance of the dorso-medial wall of the sacculus, lying just under the utriculus. The macula is sigmoid in shape and contains about 1500 hair cells, innervated by about 1000 nerve fibres. The pattern of hair cell polarization of this macula is complex, the significance of this arrangement being unknown. The frequency response of the papilla is determined primarily by the properties of the tectorial membrane and its attachment, and within the papilla frequency appears to be represented spatially. Thus, the "place" mechanism makes its first appearance in the anuran amphibian papilla (Capranica, 1978).

The basilar and amphibian papillae have their own independent nerve rami from the auditory nerve. The basilar papilla appears to lack efferent innervation (Frishkopf and Flock, 1974) but efferent synapses have been reported from the amphibian papilla (Flock and Flock, 1966).

The anurans develop a middle ear at metamorphosis as an adaptation to a terrestrial existence. A drum membrane, or tympanum on the outside

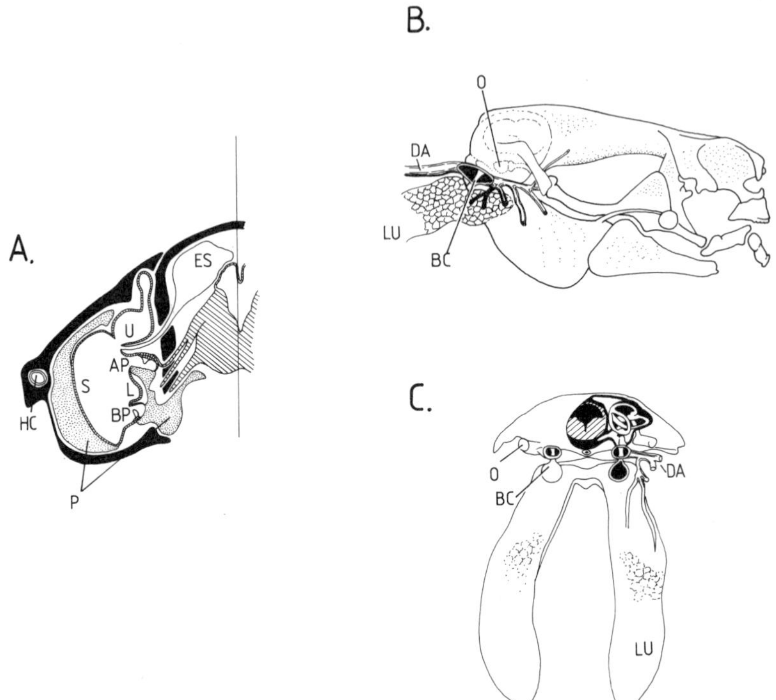

Figure 11 (A) Schematic T.S. of membranous labyrinth and perilymphatic system of *Xenopus* during metamorphosis. Note the position of the amphibian and basilar papillae (modified from Paterson, 1949).
(B) *Rana clamitans* in early metamorphosis. Lateral view showing bronchial columella passing through dorsal aorta.
(C) *R. clamitans*, posterior view with part of cranium cut away. AP, amphibian papilla. BC, bronchial columella. BP, basilar papilla. DA, dorsal aorta. ES, endolymphatic sac. HC, horizontal canal, L. lagena. LU, lung. P, perilymph. O, operculum. S, sacculus. U, utriculus.

of the head is connected by a chain of fused ossicles, the tympanic columella, to an operculum in the side of the skull. Thus, sound is conducted from the surrounding air to the perilymphatic spaces surrounding the inner ear.

The structure and operation of the terrestrial middle ear does not concern us here. What is important is that the middle ear structure is paralleled in the frog tadpole by an entirely independent aquatic middle ear. This part of the ear has been described by Witschi (1949) for *Rana clamitans* and is illustrated in Fig. 11. The lungs of the tadpole are joined by a short stiff connective tissue rod, the bronchial columella, to a round window in the otic capsule. To reach the skull, the columella pierces the dorsal aorta. Movement of the air-filled lungs is thus transmitted directly to the perilymph surrounding the ear, an oval window situated in a lateral

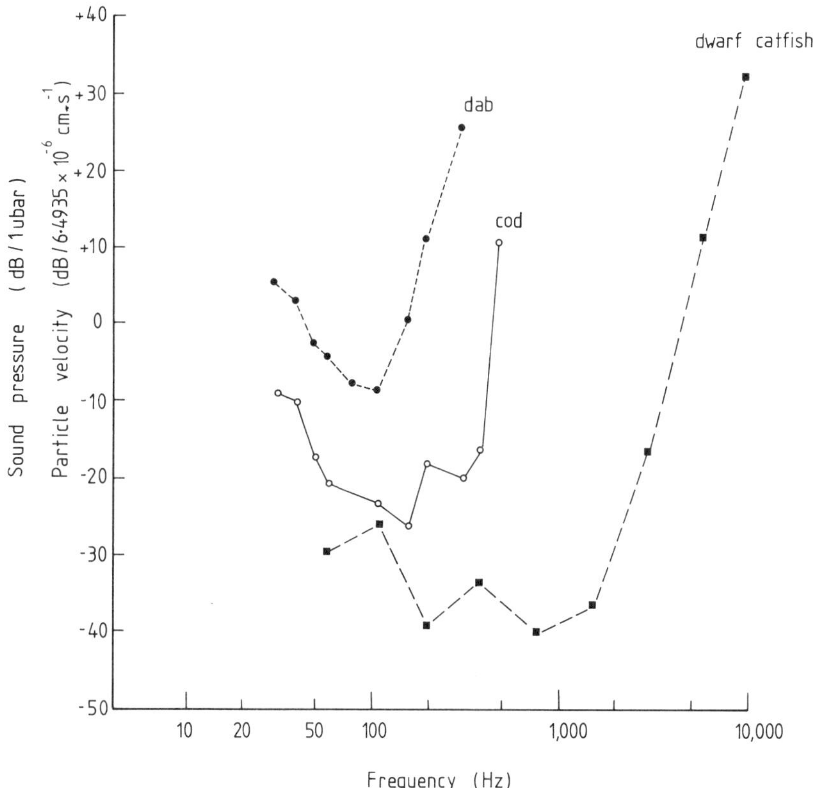

Figure 12 Audiograms for three species of teleost fish. Data for the dab from Chapman and Sand (1974), for the cod from Chapman and Hawkins (1973), and for the dwarf catfish from Poggendorf (1952).

position serving as a release window. At metamorphosis, the oval window develops an operculum, coupled to the terrestrial middle ear, while the bronchial columella degenerates, allowing the round window to serve as a release window. At metamorphosis the structure of the inner ear does not change.

Thus, though the inner ear is more developed, the aquatic ear of the tadpole has much in common with the ear of the goldfish and other fish, showing a coupling of the ear to a gas-filled space.

The functions of the inner ear

We have already commented on a fundamental difference between the inner ear and lateral line of aquatic vertebrates. The former is completely buried within the tissues of the head and is therefore independent of local water movements. Thus, though the semicircular canals of fish and amphibians bear a superficial resemblance to the lateral line organs and may indeed have developed from them in evolutionary history, their function is quite different. The former can essentially be regarded as functionally closed fluid-containing semicircular tubes, with fluid continuity being maintained via the utriculus. It has long been established that such a mechanical system is sensitive to angular motion of the head. Thus any angular acceleration in the plane of the toroidal canal will result in the fluid contained within it lagging behind by virtue of its inertia. The relative motion of the canal and fluid displaces the cupula, exciting the hair cells of the crista. Such a system is rather insensitive to translational accelerations such as those produced by linear motion, or by gravity.

The arrangement of the three semicircular canals of each ear in three orthogonal planes is clearly related to the perception of angular acceleration in three dimensional space. However, not only does each individual ear have a canal in each of three mutually perpendicular planes, but the canals on either side of the head are complementary. That is, pairs of canals on opposite sides of the skull tend to parallel one another, generating differentially organized outputs of opposite sign. Thus, counterclockwise motion of the head stimulates the crista of the left horizontal canal, producing a more frequent discharge of the regularly active canal afferent neurones, while it suppresses the activity of the right canal primary afferents. This differential action of the sense organs seems to be a fundamental feature of the vertebrate inner ear.

Just as the morphology of the semicircular canals fits them for inertial transduction of movement in the three rotational degrees of freedom, so the otolith organs are fitted for the inertial transduction of linear acceleration in the three translational degrees of freedom. We have seen that each otolith organ consists of a heavy mass—the otolith—sitting on a sensory membrane or macula. Linear acceleration of the whole body causes the heavy mass to be left behind by virtue of its own inertia, thereby exciting the hair cells of the sensory membrane. Similarly, a tilting of the head causes the otolith to move to one side under the action of gravity. The mechanics of such a system have been reviewed in some detail by Wilson and Jones (1979). The principal source of data on the movements of the otoliths is de Vries (1950), who based his observations on the otoliths of fish. De Vries derived a series of constants for the otolith organs, relating both to their static and dynamic responses to acceleration. His general conclusion was that the movement of the otolith is critically damped, giving it a rapid response to linear acceleration without any prolonged period of oscillation at the end of the acceleration.

The early work of Lowenstein and Roberts (1949) on the otolith organs of the ray, *Raja clavata*, showed clearly that all three otolith organs (those of the utriculus, sacculus and lagena) were sensitive to the gravitational stimuli generated by positional changes. It was shown that the afferent fibres of the utriculus gave an excitatory response to tilts around a wide range of axes. Like the afferents of the semicircular canals, many of the primary afferent fibres of the macular epithelia showed a high spontaneous firing rate, enabling the organ to give a bidirectional signalling of response from the morphologically polarized hair cells. Determination of the sensitivity vectors of the three separate otolith organs has been performed only for mammals (Fernandez and Goldberg, 1976). It is clear that in the monkey the saccular and utricular otolith organs both respond to static gravitational stimuli, and that the distributions of vectors shown by the two organs are quite different. The main vectors of the utriculus spread out in a fan-like way in a plane tilted some 9° from the horizontal. The vectors of the sacculus are clustered in a plane almost at right angles to the plane of the utriculus and slightly tilted from the vertical.

The otolith organs are not only sensitive to static tilting of the head but also respond to dynamic stimulation. Indeed many of the afferent fibres show an extreme degree of adaptation in a stationary position and cannot therefore constitute static position sensors (Lowenstein and Saunders, 1975). The dynamic otolith units show a low frequency random discharge and fire more rapidly in response to low frequency sinusoidal stimuli or to an applied "ramp" of linear acceleration. Wilson and Jones (1979) have stressed that there is ambiguity between measurements of gravity and linear acceleration which necessitates a separation of gravitoinertial information into static gravitational and dynamic linear accelerative components to allow the animal to distinguish between a change in attitude, or a translational movement. In fish, and perhaps also in aquatic amphibians, the otolith organs also serve as detectors of propagated sound waves (von Frisch, 1938). An explanation for the stimulation of these organs by sound was provided by Pumphrey (1950). Pumphrey pointed out that in an underwater sound field the tissues of fish were essentially transparent to sound, and tended to move back and forth in phase with the applied particle motion. However, the dense calcareous otolith, with its very different acoustic properties to water, lagged behind in its movement, giving rise to shearing forces in the macula which excited the hair cells. Such a sensor is essentially a particle motion detector.

It is now well established that fish can hear and that they can distinguish between sounds of differing quality, and sounds coming from differing directions (reviews by Griffin, 1955; Kleerekoper and Changon, 1955; Moulton, 1963; Tavolga, 1971; Popper and Fay, 1973; Hawkins, 1973; Fay and Popper, 1980). The frequency range of sounds which can be detected by individual fish varies. Some fish, for example the flatfish studied by Chapman and Sand (1974) and the salmon studied by Hawkins and Johnstone (1976), show a rather restricted frequency range, and a limited sensitivity (Fig. 12) compared to many others like the cod

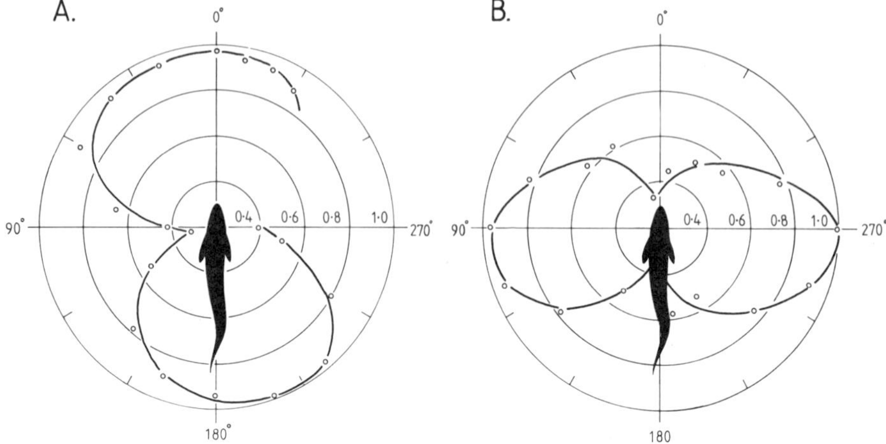

Figure 13 (A) Response of a primary unit from the anterior saccular ramus of the left auditory nerve of the cod to stimulation at different angles of azimuth. The response is shown as the mean number of spikes per unit cycle, along the radius.
(B) Response of a unit from the utricular ramus.

(Chapman and Hawkins, 1973) and dwarf catfish (Poggendorf, 1952). The main difference is that in the latter species the otolith organ is functionally coupled to the gas-filled swimbladder. Sound pressures incident upon the gas-filled swimbladder therefore force the latter organ to pulsate, The amplitude of motion at the periphery of the gas bladder is far greater than the amplitude of particle motion in the free sound field. Thus, if this amplified motion is transmitted to the otolith organs of the ear, the sensitivity of the organ is increased. Increase in sensitivity, and hence bandwidth, is not the only advantage of a sound pressure detector, however. We shall see later that the presence of a sound pressure-sensitive organ permits the resolution of ambiguities in determining the direction of a sound source.

There are two aspects of hearing in fish which have recently attracted great interest. These are the analysis of sound direction by the auditory system, and the analysis of sound quality.

It is now well established that at least some teleosts have a directional hearing sense. The cod, *Gadus morhua*, can detect a change in the direction of propagation of sound, and can discriminate between spatially separated sound sources both in the horizontal and vertical planes (Chapman and Johnstone, 1974; Schuijf, 1975; Hawkins and Sand, 1977). Indeed, the cod can discriminate direction in circumstances which are ambiguous or confusing for man (Schuijf and Buwalda, 1980).

Fish do not determine the direction of sound using differences in the time of arrival, phase and intensity at the two ears, as do man and the other large mammals. The speed of sound in water is so fast that differences in the time of arrival or phase at the two ears are too small. Moreover, fish are small in relation to the sound wavelengths of interest to them, and having the same overall properties as the surrounding water any sound shadowing is minimal, and differences in signal strength at the two ears insignificant.

As we have seen, Pumphrey (1950) suggested that the otolith organs were sensitive to the movement of the medium accompanying passage of a sound wave. Dijkgraaf (1960) pointed out that such a particle motion detector is inherently directional. Depending on the suspension of the otolith, and the orientation of the polarized hair cells, the organ will respond differently to sound waves incident from different directions. Confirmation of the directionality of the sacculus was provided by Enger *et al.* (1973), who showed that the amplitude of microphonic potentials from this otolith organ was highly dependent upon the direction of stimulation in the horizontal plane. More recently, Hawkins and Horner (1980) have shown that the primary afferent fibres of both the sacculus and utriculus of cod are strongly directional in the horizontal plane. Examples of the directional responses of a saccular and a utricular unit are given in Fig. 13.

Thus, it would seem that the direction of a sound can be determined in fish by comparison of the outputs of two or more differently aligned bidirectional receivers or vector detectors. Indeed, it looks very much as if the organization of the static receptive function of the otolith organs into orthogonally orientated vectors may well be paralleled in the auditory system.

Schuijf (1976) has pointed out that such a vector weighing procedure yields a 180° ambiguity in the determination of sound source direction. However, he suggests that the addition of a receiver sensitive to sound pressure can resolve the ambiguity. Such a receiver exists in the ears of fish like the cod, the Ostariophysans, and the Clupeids where the ear is coupled to a gas space. What is not clear for these species is to what extent the specialization of one or more of the maculae to detect sound pressure interferes with its capacity to act as a vector detector responding to particle motion. In other fish, without any obvious sound pressure receiver the means of resolution of the ambiguity is less clear. It is possible that in those fish with a macula neglecta this end organ might form a functional reference receiver. Close to an air/water interface like the water surface, where there is a strong gradient of particle motion to stimulate the organ, a reference signal is provided which is independent of the direction of propagation.

The mechanism by which sound quality is analysed by fish is a matter of conjecture. The auditory response of primary afferent nerve fibres has been recorded for a number of species of fish: goldfish, *Carassius auratus*

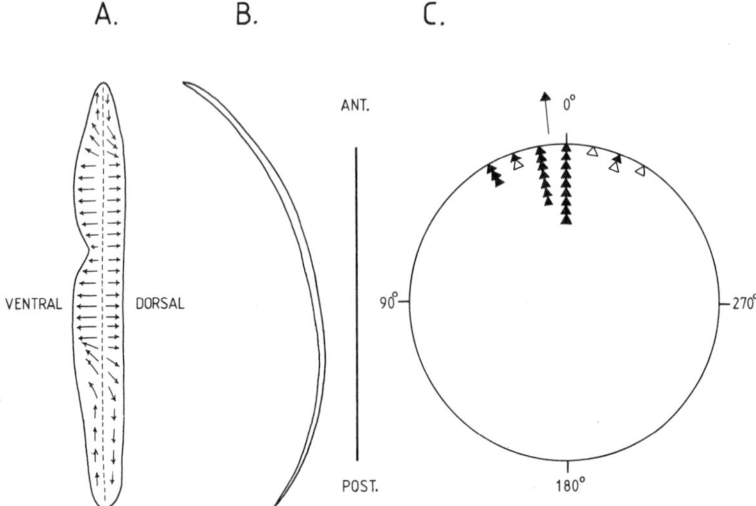

Figure 14 (i) (A) Lateral view of the left saccular macula of cod, showing the main polarization axes of the sensory hair cells.
(B) Dorsal view of the macula.
(C) The angular distribution of units from the saccular nerve. Closed arrows are units from the anterior ramus, and open arrows units from the posterior ramus.

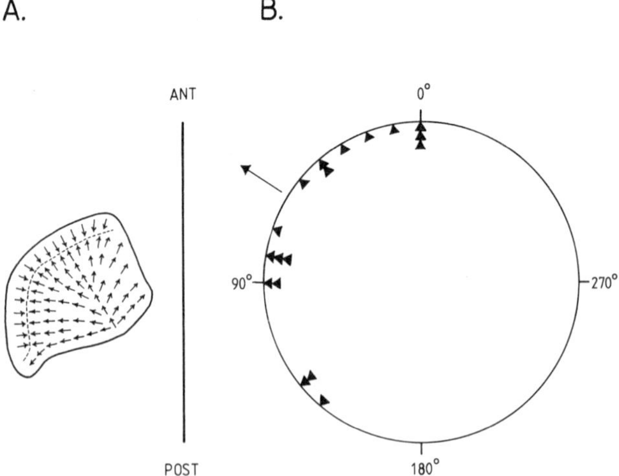

Figure 14 (ii) As (i) but for the left utricular macula.

by Furukawa and Ishii (1967); Fay (1978*a*, *b*); Fay and Olsho (1979); codfish, *Gadus morhua*, by Horner *et al.* (1980); Hawkins and Horner (1980); sculpin, *Cottus scorpius*, Enger (1963); herring, *Clupea harengus*, Enger (1967); and tench, *Tinca tinca*, Gruzinger (1967).

The general feature common to all the species above is a phase locking of spikes to the stimulus cycle. The degree of synchronization between the stimulus and the response describes the temporal error in phase locking. Fay (1978*b*) demonstrated that in goldfish the temporal error is a constant fraction of the period length. The studies on frequency discrimination, however, are not in agreement on the probable site of frequency analysis in the absence of a structure equivalent to the basilar membrane of higher vertebrates (Kiang *et al.*, 1965). The data from goldfish clearly indicates two distinct populations of fibres, high and low frequency. However the results from codfish, a non-specialist teleost, do not demonstrate the distinct difference in frequency selectivity. The high frequency tuning (up to 800 Hz) may therefore be a feature associated with specialized swimbladder-to-labyrinth connections via the Weberian ossicles.

In the amphibia, there is a clear frequency differentiation within the ear. Single unit recordings from the eighth nerve of the bullfrog have revealed three populations of auditory fibres (Feng *et al.*, 1975). These are: low-frequency inhibitable fibres, mid-frequency non-inhibitable fibres and high-frequency non-inhibitable fibres. The amphibian papilla gives rise to the low- and mid-frequency sensitive units and the basilar papilla to the high-frequency sensitive units. The mechanism of tuning of the fibres is not known. One interesting feature of the amphibian auditory system is that in different species the two auditory organs are tuned to different frequency ranges, which are related to the spectral energy in their species-specific vocal signal. Thus the peripheral auditory system is specialized towards processing the spectral and temporal properties of the calls of the species.

REFERENCES

Alexander, R. McN. (1962) The structure of the Weberian apparatus in the Cyprini *Proc. Zool. Soc. Lond.*, **139**, 451–473.

Bennett, M. V. L. (1970) Comparative physiology: electric organs *Ann. Rev. Physiol.*, **32**, 471–528.

Bennett, M. V. L. (1971) "Electroreception" in *Fish Physiology* Vol. 5 (eds. Hoar, W. S., Randall, D. S.) Academic Press, New York, 493–516.

Bergeijk, W. A. van (1967*a*) "Introductory comments on lateral line function" in *Lateral Line Detectors* (ed. Cahn, P. H.) Indiana University Press, Bloomington, 73–81.

Bergeijk, W. A. van (1967*b*) The evolution of vertebrate hearing *Contrib. Sens. Physiol.*, **2**, 1–49.

Bullock, T. H. (1974) "An essay on the discovery of sensory receptors and the assignment of their functions together with an introduction to electroreceptors" in *Handbook of Sensory Physiology* Vol. III/3 (ed. Fessard, A.) Springer Verlag, Berlin, 1–12.

Cahn, P. H., Siler, W. and Fujiya, M. (1973) "Sensory detection of environmental changes by fish" in *Responses of Fish to Environmental Changes* (ed. Charin, W.) Charles C Thomas, Springfield, 73–91.

Cahn, P. H., Siler, W. and Wodinsky, J. (1969) Acoustico lateralis system of fishes: tests of pressure and particle velocity sensitivity in grunts, *Haemulon sciurus* and *H. parrai J. Acoust. Soc. Am.*, **46**, 1572–1578.

Camp, L. (1970) *Underwater Acoustics* Wiley Interscience, New York.

Capranica, R. R. (1978) Auditory processing in anurans *Federation Proc.*, **37**, 2324–2328.

Chapman, C. J. and Johnstone, A. D. F. (1974) Some auditory discrimination experiments on marine fish *J. Exp. Biol.*, **61**, 521–528.

Chapman, C. J. and Hawkins, A. D. (1973) A field study of hearing in the cod, *Gadus morhua* L *J. Comp. Physiol.*, **85**, 147–167.

Chapman, C. J. and Sand, O. (1974) Field studies of hearing in two species of flatfish *Comp. Biochem. Physiol.*, **47A**, 371–385.

Cole, F. J. (1898) Observations on the structure and morphology of the cranial nerves and lateral sense organs of fishes with special reference to the genus *Gadus*. *Trans. Liverpool Biol. Soc.*, **20**, 162.

Corwin, J. T. (1977) Morphology of the macula neglecta in sharks of the genus *Carcharhinus J. Morph.*, **152**, 341–361.

Corwin, J. T. (1980) "Audition in elasmobranchs" in *Hearing and Sound Communication in Fishes* (eds. Fay, R. R., Popper, A. N., Tavolga, W. N.) Springer Verlag, New York.

Dale, T. (1976) The labyrinthine mechanoreceptor organs of the cod (*Gadus morhua*) *Norw. J. Zool.*, **24**, 85–128.

Denton, E. J. and Blaxter, J. H. S. (1976) The mechanical relationships between the clupeid swimbladder, inner ear and lateral line *J. Mar. Biol. Ass. U.K.*, **56**, 787–807.

Dijkgraaf, S. (1934) Untersuchungen über die Funktion der Seitenorgane an Fischen *Z. vergl. Physiol.*, **20**, 162–214.

Dijkgraaf, S. (1947) Über die Reizung des Ferntastsinns bei Fischen und Amphibien *Experientia*, **3**, 206–208.

Dijkgraaf, S. (1956) Elektrophysiologische Untersuchungen an der Seitenlinie von *Xenopus laevis Experientia*, **12**, 276–278.

Dijkgraaf, S. (1960) Hearing in bony fishes *Proc. Roy. Soc. Lond.* B, **152**, 51–54.

Dijkgraaf, S. (1963) The functioning and significance of the lateral line organs *Biol. Rev.*, **38**, 51–105.

Dijkgraaf, S. (1967) "Biological significance of the lateral line organs" in *Lateral Line Detectors* (ed. Cahn, P. H.) Indiana University Press, Bloomington, 83–96.

Enger, P. S. (1963) Single unit activity in the peripheral auditory system of a teleost fish *Acta Physiol. Scand.* 59, Suppl. 3, 9–48.

Enger, P. S. (1967) Hearing in herring *Comp. Biochem. Physiol.*, **22**, 527–538.

Enger, P. S., Hawkins, A. D., Sand, O. and Chapman, C. J. (1973) Directional sensitivity of saccular microphonic potentials in the haddock *J. Exp. Biol.*, **59**, 425–433.

Fay, R. R. (1978*a*) Coding of information in single auditory nerve fibres of the goldfish *J. Acoust. Soc. Am.*, **63**, 136–146.

Fay, R. R. (1978*b*) Phase-locking in goldfish saccular nerve fibres accounts for frequency discrimination capacities *Nature*, **275**, 320–322.

Fay, R. R., Kendall, J. I., Popper, A. N. and Tester, A. L. (1974) Vibration detection by the macula neglecta of sharks *Comp. Biochem. Physiol.*, **47A**, 1235–1240.

Fay, R. R. and Olsho, L. W. (1979) Discharge patterns of lagenar and saccular neurons of the goldfish eighth nerve: displacement sensitivity and directional characteristics *Comp. Biochem. Physiol.*, A, **62**, 377–387.

Fay, R. R. and Popper, A. N. (1980) "Structure and function in teleost auditory systems" in *Comparative Studies in Hearing in Vertebrates* (eds. Popper, A. N., Fay, R. R.) Springer Verlag, New York, 7.

Feng, A. S., Narins, P. M. and Capranica, R. R. (1975) Three populations of primary auditory fibres in the bullfrog (*Rana catesbeiana*): Their peripheral origins and frequency sensitivities *J. Comp. Physiol.*, **100**, 221–229.

Fernandez, C. and Goldberg, J. M. (1976) Physiology of peripheral neurons innervating otolith organs of the squirrel monkey *J. Neurophysiol.*, **39**, 970–984.

Flock, Å. (1964) Structure of the macula utriculi with special reference to directional interplay of sensory responses as revealed by morphological polarisation *J. Cell Biol.*, **22**, 413–426.

Flock, Å. (1965) Transducing mechanisms in lateral line canal organ receptors *Cold Spring Harbor Symp. Quant. Biol.*, **30**, 133–145.

Flock, Å. (1967) "Ultrastructure and function in the lateral line organs" in *Lateral Line Detectors* (ed. Cahn, P. H.) Indiana University Press, Bloomington, 163–197.

Flock, Å. (1971) "Sensory transduction in hair cells" in *Handbook of Sensory Physiology* Vol. 1 (ed. Lowenstein, W.) Springer Verlag, Berlin, 396–441.

Flock, Å. and Flock, B. (1966) Ultrastructure of the amphibian papilla in the bullfrog *J. Acoust. Soc. Amer.*, **40**, 1262.

Flock, Å., Flock, B. and Murray, E. (1977) Studies on the sensory hairs of receptor cells in the inner ear *Acta Oto-laryngol.*, **83**, 85–91.

Flock, Å. and Russell, I. (1973) The postsynaptic action of efferent fibres in the lateral line organ of the burbot, *Lota lota J. Physiol.*, **235**, 591–605.

Flock, Å. and Russell, I. (1976) Inhibition by efferent nerve fibres: Action on hair cells and afferent synaptic transmission in the lateral line canal organ of the burbot, *Lota lota J. Physiol.*, **257**, 45–62.

Frisch, K. von (1938) Über die Bedeuting der Sacculus und der Lagena für den Gehörsinn der Fische *Z. vergl. Physiol.*, **25**, 703–747.

Frishkopf, L. S. and Flock, Å. (1974) Ultrastructure of the basilar papilla, an auditory organ in the bullfrog *Acta Oto-laryngol.*, **77**, 176–184.

Furukawa, T. (1978) Sites of termination on the saccular macula of auditory nerve fibres in the goldfish as determined by intracellular injection of procion yellow *J. Comp. Neurol.*, **180**, 807–814.

Furukawa, T. and Ishii, Y. (1967) Neurophysiological studies on hearing in goldfish *J. Neurophysiol.*, **30**, 1377–1403.

Gertychowa, R. (1970) Studies on the ethology and space orientation of the blind cave fish *Anoptichthys jordani Folia Biol.*, **18**, 4–69.

Görner, P. (1963) Untersuchungen zur Morphologie und Elektrophysiologie des Seitenorgans vom Krallenfrosch (*Xenopus laevis*) *Z. vergl. Physiol.*, **47**, 316–338.

Gray, J. A. B. and Denton, E. J. (1979) The mechanics of the clupeid acoustico-lateralis system: low frequency measurements *J. Mar. Biol. Ass. U.K.*, **59**, 11–26.

Griffin, D. R. (1955) Hearing and acoustic orientation in marine animals *Deep Sea Res.*, Suppl., 3, 406–417.

Gruzinger, B. (1967) Elektro-Physiologische Untersuchungen an der Horbahn der Schleie *Tinca tinca Z. vergl. Physiol.*, **57**, 44–76.

Harris, G. G. (1967) "Comments on the lateral line" in *Lateral Line Detectors* (ed. Cahn, P. H.) Indiana University Press, Bloomington, 231–236.

Harris, G. G. and Bergeijk, W. A. van (1962) Evidence that the lateral line organ responds to near-field displacements of sound sources in water *J. Acoust. Soc. Am.*, **34**, 1831–1841.

Harris, G. G. and Flock, Å. (1967) "Spontaneous and evoked activity from the *Xenopus laevis* lateral line" in *Lateral Line Detectors* (ed. Cahn, P. H.) Indiana University Press, Bloomington, 135–161.

Harris, G. G. and Milne, D. C. (1966) Input–output characteristics of the lateral line sense organs of *Xenopus laevis J. Acoust. Soc. Am.*, **40**, 32–42.

Hawkins, A. D. (1973) The sensitivity of fish to sounds *Oceanogr. Mar. Biol. Ann. Rev.*, **11**, 291–340.

Hawkins, A. D. and Horner, K. (1980) "Directional characteristics of primary auditory neurones from the codfish ear" in *Hearing and Sound Communication in Fishes* (eds. Fay, R. R., Popper, A. N., Tavolga, W. N.) Springer Verlag, New York.

Hawkins, A. D. and Johnstone, A. D. F. (1978) The hearing of the Atlantic salmon, *Salmo salar. J. Fish. Biol.*, **13**, 655–673.

Hawkins, A. D. and MacLennan, D. N. (1976) "An acoustic tank for hearing studies on fish" in *Sound Reception in Fish* (eds. Schuijf, A., Hawkins, A. D.) Elsevier, Amsterdam, 149–169.

Hawkins, A. D. and Sand, O. (1977) Directional hearing in the median vertical plane by the cod *J. Comp. Physiol.*, **122**, 1–8.

Hoagland, H. (1933) Electrical responses from the lateral line nerve of the catfish *J. Gen. Physiol.*, **16**, 695–714.

Hofer, B. (1908) Studien über die Hautsinnesorgane der Fische. I. Die Funktion der Seitenorgane bei den Fischen *Ber. Kgl. Bayer. biol. Versuchsstation München*, **1**, 115–168.

Horner, K., Hawkins, A. D. and Fraser, P. J. (1980) "Frequency characteristics of primary auditory neurons from the ear of codfish" in *Hearing and Sound Communication in Fishes* (eds. Fay, R. R., Popper, A. N., Tavolga, W. N.) Springer Verlag, New York.

Horner, K., Sand, O. and Enger, P. S. (1980) Binaural interaction in the cod *J. Exp. Biol.*, **85**, 323–331.

Hudspeth, A. J. and Corey, D. P. (1977) Sensitivity, polarity and conductance change in the response of vertebrate hair cells to controlled mechanical stimuli *Proc. Natl. Acad. Sci.*, **74**, 2407–2411.

Jande, S. S. (1966) The structure of lateral line organs of frog tadpoles *J. Ultrastruct. Res.*, **15**, 496–509.

Jenkins, D. B. (1979) A transmission and scanning electron microscopic study of the saccula in five species of catfishes *Amer. J. Anat.*, **154**, 81–101.

Jorgensen, J. M. (1976) Hair cell polarization in the flatfish inner ear *Acta Zool.*, **57**, 37–39.

Kiang, N. Y. S., Watanabe, T., Thomas, E. G., Clarke, L. (1965) *Discharge patterns of single fibers in the cat's auditory nerve. Res. Monogr.* **35**, M.I.T. Press, Cambridge, Mass.

Kleerekoper, H. and Changon, E. C. (1954) Hearing in fish, with special reference to *Semotilus atromaculatus* (Mitchell) *J. Fish. Res. Bd. Can.*, **11**, 130–152.

Kroese, A. B. A., van der Zalm, J. M. and van den Bercken, J. (1978) Frequency response of the lateral line organ of *Xenopus laevis Pflügers Arch.*, **375**, 167–175.

Kuiper, J. W. (1967) "Frequency characteristics and functional significance of the lateral line organ" in *Lateral Line Detectors* (ed. Cahn, P. H.) Indiana University Press, Bloomington, 105–121.

Kuroki, T. (1967) "Theoretical analysis of the role of the lateral line in directional hearing" in *Lateral Line Detectors* (ed. Cahn, P. H.) Indiana University Press, Bloomington, 217–231.

Lewis, E. R. and Li, C. W. (1973) Evidence concerning the morphogenesis of saccular receptors in the bullfrog (*Rana catesbeiana*) *J. Morph.*, **139**, 351–362.

Lissman, H. W. and Mullinger, A. M. (1968) Organisation of ampullary electric receptors in Gymnotidae (Pisces) *Proc. Roy. Soc. B.*, **169**, 345–378.

Lowenstein, O. (1967) "The concept of the acousticolateral system" in *Lateral Line Detectors* (ed. Cahn, P. H.) Indiana University Press, Bloomington, 3–12.

Lowenstein, O., Osborne, M. P. and Thornhill, R. A. (1968) The anatomy and ultrastructure of the labyrinth of the lamprey (*Lampetra fluviatilis*) *Proc. Roy. Soc. B.*, **1970**, 113–134.

Lowenstein, O., Osborne, M. P. and Wersäll, J. (1964) Structure and innervation of the sensory epithelia of the labyrinth in the thornback ray (*Raja clavata*) *Proc. Roy. Soc. Lond. B.*, **160**, 1–54.

Lowenstein, O. and Roberts, T. D. (1949) The equilibrium function of the otolith organ of the thornback ray, *Raja clavata J. Physiol.*, **110**, 392–415.

Lowenstein, O. and Saunders, R. D. (1975) Otolith controlled responses from the first order neurons of the labyrinth of the bullfrog (*Rana catesbeiana*) to changes in linear acceleration *Proc. Roy. Soc. Lond. B.*, **191**, 475–505.

Lowenstein, O. and Thornhill, R. A. (1970) The labyrinth of *Myxine*: anatomy, ultrastructure and electrophysiology *Proc. Roy. Soc. Lond. B.*, **176**, 21–42.

Lowenstein, O. and Wersäll, J. (1959) A functional interpretation of the electron microscopic structure of the sensory hairs in the cristae of the elasmobranch, *Raja clavata*, in terms of directional sensitivity *Nature*, **184**, 1807.

Mayser, P. (1882) Vergleichend anatomische Studien über das Gehirn der Knochenfische mit besonderer Berucksichtigung der Cyprinoiden *Z. Wiss. Zool.*, **36**, 259–364.

Moulton, J. M. (1963) "Acoustic behaviour of fishes" in *Acoustic Behaviour of Animals* (ed. Busnel, R. G.) Elsevier, Amsterdam, 655–693.

Murray, R. W. (1955) The lateralis organs and their innervation in *Xenopus laevis Quart. J. Microscop. Sci.*, **96**, 351–361.

Nakajima, Y. and Wang, D. W. (1974) Morphology of afferent and efferent synapses in the hearing organ of goldfish *J. Comp. Neurol.*, **156**, 403–416.

O'Connell, C. P. (1955) The gas bladder and its relation to the inner ear in *Sardinops caerulea* and *Engraulis mordax U.S. Fisheries Bull.*, **56**, 505–533.

Pabst, A. (1977) Number and location of the sites of impulse generation in the lateral line afferents of *Xenopus laevis J. Comp. Physiol.*, **114A**, 51–67.

Parker, G. H. (1904) The function of the lateral line organs in fishes *Bull. Bur. Fisheries*, **24**, 43–57.

Paterson, N. (1949) The development of the inner ear of *Xenopus laevis* *Proc. zool. Soc. Lond.*, **119**, 269–291.

Poggendorf, D. (1952) The absolute auditory thresholds of the dwarf catfish *Amiurus nebulosus* *Z. vergl. Physiol.*, **34**, 222–257.

Popper, A. N. (1977) A scanning electron microscopic study of the sacculus and lagena in the ears of fifteen species of teleost fishes *J. Morph.*, **153**, 397–418.

Popper, A. N. (1978) A comparative study of the otolithic organs in fishes *Scanning Electron Microscopy*, **2**, 405–416.

Popper, A. N. and Fay, R. R. (1973) Sound detection and processing by teleost fishes: a critical review. *J. Acoustic. Soc. Am.*, **53**, 1515–1529.

Popper, A. N. and Platt, C. (1979) The herring ear has a unique receptor pattern *Nature*, **280**, 832–833.

Pumphrey, R. J. (1950) Hearing *Symp. Soc. Expl. Biol.*, **4**, 3–18.

Roberts, B. L. (1972) Activity of lateral line sense organs in swimming dogfish *J. Exp. Biol.*, **56**, 105–118.

Roberts, B. L. and Ryan, K. P. (1971) The fine structure of the lateral line sense organs of dogfish *Proc. Roy. Soc. Lond. B.*, **129**, 157–169.

Russell, I. (1971) The role of the lateral line efferent system in *Xenopus laevis* *J. Exp. Biol.*, **54**, 621–641.

Russell, I. (1974) Central inhibition of lateral line input in the medulla of the goldfish by neurones which control active body movements *J. Comp. Physiol.*, **111**, 335–358.

Russell, I. and Roberts, B. L. (1972) The activity of lateral line efferent neurons in stationary and swimming dogfish *J. Exp. Biol.*, **57**, 435–448.

Saito, K. (1973) Fine structure of the macula of the lagena in the teleost inner ear *Acta Anat. Nipponica*, **48**, 1–18.

Sand, A. (1937) The mechanism of the lateral sense organs of fishes *Proc. Roy. Soc. B.*, **123**, 427–495.

Schuijf, A. (1975) Directional hearing in cod under approximate free field conditions *J. Comp. Physiol.*, **98**, 307–332.

Schuijf, A. (1976) "The phase model of directional hearing in fish" in *Sound Reception in Fish* (eds. Schuijf, A., Hawkins, A. D.) Elsevier, Amsterdam, 63–86.

Schuijf, A. and Buwalda, R. (1980) "Underwater localisation—a major problem in fish acoustics" in *Comparative Studies of Hearing in Vertebrates* (eds. Popper, A. N., Fay, R. R.) Springer Verlag, New York.

Schulze, F. E. (1870) Über die Sinnesorgane der Seitenlinie bei Fischen und Amphibien *Arch. mikr. Anat.*, **6**, 62–88.

Schwartz, E. (1965) Bau und Funktion der Seitenlinie des Streifenhechtlings, *Aplocheilus lineatus* *Z. vergl. Physiol.*, **50**, 55–87.

Schwartz, E. (1967) "Analysis of surface-wave perception in some teleosts" in *Lateral Line Detectors* (ed. Cahn, P. H.) Indiana University Press, Bloomington, 123–133.

Schwartz, E. (1971) Die Ortung von Wasserwellen durch Oberflächenfische *Z. vergl. Physiol.*, **74**, 64–80.

Schwartz, E. and Hasler, A. D. (1966) Perception of surface waves by the blackstripe topminnow, *Fundulus notatus* *J. Fish. Res. Bd. Canada*, **23**, 1331–1352.

Shelton, P. (1971) The structure and function of the lateral line system in larval *Xenopus laevis* *J. Exp. Zool.*, **178**, 211–231.

Stipetic, E. (1939) Über das Gehörorgan der Mormyriden *Z. vergl. Physiol.*, **26**, 740–752.

Strelioff, D. and Honrubia, V. (1978) Neural transduction in *Xenopus laevis* lateral line system *J. Neurophysiol.*, **41**, 432–443.

Suckling, E. E. and Suckling, J. A. (1951) The electrical response of the lateral line system of fish to tone and other stimuli *J. gen. Physiol.*, **34**, 1–8.

Szabo, T. (1972) Ultrastructural evidence for a mechanoreceptor function of the ampullae of Lorenzini *J. Microsc.*, **14**, 343–350.

Szabo, T. (1974) "Anatomy of the specialised lateral line organs of electroreception" in *Handbook of Sensory Physiology* Vol. III/3 (ed. Fessard, A.) Springer Verlag, Berlin, 13–58.

Tavolga, W. N. (1971) "Sound production and detection" in *Fish Physiology* Vol. 5 (eds. Hoar, W. S., Randall, D. J.) Academic Press, New York, 135–205.

Tester, A. L., Kendall, J. I. and Milisen, W. B. (1972) Morphology of the ear of the shark genus *Carcharhinus*, with particular reference to the macula neglecta *Pacific Sci.*, **76**, 264–274.

Thompson, K. S. (1977) "On the individual history of cosmine and a possible electroreceptive function of the pore-canal system in fossil fishes" in *Problems in Vertebrate Evolution* (eds. Andrews, S. M., Miles, R. S., Walker, A. D.) Academic Press, London, 247–270.

Vries, H. de (1950) The mechanics of the labyrinth otoliths *Acta Otolaryngol.*, **38**, 262–273.

Watson, D. M. S. (1938) On the Acanthodian fishes *Phil. Trans. R. Soc., B.*, **228**, 39–146.

Wilson, V. J. and Jones, G. M. (1979) *Mammalian Vestibular Physiology* Plenum Press, New York, 365 pp.

Witschi, E. (1949) The larval ear of the frog and its transformation during metamorphosis *Z. Naturforschg.*, **4b**, 230–242.

Wodinsky, J. and Tavolga, W. N. (1964) "Sound detection in teleost fishes" in *Marine Bioacoustics* (ed. Tavolga, W. N.) Pergamon, Oxford, 269–279.

Wohlfahrt, T. A. (1936) Das Ohrlabyrinth der Sardine (*Clupea pilchardus* Walb) und seine Beziehungen zur Schwimmblase und Seitenlinie *Z. Morphol. Oekol. Tiere*, **31**, 371–410.

CHAPTER FOURTEEN

RETINAL FIBRE PROJECTION PATTERNS IN THE PRIMARY VISUAL PATHWAYS TO THE BRAIN

J. H. SCHOLES

Introduction

Both the retina and its target visual areas in the brain are epithelial in embryonic origin, and they become connected together during development as growing retinal axons order their synaptic terminals to form neurological maps of the image in the eye. Some kind of embryological *correspondence* must determine the fixed layout of the maps relative to the rest of the brain and the outside world, and the curiosity I will examine here is that this correspondence is never a simple one. In all animals with advanced eyes, retinal axons do not run parallel with one another from the eye to the brain, but systematically become laid out in more complicated ways, whose outcome is always to *reverse* the neighbourly spatial order in which they first left the eye.

Just three groups of animals, in fact, possess eyes sufficiently refined to resolve visual angles of less (and usually much less) than a degree of arc. They are the arthropods (crustaceans and insects in particular), the cephalopod molluscs (e.g. squid and octopus) and the vertebrates. In all of these organisms, retinal nerve fibres interleave in conspicuous pleated structures in the visual pathway, best called *internal* chiasms or crossovers to distinguish them from the mid-line crossings of the two optic nerves in vertebrates. These internal crossings reverse the spatial ordering of retinal axons, but in each of the three groups the geometrical nature of the reversal so achieved is quite different.

Among the two invertebrate groups, axonal crossings associated with the optic lobes of the brain reverse one or other of the two *Cartesian* co-ordinates of the retinal fibre array. In arthropods, the *horizontal* ordering of retinal axons is reversed in a structure called the first chiasm of the optic lobe (Zawarzin, 1913), while, in cephalopods, a different kind of fibre crossing reverses order along the *vertical* axis of the eye (Kopsch, 1899). Vertebrate animals also possess an internal fibre crossing in the visual projection to the contralateral tectum of the mid-brain (Lubsen, 1921), and this, by contrast, operates a reversal on one of the *polar* co-ordinates of the retinal disc (Scholes, 1979).

In this chapter I will try to make some sense of these conspicuous differences in the organization of the primary neural pathways underlying vision. I will show how they can be related to the radically different principles of optical design and eye construction which, between them, these animals have separately come to exploit. In turn, this uncovers an intriguing generalization, that in each case the outcome of these fibre reversals is the same, as far as the central representation of visual space is concerned. Some deep significance could attach to this observation, and it certainly provides a mnemonic tool for understanding the difficult topology of the primary visual pathway in vertebrates.

Optical design and eye construction

The argument rests on two basic distinctions which can be drawn between the various forms of eyes which animals in the three groups possess. First of all, arthropods are exceptional in the optical design of their eyes (see Land, this volume). Compound eyes function like straw-box collimators, so that receptors in the retinal surface capture light just from their own angular subtense into the outside world (Müller, 1826). If one can think of this mechanism as a kind of image formation, then compound eyes form *erect* images of the visual field in their retinas, and when their optical elements act co-operatively, as they do in superposition eyes (Exner, 1891; Kunze, 1972; Vogt, 1975; Land, 1976), the resultant true image is also congruent with the visual scene it represents. On the other hand, both cephalopods and vertebrates have camera eyes—this means their retinal surfaces sample an image which is rotated through 180° relative to the visual field, usually called an *inverted* image.

Secondly, vertebrate animals are exceptional among the three groups so far as a second, quite separate feature of eye construction is concerned. For reasons to do with the way the vertebrate eye arises as an outgrowth of the anterior neural tube during development, rods and cones face away from the direction of incident light, towards the sclera. Optic nerve fibres originate on the outward-facing surface of the retina, and must negotiate this epithelium in order to reach their central destinations. This has geometrical consequences, not for the retinal image itself, but for the fibre map of the retinal surface which the optic nerve conveys towards the brain. The important consequence is that the array of optic nerve fibres leaving the eye inescapably becomes bodily reversed relative to its origin on the retinal surface.

By contrast, retinal receptors point towards incident light in both compound eyes and cephalopod camera eyes, and retinal axons originate on the proximal surface, already aimed at their targets in the brain. Therefore, visual fibre arrays are congruent with the retinal image as they leave the eye in invertebrates, and are superimposable with the visual field, either directly, as in arthropods, or by rotation through π, as in cephalopods. However, as we have seen, this congruence is not preserved as retinal axons penetrate deeper into the invertebrate visual pathway.

Internal chiasms in invertebrate visual pathways

In both arthropods and cephalopods, primary retinal nerve fibres enter a synaptic plexus directly apposed to the back of the receptor layer. This has a status analogous with that of the neural retina in the vertebrate eye, to the extent that its layout is directly congruent with the mosaic of receptors in front. In cephalopods, receptor axons simply traverse the plexus directly, forming synapses collaterally (Cajal, 1917; Cohen, 1973). In arthropods, most of them terminate in an analogous structure, the *lamina ganglionaris* of the optic lobe of the brain, whose neuronal mosaic is exactly congruent with the retinal array of facets (Cajal and Sanchez, 1915; Braitenberg, 1967; Strausfeld, 1971). However, in both sorts of animals, the fibre map becomes drastically transformed at the next level of

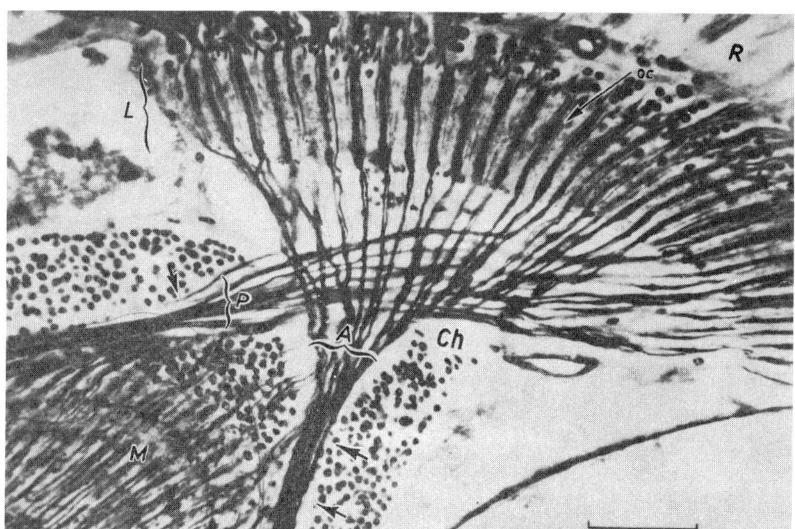

Figure 1 N. J. Strausfeld's (1971) horizontal plane micrograph of the first visual chiasm in the fly *Musca*, showing how visual fibres from the lamina (L) cross one another to reverse the antero-posterior axis (left to right) of the visual map formed in the medulla (M, bottom left). Reproduced with permission.

the visual pathway, on the way to the medulla of the optic lobe, which is the first synaptic relay in the cephalopod brain, and the second in arthropods.

In arthropods, visual fibres cross over one another between the lamina and the medulla (see Fig. 1, reproduced from Strausfeld, 1971), reversing their order along the horizontal axis of the optic lobe (Zawarzin, 1913; Cajal and Sanchez, 1915; Hanström, 1928). In dipteran insects, for example, the crossing takes the form of a twist through 180° applied to individual sheets of axons from each of the horizontal rows of facets in the eye (Strausfeld, 1971), and the exactitude of these horizontal exchanges of position leaves the vertical axis of the pathway unchanged. The reversal, one of the most conspicuous features of the arthropod visual pathway and absent only in certain decapod crustaceans (Eloffson and Dahl, 1970), is accurate to the level of single axons (Strausfeld, 1971; Meinertzhagen, 1976), and results in a visual map in the medulla which is an exact mirror reflexion of the retinal image.

In cephalopods, retinal axons re-order themselves in a different way. Leaving the retinal plexus, they tunnel locally through the sclera to emerge from the back of the eye. They run from their origins over the surface of the eye-globe to the horizontal meridian, where they cross over, dorsal to ventral and *vice versa*, as shown in Fig. 2, which is reproduced from J. Z. Young's (1962*a*) account of the *Octopus* visual system. This

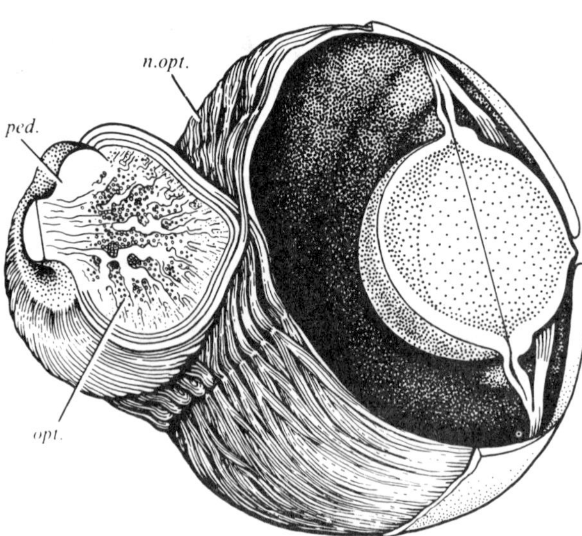

Figure 2 View of the opened *Octopus* eye, reproduced with permission from Young (1962*a*), to show how retinal fibre bundles cross at the horizontal meridian of the globe to achieve a systematic inversion, along the vertical axis, of the visual map in the optic lobe of the brain (*opt*). Dorsal is upwards in the drawing.

chiasm, as Kopsch (1899) and Cajal (1917) clearly understood, reverses the visual map dorsiventrally with respect to the retinal image, thus contrasting with the horizontal reflexion found in arthropods. It is mediated with an accuracy which extends to the level of single fibres (Young, 1962*a*), and this visible precision of connectivity, measured against the vast receptor populations in the eyes of large oceanic cephalopods (Young, 1962*b*) must by far exceed any yet inferred in the visual systems of vertebrates (Gaze, 1970; Hunt and Jacobson, 1974; Horder and Martin, 1978).

Young (1962*b*) has related the curious story of how Cajal announced, in 1917, his intention to adduce the significance of these internal fibre crossings in invertebrate visual systems, and relate them to the disposition of the visual pathway in vertebrates, going so far as to entitle the paper he planned to publish. But whatever his insights were, they remained private, for the work never appeared in the literature.

Consequences

This brief sketch of optical function and neural connectivity in the two principal sorts of invertebrate eyes brings us to the point where a provisional synthesis can be made. It is one of such intriguing simplicity that I have been surprised to find it overlooked in the literature on visual chiasms which has accumulated since the turn of the century (Cajal, 1898; Szentagothai and Szekely, 1956; Polyak, 1957; Young, 1962*b*; Braitenberg, 1970; Strausfeld, 1971; Meinertzhagen, 1973).

The visual map in the medulla of the optic lobe in arthropods is oriented in the *same* way as that in cephalopods, with respect to body co-ordinates and the outside world. It is the right way up, but reversed along the horizontal axis of this brain structure, from front to back. This equivalence, illustrated by the sketches in Fig. 3, comes about in no more mysterious way than that *image rotation through* π in the cephalopod eye, followed by *vertical neural reflexion*, has the same geometrical outcome as *no change* optically in the compound eye, followed by *horizontal neural reflexion*. This can be verified, best in private, by inspecting the results of rotating and reflecting one's hands appropriately.

Other invertebrates

Is there something special about building a primary visual map which is the right way up, but reversed from front to back—or is this single organizational feature which the two kinds of visual system share in common merely a seductive coincidence? What about other animals? Despite their more rudimentary visual facilities, annelids are interesting because some of them have quite reasonable camera eyes, while others

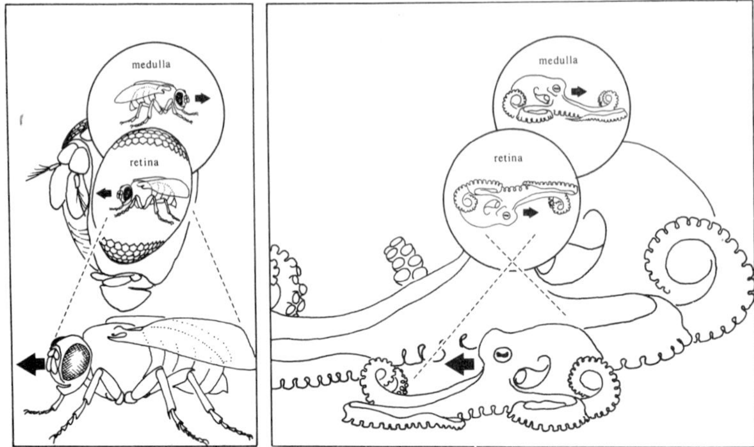

Figure 3 The left-hand scene represents a fly's head, with its left eye looking at another, smaller, fly. The image in the eye is "erect", but by virtue of the nerve fibre chiasm (Fig. 1), the visual map in the ipsilateral optic lobe medulla is reversed along the horizontal axis (left to right).

The sketch on the right represents an octopus looking at another with its left eye. The retinal image is rotated through 180°, but the fibre chiasm (Fig. 2) reinstates the vertical axis, with the same outcome for the map in the ipsilateral medulla as achieved in arthropods (*left*).

possess structures which resemble compound eyes. Hanström's (1928) drawing of the neural structures in the optic lobe behind the camera eye of *Leodice* (see Bullock and Horridge, 1965) is encouraging; it depicts what appears to be a dorsiventral (cephalopod-like) crossing of retinal nerve fibres. Unfortunately, however, I have found no comparable account of the visual pathway in such polychaetes as *Branchiomma*, which has a faceted type of compound eye (Hesse, 1899; Bullock and Horridge, 1965). Nor have I been able to grasp the geometry of the visual fibre chiasms in spiders (Hanström, 1928; Oberdorfer, 1977), which often possess frontal camera eyes (Land, 1969) in addition to lateral ocelli.

That animals as different as insects and octopi share a similarly oriented visual map (Fig. 3) is certainly interesting, and it would merit serious thought if other animals with camera or compound eyes prove to use similar tricks to build similar primary visual representations. However, one must observe the caution that arthropods are profligate in the differentiation of internal visual chiasms (Hanström, 1928; Eloffson and Dahl, 1970). The variety of internal fibre crossings in between the various neuropile structures behind the crustacean external medulla and its equivalent in the insect optic lobe suggests that it may be optimistic to search for any single principle to explain them all. But what about vertebrate visual pathways?

The vertebrate visual projection to the mid-brain

An obstacle to thinking about the vertebrate visual system along the same lines is that at least half of the fibre projection from one eye runs to the opposite side of the brain (Cajal, 1899; Polyak, 1957), so the visual maps represent the contralateral hemifields of view almost exclusively. Moreover, since retinal axons project to the diencephalon and the mid-brain in parallel, there is no special reason for allocating primary status to any of the maps in particular. As a beginning, however, it makes sense to consider the projection to the tectum of the mid-brain, if only because it is phylogenetically archaic and more is known of the layout of visual fibres within this pathway than in the thalamo-cortical branch of the visual system.

The development and layout of the tectal pathway is best understood in amphibia, particularly *Xenopus laevis* (Gaze, 1970; Gaze, Keating and Chung, 1974; Gaze and Grant, 1978; Steedman *et al.*, 1979). Unlike that in certain other lower vertebrates (Repérant, 1973; Northcutt and Butler, 1974; Caldwell and Berman, 1977; Cruce and Cruce, 1977; Kennedy and Rubinson, 1977), the projection is completely crossed and no retinal axons innervate the ipsilateral tectum directly. Nevertheless, amphibians, like other vertebrates, possess an ipsilateral visual field representation, but mediated indirectly by commissural fibres from the other side of the mid-brain (Keating, 1968, 1975; Keating *et al.*, 1975). This map represents just the frontal binocular field, imaged on a narrow temporal crescent of the retina. It is restricted to the rostral pole of the tectum, where it superimposes with the complete map formed by the direct contralateral projection from the opposite eye.

To achieve this superimposition in such a way that visual points seen in common by the two eyes project to the same tectal loci, the ipsilateral retinal surface must be mapped in the tectum according to different anatomical rules of connectivity (correspondence) from those which order the contralateral pathway (Keating and Kennard, 1976; Thompson, 1979). Moreover, binocular visual experience determines the disposition of the ipsilateral tectal map during the normal course of development, while the lines of sight of the two eyes are continually changing (Keating and Gaze, 1975; Keating *et al.*, 1975).

Notwithstanding their phylogenetic status, the situation is simpler in mammals, particularly in those with laterally placed eyes and a limited frontal field of binocular overlap. Ganglion cell fibres from the binocular crescent of the temporal retina diverge at the optic chiasm to innervate both the ipsilateral and the contralateral superior colliculi (tecta) directly (Lund and Lund, 1976; Tiao and Blakemore, 1976). Taking rodents as representative, development of this direct ipsilateral tectal projection does not require binocular visual experience (Thompson, 1979). However, the

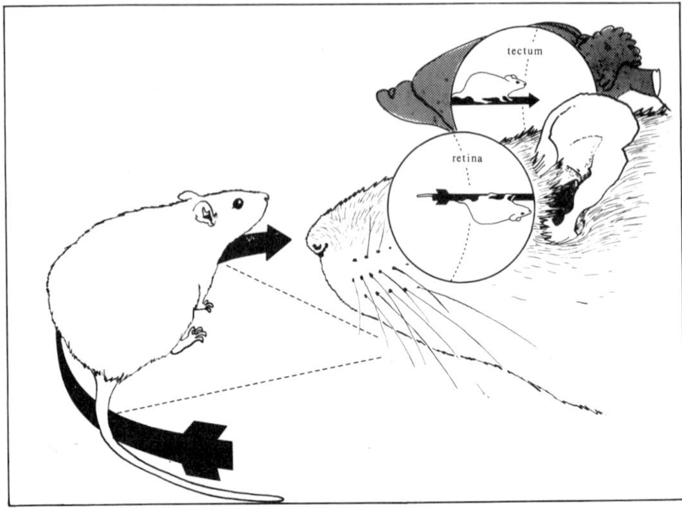

Figure 4 A rat (*right*) surveys another in its binocular field. The image in its left retina is shown, with the dashed line marking the boundary of the binocular temporal crescent (exaggerated). Behind, the map in the ipsilateral superior colliculus is aligned with a sketch of the brain, with the medial border pointing upwards. Temporal retina maps on to ipsilateral tectal rostrum with the same results as in invertebrate visual systems (cf. Fig. 3).

organization of the resultant map on the tectum exactly resembles that of the indirect projection in amphibia. It is restricted to the tectal rostrum, and it superimposes on the map from the contralateral eye, bringing into register identical visual points in the binocularly shared frontal field, rather than corresponding retinal locations (Thompson, 1979).

Now, outside the few vertebrate animals like primates with nearly complete frontal binocular overlap (Polyak, 1957), the contralateral pathway to the mid-brain (and thalamus) is the dominant visual projection from the retina. Here, on the other hand, I have considered the minor, ipsilateral, tectal representation first, not for awkwardness' sake, but because I am intent on forcing a comparison. Invertebrate visual systems entirely lack direct contralateral pathways, so to begin with one can only seek parallels with the ipsilateral maps of vertebrates. By coincidence or otherwise, this comparison, like that between arthropods and cephalopods (Fig. 3), proves to be a rewarding one, again overlooked in the literature so far as I am aware.

Considered on its own, the ipsilateral visual field map in the vertebrate optic tectum is laid out in the same unreasonable way as that in the medulla of the optic lobes of invertebrate brains. Like them, it is the right way up in body co-ordinates but reversed from front to back, as illustrated by Fig. 4. The only qualification is that the vertebrate ipsilateral map originates just from the temporal crescent of the retina, and is restricted to the rostral pole of the tectum.

Neighbourly ordering in the vertebrate optic nerve

If the visual map in the vertebrate ipsilateral mid-brain is laid out in the same way as the primary visual representations in advanced invertebrates, are the retinal axons involved also organized in similar ways? Unfortunately, nothing is yet known of nerve fibre layout in the ipsilateral tectal projection, so it will be necessary to develop the argument in a less direct way. In fact, it is only recently that axonal retinotopicity has been examined in any detail, even in the contralateral tectal pathway of lower vertebrates (Scalia and Fite, 1974; Bunt and Horder, 1977; Gaze and Grant, 1978; Scholes, 1979; Levinthal and Bodick, 1979; Rusoff and Easter, 1980).

This neglect has its historical context, for most work on the mid-brain projection over the last 20 years has been concerned with developmental questions. R. W. Sperry's classical experiments on visual regeneration in lower vertebrates (see Sperry, 1963), and the enigmatic branch of developmental neurobiology (see Edds, 1975) which has grown on their foundation, seem to exclude that retinal fibre ordering *en route* to the brain plays any necessary, and therefore interesting, role in the development of the visual map. Moreover, observations of the amphibian optic nerve seem to show that retinal axons are laid out there in a disorderly manner (Maturana, 1960; Fawcett, 1980), as they are also in the cat (Horton, Greenwood and Hubel, 1979).

Tangled systems of wiring generate their own problems, and this alone should suggest that the vertebrate visual system becomes connected up in a more orderly fashion than these influential findings have indicated. The chick visual system (Goldberg and Coulombre, 1972; Goldberg, 1974; Rager and Rager, 1978) illustrates the scope of the problems involved. In the chick embryo, the tectal pathway is substantially completed between days 8 and 12 of incubation, with overkill since many more fibres grow from the eye to the brain (4×10^6 from each retina: Rager and Rager, 1978) than will ultimately survive an ensuing episode of retinal cell death. Thus, growing axons leave the eye at an average rate in excess of 10 per second, and the peak rate must presumably be many times this alarming figure. Marshalling them into an orderly tectal representation would seem to predicate special and unfamiliar mechanisms, which the textile industry might be best qualified to elucidate.

Many visual systems develop much more slowly, however, and fish are exemplary in this respect, starting their free-swimming life very small and bringing it to a conclusion, often many years later, very large. Retinal growth continues throughout life, in a tree-ring mode sustained by a narrow annulus of dividing neuroblasts around the iris margin (Johns and Easter, 1977). Thus retinal ganglion cell fibres continually accrue to the visual pathway, though orders of magnitude more slowly than in the chick embryo.

Like the retinal surface, the cross-section of the optic nerve assumes a natural chronological ordering, and the most spectacular example of this organization occurs in fishes which possess ribbon optic nerves (Anders and Hibbard, 1974; Scholes, 1979). Retinal axons and their satellite cells are arranged in a continuous thin sheet (Fig. 5a), longitudinally pleated into the cylindrical outline of the nerve, and this structure widens into increasingly elaborate folds as retinal area increases during growth. It contains myelinated fibres exclusively, except for a small tract of unmyelinated axons along one edge of the ribbon. This tract is the key to the organization of the nerve, comprising as it does, axons engaged in growth towards the brain from the most recent annulus of ganglion cells added by cell division to the margin of the retina. Thus successive annuli of ganglion cells which accrue during growth come to dispose their axons in chronological order across the width of the ribbon, mapping the radius of the retinal disc. Conversely, retinal sectors are mapped orthogonally through the thickness of the ribbon, in their natural circumferential order (Scholes, 1979).

Forming this rectangular map means that the closed circumference of the fibre projection from the retinal disc must be opened at some point (cf.

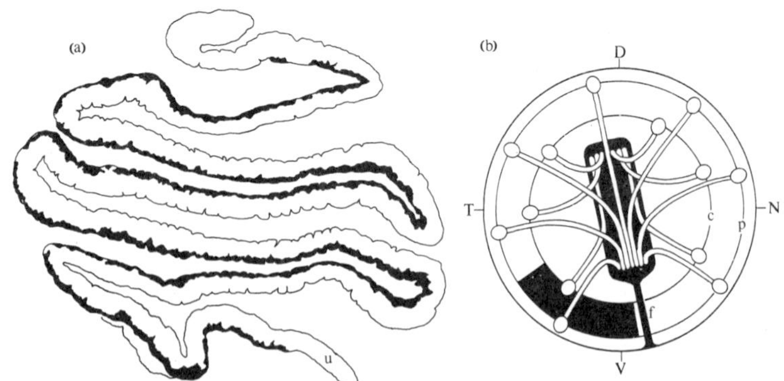

Figure 5 The retinal fibre map in the ribbon optic nerve of perciform fish.

(a) *Camera lucida* drawing of the cross-section of the right optic nerve (*Aquidens* sp.), with black marking the extent of fibre degeneration after an ocular lesion which severed axons from the ventro-temporal sector of the retina. The approximate retinal area involved is shown in (b), and *u* denotes the unmyelinated fibre tract.

(b) Schematic diagram of the way fibres run over the right retinal surface to enter the ribbon optic nerve. Extreme central (*c*) and peripheral (*p*) annuli only of ganglion cells are shown. Axons run with their neighbours throughout, and new ones accrue to the ventral edge of the nerve. *T* is temporal: *N*, nasal: *V*, ventral and *D* is dorsal. *f* is the choroid fissure, and the black sector relates to (a).

Gaze and Grant, 1978) to establish the boundary surfaces of the ribbon. It is characteristic of fish with ribbon nerves that the choroidal fissure of the embryonic eye vesicle survives throughout life as a radial cleft in the ventral retina. Fibres from the two margins of the fissure respectively populate the two surfaces of the ribbon, and this enables the retinal projection to deform, like a fluid, into the folded outline of the optic nerve. Fig. 5(b) shows how retinal axons enter the ribbon in this way, without exchanging their local neighbour relations.

There are many indications of similar temporal ordering in other vertebrate visual pathways, particularly where the optic nerve becomes apposed to the ventral and contralateral walls of the diencephalon, to form the optic tract, as was elegantly shown in amphibia by Gaze and Grant (1978). Whether ribbons exist cryptically within the conventional cylindrical outlines of other optic nerves is an open question. Something of the sort seems likely in the goldfish (Dawnay, 1979), where Rusoff and Easter (1980) have shown in a simple and direct way how small bundles of fibres in the optic nerve always originate from annuli of ganglion cells on the retinal surface.

Internal crossings in the contralateral tectal pathway

Ribbons illustrate how a seemingly elaborate pattern of fibre ordering in the optic nerve can be generated by rather simple developmental constraints, related to the mode of growth of the retina itself and the resultant substrate presented to newly extending axons—a template surface of older fibres and their satellite cells (Scholes, 1979). It would be satisfying if these constraints were the only ones to operate throughout the growing visual pathway, and retinal axons maintained their neighbourly order all the way onto the tectal surface.

The reality, as in invertebrates, is otherwise, and this is best seen by considering first the retinotopic arrangement of the amphibian optic tract. In amphibia, the tract has a wedge-shaped cross-section embedded in the wall of the contralateral diencephalon. Scalia and Fite (1974) showed that the array of fibres parallel to this surface maps the retinal circumference, in the sequence $n : v : t : d$, where $n =$ nasal, etc., as in Fig. 5(b). Moreover, tract fibres are chronologically ordered normal to the diencephalic surface, mapping retinal eccentricity (Gaze and Grant, 1978), with old fibres running deep and new ones superficially.

Gaze and Grant reasoned that this organization could be achieved by a simple deformation of the retinal fibre projection, if it were opened (in the sense used in connection with Fig. 5(b)) naso-dorsally to enable nasal and dorsal axons to form the tract boundaries. This cannot be correct, since their comparison of retina and tract neglected the handedness of the projection, conferred by a z axis, the direction of fibre growth. Viewing the cross-section of the tract upstream necessitates viewing the corresponding retina from behind, because axons originate on its *outward* surface. Looking at the two levels of the right eye projection in this way, we see two strings of circumferential positions:

$$\frac{N}{n}:\frac{V}{v}:\frac{T}{t}:\frac{D}{d}\ \text{(tract)} \neq \frac{N}{n}:\frac{D}{d}:\frac{T}{t}:\frac{V}{v}\ \text{(retina)},$$

where upper case are peripheral fibres and lower case are central ones. Because the two strings have opposite handedness, running anticlockwise and clockwise, the projection must pass through an internal reversal, like those in invertebrates. Where this is mediated in amphibia, and what form it takes, remains to be discovered.

The situation is clearer in cichlid fish, where the tract is a more abbreviated structure in the contralateral pathway, into which the ribbon condenses just before fibres invest the tectal surface. The ribbon arrives at this point with new fibres arranged laterally, as they are on the amphibian diencephalon, but retaining the retinal circumferential ordering adopted at the head of the optic nerve ($v : n : d : t : v$, see Fig. 5b). This order is re-shuffled into that seen in the amphibian tract ($n : v : t : d : n$) by an internal fibre chiasm which operates across the thickness of the ribbon (Fig. 6a) as its folds begin to coalesce with the simpler outline of the optic tract.

Like the invertebrate visual chiasms, this crossing reverses the handedness of the fibre map, but its significance is different because a further rearrangement, hitherto unrecognized, results from the pattern in which axons radiate from the tract onto the tectal surface. The pattern of fibre radiation over this convex mid-brain structure, shared by other lower vertebrates (Leghissa, 1955; Attardi and Sperry, 1963; Steedman *et al.*, 1979; Goldberg, 1974; Horder, 1974), differs in principle from that in which retinal axons converge on the head of the optic nerve. The radiation runs *circumferentially* around the margins of the tectum (cf. Cook and Horder, 1977), resulting in another reversal of map order, orthogonal to that effected in the ribbon. One can verify in Fig. 6b that rostrocaudal order would be opposite if the tectal fibre radiation took the pattern seen in the retina. Two reversals of this kind, like two mirror reflections at right angles, are geometrically equivalent to a rotation through 180°, so in this way, the organization of the contralateral tectal pathway effectively removes from the projection the optical image inversion mediated in the eye (Fig. 6b). Because the tectal map is oriented in the same way in all known vertebrates, this rotation must be a general feature of the projection, to what end we shall consider later.

To achieve the same thing with a fibre optic bundle, the natural strategy would be to twist it through 180°. The contralateral tectal pathway uses the more devious solution of pleating fibres through one another, and this

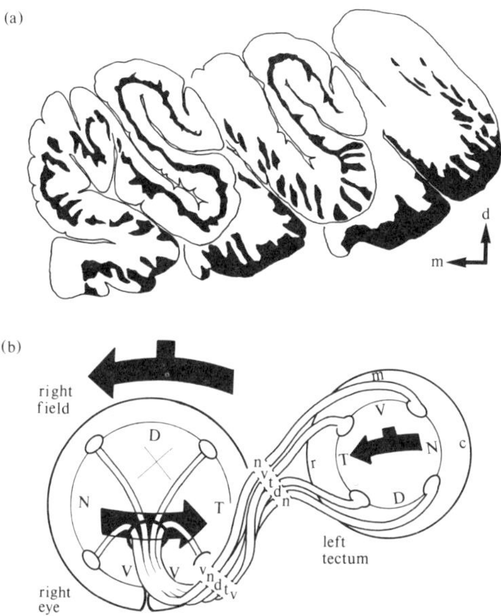

Figure 6 (a) Three successive sections through the ribbon nerve of the right eye as it approaches the left tectum. Black areas show the extent of fibre debris following a lesion which severed axons from the dorsal (and slightly nasal) retinal sector. Initially arranged in a continuous strip at the centre of the ribbon (cf. Fig. 5b) these fibres segregate into blocks and exchange position with others at the lateral boundary of the ribbon. *m* points medially, and *d*, dorsally.

(b) The contralateral projection from the right eye to the left tectum. The direction of view in this diagram is from the left side of the body, so the eye is seen from behind. Two separate reversals of fibre order rotate the retinal fibre map (see black arrows). One is mediated as the ribbon runs around the (nearest) side of the brain to approach the tectum (cf. a), and the other in the fibre radiation on the tectal surface (see text). Labels as in Fig. 5, except *m*, *c* and *r* which denote the medial, caudal and rostral poles of the tectum. See text.

reflects a developmental constraint likely to be fundamental to all fibre projections in the nervous system. The constraint is that growing neurites extend only over physical surfaces (see, for example, Bray, 1979)—in this case, over the continuous neural epithelium of which the embryonic eye is still a part (Silver and Robb, 1979; Cima and Grant, 1980; Holt, 1980), and then later over differentiated axons which have meanwhile accrued to the projection. Bodily twisting the pathway relative to its substrate could only be achieved at the expense of breaking this contact and the orderly chronological stratification it underlies.

The ipsilateral tectal pathway

The foregoing analysis of the geometry of the contralateral tectal projection dealt only with internal reordering of fibres *within* the cross-section

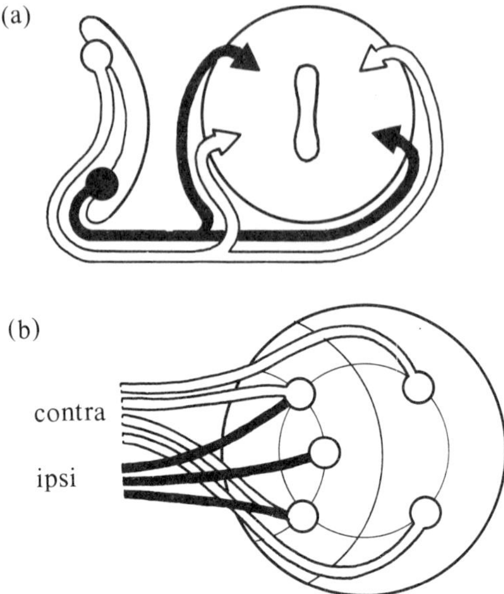

Figure 7 (a) Schematic diagram of an imaginary vertebrate visual system to show how, just as one bodily reversal of order results as fibres leave the retina (*left*), another opposite reversal inheres in innervating the opposite side of the brain (*right*). (*See text, and note that the real contralateral tectal projection achieves a rotation on the way to the mid-brain:* cf. Fig. 6.) However, the ipsilateral projection (*left*), if it preserves neighbour ordering, naturally achieves the dorsoventral map inversion found in reality (Fig. 4).

(b) contrasts the known contralateral tectal radiation pattern (white profiles) with a hypothetical one for ipsilateral fibres (black profiles), which would achieve binocular superimposition.

of the pathway. It did not invoke the *bodily* reversal of retinotopic order, considered earlier, which results when fibres turn from the outer surface of the retina to enter the head of the optic nerve. This reversal, unique to vertebrate eyes and a consequence of their inside-out construction, was irrelevant to the argument, in fact, because it is cancelled by an opposite one which inheres in crossing the mid-line to innervate the contralateral side of the brain. However, it follows from this natural bilateral symmetry, shown in Fig. 7a, that the reversal must have consequences for the arrangement of the ipsilateral tectal pathway, in animals which possess a direct visual projection to this side of the mid-brain.

It is interesting that Bunt and Horder (1977) were very close to understanding this point and its implications, when they considered the relation between the embryonic choroid fissure in the eye and the disposition of the contralateral tectal map. But, failing to adopt a consistent standpoint for viewing different levels of the projection, they were led to the erroneous conclusion that it is the contralateral map which is reversed (rather than rotated through 180°, as we have seen it to be) relative to the retinal image, and attributed this to the bodily reversal at the head of the optic nerve.

The reversal at the head of the optic nerve takes a definite form which is determined by the embryonic choroid fissure in the ventral part of the retina. The dorsal apex of the fissure is the exit for fibres leaving the retina, and this means that the array of axons turning back towards the brain over the template surface it forms, naturally reverse their order in the vertical plane (Fig. 5b; Bunt and Horder, 1977; Scholes, 1979; Levinthal and Bodick, 1979). That is to say, the structure of the eye in vertebrates necessarily places retinal axons of the optic nerve in the same order relative to body co-ordinates as is achieved by the visual chiasm at the back of the eye-globe in cephalopods.

This means that where vertebrate retinal fibres connect directly with the ipsilateral tectum, and if they do so in a topologically continuous manner, the map they form should carry the same reversal of the retinal image found in the cephalopod optic lobe. This we have already seen to be the case (Fig. 4), but what is meant here by a topologically continuous projection to the ipsilateral tectum needs careful definition, as long as no information exists on the layout of retinal fibres in this pathway.

Fig. 7a showed an imaginary vertebrate visual pathway in which retinal axons run parallel with one another to their destinations in the nervous system. Its purpose was to decompose the tectal projection geometrically, in order to understand the bodily reversals of fibre order naturally entailed in connecting the retina to the two sides of the brain. As we have seen, however, the contralateral projection contains two further internal rearrangements of fibre order, one in the optic nerve, and the other in the tectal radiation. Their joint outcome is equivalent to rotating the fibre map through π (arrow in Fig. 6b), with the result that the representation on the contralateral tectum is congruent with the visual field.

In animals which have a direct projection to the same side of the mid-brain (Fig. 4), no such rotation is necessary for retinal fibres to reach their destinations in the ipsilateral map (Fig. 7a), and this point has an interesting corollary. Since the rotation is absent from the ipsilateral pathway, so, obviously, must be the internal fibre reversals which mediate it in the contralateral pathway. One of these is on the tectal surface, and it follows, therefore, that the fibre radiation on the ipsilateral tectum must be different, and geometrically equivalent to that whereby fibres converge on the head of the optic nerve inside the eye (Fig. 5b).

This prediction is shown in Fig. 7b, and its interest, if correct, is that it provides a structural description of the way in which fibres from the ipsilateral retina can superimpose with the contralateral map, matching binocular visual directions rather than retinal locations (Thompson, 1979). Such a pattern, then, would represent the way in which the different ontogenetic rules for the ipsilateral and contralateral projections find their expression.

Conclusions

It may afford some teleological satisfaction to see that the contralateral tectal pathway in lower vertebrates rotates the fibre map through 180° and sets the brain's image of the world the right way up again, especially as this is achieved by such complicated means (Fig. 6b). There is, however, a more satisfactory way of exploring this observation. Imagine, in an animal with partial binocular overlap, cutting the anterior neural tube along the dorsal mid-line, so that it can be opened and spread out into the original configuration of the embryonic neural plate. Since, in origin, the two retinas are continuous parts of this epithelium, the operation makes it possible to visualize them both at the same time, and see, from the common standpoint of nerve fibre growth, the geometrical relation between the two retinal images of the frontal binocular field. This is done in Fig. 8a, where it becomes obvious that the two images, located temporally in both retinas, are simply related by rotation through π. It is a clear demonstration that it is necessary, in order to achieve binocular superimposition of the two retinal projections in the brain, for one of them to rotate through 180° relative to the other *en route* from the eyes. The

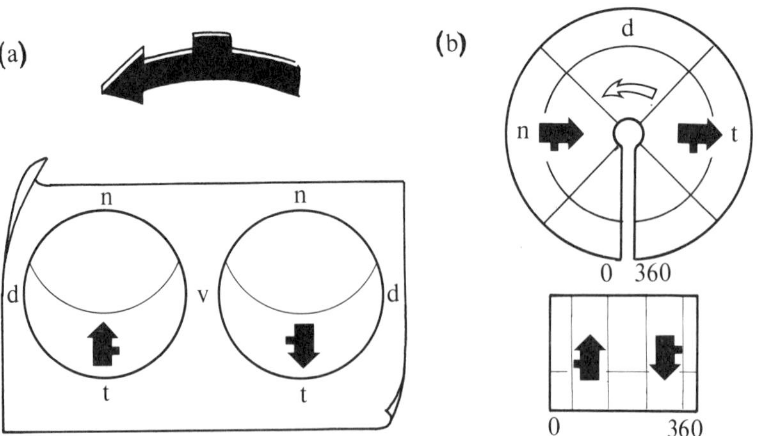

Figure 8 (a) The neural tube is opened from an incision along the dorsal mid-line and spread out flat, so that it is possible to visualize both retinas from a common standpoint (relative to nerve fibre growth). The images in the two binocular crescents (smaller black arrows) are related to one another by rotation through 180°. Labels as Fig. 5b.

(b) Illustrates how translating a binocular image (black arrow) from the temporal half of the eye to the nasal one involves a 180° rotation within the polar co-ordinates of the retina, shown for clarity as rectangular below (cf. Fig. 5b).

subtlety is that achieving binocular superimposition thus necessarily *entails* setting the map in some sense the right way up again.

Looking at the projection in this way puts us in the position to consider the implications of achieving, as primates and certain other animals have done (Polyak, 1957), complete frontal binocular overlap. Moving the eyes frontally means that binocular visual directions, previously imaged on both temporal retinas, are now imaged in the temporal half of one eye but the nasal half of the other. Only the nasal hemi-retina projects contralaterally through the partial decussation at the mid-line optic chiasm, so the visual maps each represent half of the field of view. In the mid-brain, however, they remain in principle oriented in the same way relative to body co-ordinates as in animals with partial binocular overlap—the vertical field meridian lies rostrally (Cynader and Berman, 1972). Thus the only change of importance is that the contralateral projection now conveys a map of the binocularly shared image which has been simply translocated horizontally across the eye onto the nasal hemi-retina. The geometrical consequence is an interesting one: it is that the image translocation from temporal to nasal is actually equivalent to a rotation through π, when considered in relation to the natural circular co-ordinates of the retina. This equivalence, shown in Fig. 8b, is especially clearly seen if the retinal disc is transformed into rectangular co-ordinates, as we have seen can happen to the fibre map in the visual pathway, as a natural consequence of its mode of growth (Fig. 5). It follows as a prediction, then, that no fibre crossings will be found in animals with full binocular overlap: the map rotation they mediate where the eyes face sideways is now effected on the retinal surface.

By virtue of these necessary fibre crossings in animals with partial binocularity, the contralateral pathway is topologically more complex than the ipsilateral one, where such exists as a direct projection from the retina. The ipsilateral map has the same orientation and handedness as the array of fibres leaving the eye (cf. Figs. 4 and 7), so it is likely that no internal fibre re-orderings are mediated in this pathway. It is as if the ipsilateral projection, although numerically the minor one, placed on the contralateral pathway the full onus of the fibre manoeuvres necessary for binocular superimposition. This impression of ipsilateral primacy is strengthened by the evidently archaic layout of the ipsilateral tectal map, oriented as it is in the same way as the primary visual maps in invertebrates (Figs. 3 and 4).

What would be the implications of arranging the vertebrate primary visual pathway in alternative ways to achieve neural superimposition of *partial* binocular fields? The simplest alternative among the two or three that come to mind would be to place the rotation and its attendant fibre manoeuvres in the ipsilateral rather than the contralateral pathway, thus altering by 180° the orientation of the tectal maps. On the face of it, this strategy and other similar ones are neither more nor less complicated than that adopted in reality: certainly the rotation is geometrically inescapable (Fig. 8a) and can only be achieved in different ways. However, interesting implications appear if one considers the problem of achieving *full* binocularity from such a hypothetical evolutionary basis, adopted for the sake of argument.

Translating the binocular image from the temporal to the nasal hemiretina of one eye, which is the result of full binocular overlap, amounts, as we have seen, to a rotation through 180° in the natural circular coordinates of the visual pathway (Fig. 8b). Therefore, to achieve binocular neural superposition now, from the alternative organizational basis proposed above, it would be necessary that a further map rotation be mediated in the contralateral pathway: there is no existing one there to delete. The only alternative to such a gratuitous increase in the net complexity of the visual pathway would, by symmetry, be to delete the rotation from the ipsilateral pathway, where it was placed for argument's sake. Doing so, of course, returns the organization of the visual pathway from the hypothetical form proposed to that actually extant. Could such simple considerations of economy have anything to do with the surprisingly conservative disposition we have seen to be adopted by primary visual maps in various organisms?

Acknowledgements

I am indebted to Dr B. C. Goodwin for much encouragement, and particularly grateful to Professor J. Z. Young, F.R.S., who informed me of the *Octopus* chiasm and thus stimulated the line of thought developed here. I thank Professor B. B. Boycott, F.R.S. and Christine Holt for helpful suggestions and discussions.

REFERENCES

Anders, J. J. and Hibbard, E. (1974) The optic system of the teleost *Cichlasoma biocellatum J. comp. Neur.*, **158**, 145–154.

Attardi, D. G. and Sperry, R. W. (1963) Preferential selection of central pathways by regenerating optic fibres *Exptl. Neurol.*, **7**, 46–64.

Braitenberg, V. (1967) Patterns of projection in the visual system of the fly. I. Retina-lamina projections *Exptl. Brain Res.*, **3**, 271–298.

Braitenberg, V. (1970) Ordnung und Orientierung der Elemente im Sehsystem der Fliege *Kybernetik*, **7**, 235–242.

Bray, D. (1979) Mechanical tension produced by nerve cells in tissue culture *J. Cell Sci.*, **37**, 391–410.

Bullock, T. H. and Horridge, G. A. (1965) *Structure and Function in the Nervous Systems of Invertebrates* W. H. Freeman, San Francisco-London.

Bunt, S. M. and Horder, T. J. (1977) A proposal regarding the significance of simple mechanical events, such as the development of the choroid fissure, in the organisation of central visual projections *J. Physiol.*, **272**, 10–11P.

Cajal, S Ramon y. (1898) Estructura del kiasm óptico y teoría general de los entrecruzamientos de las vias nerviosas *Rev. trimest. micrográf.*, Núm. 1.

Cajal, S Ramon y. (1917) Contribución al conocimiento de la retina y centros opticos de los cefalópodos *Trab. Lab. Invest. biol. Univ. Madrid*, **15**, 1–82.

Cajal, S Ramon y. and Sanchez, D. (1915) Contribución al conocimiento de los centros nerviosos de los insectos *Trab. Lab. Invest. biol. Univ. Madrid*, **13**, 1–164.

Caldwell, J. H. and Berman, N. (1977) The central projections of the retina in *Necturus maculosus J. comp. Neur.*, **171**, 455–464.

Cima, C. and Grant, P. (1980) Ontogeny of the retina and optic nerve of *Xenopus laevis*. IV. Ultrastructural evidence of early ganglion cell differentiation *Developmental Biol.*, **76**, 229–237.

Cohen, A. I. (1973) An ultrastructural analysis of the photoreceptors of the squid and their synaptic connections. II. Intraretinal synapses and plexus *J. comp. Neur.*, **147**, 379–398.

Cook, J. E. and Horder, T. J. (1977) The multiple factors determining retinotopic order in the growth of optic fibres into the optic tectum *Phil. Trans. R. Soc. Lond. B.*, **278**, 261–276.

Cruce, W. L. R. and Cruce, J. A. F. (1977) Projections from the retina to the lateral geniculate nucleus and the mesencephalic tectum in a reptile *Tupinambis nigropunctatus*: a comparison of anterograde transport and anterograde degeneration *Brain Res.*, **85**, 221–228.

Cynader, M. and Berman, N. (1972) Receptive field organisation of the monkey superior colliculus *J. Neurophysiol.*, **35**, 187–201.

Dawnay, N. A. H. (1979) Chronotopic organisation of the goldfish optic pathway *J. Physiol.*, **296**, 13P.

Edds, M. V. (1975) "Plasticity of retino-tectal connections in fishes and amphibians" in *Specificity and Plasticity of Retinotectal Connections* (eds. Edds, M. V., Gaze, R. M., Schneider, G. E., Irwin, L. N.) *N.R.P. Bulletin* 17, M.I.T. Press, Cambridge, Mass., 251–272.

Eloffson, R. and Dahl, E. (1970) The optic neuropiles and chiasmata of crustacea *Zeit. Zellforsch. u. mikros. Anat.*, **107**, 343–360.

Exner, S. (1891) *Die Physiologie der facetirten Augen von Krebsen und Insekten* Franz Deuticke, Leipzig and Wien.

Fawcett, J. (1980) Fibre organisation in the optic nerve of *Xenopus laevis J. Physiol.*, **303**, 38P.

Gaze, R. M. (1970) *The Formation of Nerve Connections* Academic Press, London.

Gaze, R. M., Keating, M. J. and Chung, S.-H. (1974) The evolution of the retinotectal map during development in *Xenopus Proc. R. Soc. Lond. B.*, **185**, 301–330.

Gaze, R. M. and Grant, P. (1978) The diencephalic course of regenerating retinotectal fibres in *Xenopus* tadpoles *J. Emb. exp. Morph.*, **44**, 201–216.

Goldberg, S. (1974) Studies on the mechanics of development of the visual pathway in the chick embryo *Developmental Biol.*, **36**, 24–43.

Goldberg, S. and Coulombre, A. J. (1972) Topographical development of the nerve fibre layer in the chick retina. A whole mount study *J. comp. Neur.*, **146**, 507–518.

Hanström, B. (1928) *Vergleichende Anatomie des Nervensystems der wirbellosen Tiere, unter Berücksichtigung seiner Funktion* Springer Verlag, Berlin.

Hesse, R. (1899) Untersuchungen über die Organe der Lichtempfindung bei niederen Thieren. V. Die Augen der polychäten Anneliden *Zeit. wiss. Zool.*, **65**, 446–516.

Holt, C. (1980) Cell movements in *Xenopus* eye development *Nature*, **287**, 850–852.

Horder, T. J. (1974) Changes in fibre pathways in the goldfish optic tract following regeneration *Brain Res.*, **72**, 41–52.

Horder, T. J. and Martin, K. A. C. (1978) "Morphogenetics as an alternative to chemospecificity in the formation of nerve connections" in *S.E.B. Symp.* **32**: *Cell-cell recognition* (ed. Curtis, A. S. G.) Cambridge University Press, Cambridge, 275–358.

Horton, J. C., Greenwood, M. M. and Hubel, D. H. (1979) Non-retinotopic arrangement of fibres in cat optic nerve *Nature*, **282**, 720–722.

Hunt, R. K. and Jacobson, M. (1974) Neuronal specificity revisited *Curr. Topics dev. Biol.*, **9**, 203–259.

Johns, P. R. and Easter, S. S. (1977) Growth of the adult goldfish eye. II. Increase in retinal cell number *J. comp. Neur.*, **176**, 331–342.

Keating, M. J. (1968) Functional interaction in the development of specific neuronal connections *J. Physiol.*, **198**, 75–77P.

Keating, M. J. (1975) The time course of experience-dependent switching of visual connections in *Xenopus laevis Proc. R. Soc. Lond. B.*, **189**, 603–610.

Keating, M. J. and Gaze, R. M. (1975) Visual deprivation and inter-tectal connections in *Xenopus Proc. R. Soc. Lond. B.*, **191**, 467–475.

Keating, M. J., Beazley, L., Feldman, J. D. and Gaze, R. M. (1975) Binocular interaction and inter-tectal neuronal connections: dependence on developmental stage *Proc. R. Soc. Lond. B.*, **191**, 445–446.

Keating, M. J. and Kennard, C. (1976) Binocular visual neurones in the frog thalamus *J. Physiol.*, **258**, 69–70P.

Kennedy, M. C. and Rubinson, K. (1977) Retinal projections in larval, transforming and adult sea lamprey *Petromyzon marinus J. comp. Neur.*, **171**, 465–480.

Kopsch, Fr. (1899) Mitteilungen über das Ganglion opticum der Cephalopoden *Int. Mschr. Anat. Physiol.*, **16**, 33–54.

Kunze, P. (1972) Comparative studies of arthropod superposition eyes *Zeit. vergl. Physiol.*, **76**, 347–357.

Land, M. F. (1969) Structure of the retinae of the principal eyes of jumping spiders (Salticidae: Dendryphantinae) in relation to visual optics *J. exp. Biol.*, **51**, 443–470.

Land, M. F. (1976) Superposition images are formed by reflection in the eyes of some oceanic decapod crustacea *Nature*, **263**, 764–765.

Leghissa, S. (1955) La structura microscopia e la ciloarchitettonica del tetto ottico dei pesci teleostei *Z. Anat. Entw. Gesch.*, **118**, 427–463.

Levinthal, C. and Bodick, N. (1979) in *Cell Lineage, Stem Cells and Cell Determination* (I.N.S.E.R.M. Symposium No. 10).

Lubsen, J. (1921) Over het projectie het netvlies of het tectum opticum by een beenvisch *Ned. T. Geneesk.*, **67**, 1258–1260.

Lund, R. D. and Lund, J. S. (1976) Plasticity in the developing visual system: the effects of retinal lesions made in young rats *J. comp. Neur.*, **169**, 133–154.

Maturana, H. (1960) The fine anatomy of the optic nerve of Anurans: an electron microscope study *J. Biophys. biochem. Cytol.*, **7**, 107–120.

Meinertzhagen, I. A. (1973) "Development of the compound eye and optic lobe of insects" in *Developmental Neurobiology of Arthropods* (ed. Young, D.) Cambridge University Press, Cambridge, 51–104.

Meinertzhagen, I. A. (1976) The organisation of the perpendicular fibre pathways in the insect optic lobe *Phil. Trans. R. Soc. Lond. B.*, **274**, 555–596.

Müller, J. (1826) *Zur vergleichenden Physiologie des Gesichtsinnes* Cnobloch, Leipzig.

Northcutt, R. G. and Butler, A. B. (1974) Evolution of reptilean visual systems: Retinal projections in a nocturnal lizard, *Gecko gecko* (Linnaeus) *J. comp. Neur.*, **157**, 453–466.

Oberdorfer, M. (1977) The neural organisation of the first optic ganglion of the principal eyes of jumping spiders (Salticidae) *J. comp. Neur.*, **174**, 95–118.

Polyak, S. (1957) *The Vertebrate Visual System* University of Chicago Press, Chicago.

Rager, G. and Rager, U. (1978) Systems matching by degeneration: a quantitative E.M. study *Exptl. Brain. Res.*, **33**, 55–78.

Repérant, J. (1973) Les voies et les centres optiques primaire chez la vipère (*Vipera aspis*) *Arch. Anat. micr. Morph. Exp.*, **62**, 323–352.

Rusoff, A. and Easter, S. S. (1980) Order in the optic nerve of goldfish *Science*, **208**, 311–312.

Scalia, F. and Fite, K. (1974) A retinotopic analysis of the central connections of the optic nerve in the frog *J. comp. Neur.*, **158**, 455–478.

Scholes, J. H. (1979) Nerve fibre topography in the retinal projection to the tectum *Nature*, **278**, 620–624.

Silver, J. and Robb, R. M. (1979) Studies on the development of the eye cup and optic nerve in normal mice and in mutants with congenital optic nerve aplasia *Developmental Biol.*, **68**, 175–190.

Sperry, R. W. (1963) Chemoaffinity in the orderly growth of nerve fibre patterns and connections *Proc. Nat. Acad. Sci. U.S.*, **50**, 703–709.

Steedman, J. G., Stirling, R. V. and Gaze, R. M. (1979) The central pathways of optic fibres in *Xenopus* tadpoles *J. Emb. exp. Morph.*, **50**, 199–215.

Strausfeld, N. J. (1971) The organisation of the insect visual system (light microscopy). II. The projection of fibres across the first optic chiasma *Zeit. Zellforsch. u. mikros. Anat.*, **121**, 442–454.

Szentagothai, J. and Szekely, G. (1956) Zum Problem der Kreuzung der Nervenbahnen *Acta. Biol. Acad. Sci. Hung.*, **6**, 215–229.

Thompson, I. D. (1979) Changes in the uncrossed retinotectal projection after removal of the other eye at birth *Nature*, **279**, 63–66.

Tiao, Y.-C. and Blakemore, C. (1976) Functional organisation in the superior colliculus of the Golden Hamster *J. comp. Neur.*, **168**, 483–504.

Vogt, K. (1975) Zur Optik des Flusskrebsauges *Zeit. Naturforsch.*, **30C**, 691.

Young, J. Z. (1962*a*) The optic lobes of *Octopus vulgaris Phil. Trans. R. Soc. Lond. B.*, **245**, 19–58.

Young, J. Z. (1962*b*) "Why do we have two brains?" in *Interhemispheric Relations and Cerebral Dominance* (ed. Mountcastle, V. B.) Johns Hopkins Press, Baltimore, 7–24.

Zawarzin, A. (1913) Histologische studien über Insekten. IV. Die optischen Ganglien der *Aeschna*-Larven *Zeit. wiss. Zool.*, **108**, 175–257.

CHAPTER FIFTEEN

EQUILIBRIUM AND PROPRIOCEPTIVE SYSTEMS, AND THE CENTRAL NERVOUS SYSTEM OF ARTHROPODS

DAVID C. SANDEMAN

Introduction

Animals frequently face situations during their lives in which they must rapidly and correctly reorient themselves in order to maintain their normal posture and balance. When examined closely, this commonplace activity proves to be extraordinarily complex and interesting. Not only are a variety of highly sophisticated sensory systems associated with compensatory reactions, but the systems themselves are remarkably accessible to study. Stimuli can often be carefully quantified and the behavioural reactions easily measured. Compensatory reflexes are ideal for the investigation of the central processing of discrete stimuli which lead to predictable activity in known motor systems. The sensory input and the motor output of most compensatory reflexes are easily identified and characterized and the components of the system, including the anatomy of the central nervous projections, can be accurately described.

An essential feature of compensatory reactions is that they should act rapidly, and perhaps it is this which has led to the specialization of sensory systems in which considerable filtering of the input occurs. This is often followed by the direct transfer of the information to the motor neurones. Compensatory systems thus give the impression of being entirely automatic and fully determined by the sensory input.

Stability can be achieved only at the expense of manoeuvrability. The animal might therefore be said to be in a "trade-off situation" and it is interesting to see how the compensatory systems enter it. Long-bodied arthropods (lobsters, locusts) are more stable about the yaw axis than are the short-bodied forms (crabs, flies), and are not able to make the rapid turns about this axis that the short-bodied forms can. Concurrent with the greater manoeuvrability of the short-bodied forms is the presence of a high degree of refinement of the peripheral sensory systems concerned with equilibrium and proprioception. It would appear that the decrease in stability afforded by shortening the body must be accompanied by the evolution of more sophisticated equilibrium systems.

A drawback to total automatic control by the compensatory system is that the animal could become a slave to it. When at rest the compensatory systems which may be appropriate during locomotion are sometimes irrelevant and need to be switched off or at least made less sensitive. Conversely, active animals need to have the compensatory systems standing by, perhaps inactive, but ready to respond at full sensitivity if necessary.

In this review a few of the many known compensatory systems will be described which use either visual, angular accelerational, or proprioceptive information as their prime inputs. Not all of these examples are completely known in terms of their peripheral and central components, but the physical principles governing their sense organs are quite well understood and the behavioural responses have been described. Despite the relative diversity of the chosen examples a common principle relating to the organization of compensatory systems emerges, leading to the suggestion of a way in which the central nervous system could produce these and perhaps other behavioural acts.

Compensatory systems with a visual input

Compound eyes

The compound eyes of arthropods are used for the detection of shapes, contrast and movement of the entire visual field, or of smaller objects within it. The essential component in the compensatory reactions released by compound eyes is the detection of the velocity and direction of relative motion between the eyes and the visual surround. The single receptor cells arrayed at the periphery of the eye are sensitive only to changes in light intensity and are therefore not able to perform the task of movement perception. This is computed in the deeper layers of the neuropile behind the retina from the sequential stimulation of the peripheral receptors as the image of the visual world moves across the surface of the eye. It follows that for movement perception to occur there must be relative motion between the eye and the target (sometimes referred to as the *slip*). The actual neural mechanism underlying visual motion perception is not yet known.

Visually-induced compensatory or optokinetic reactions can usually be released by surrounding a stationary animal with a contrast-rich visual field, and then rotating the entire visual field around the animal. This is not the equivalent of the natural situation where the animal turns about its vertical axis, but the method has the advantage of selectively stimulating the visual receptors and excluding the inputs from proprioceptors and angular acceleration detectors. When presented with such a stimulus an animal's usual response is to turn the head or eyes in the direction of the moving visual world in an attempt to stabilize the image of the environment on the eye.

In many animals two phases of the optokinetic response can be recognized, a slow following phase and a rapid return phase in which the direction of gaze is moved abruptly against the direction of the moving surround. Slow and fast phases follow one another sequentially as long as the visual world continues to turn or until the response adapts. Adaptation is variable; some animals will make only one or two fast phases and then hold the head or eyes pointing in the direction of the movement, whilst others will continue to respond for many minutes.

The slow phase movements of the optokinetic response can be modelled as a simple negative feedback system (Fig. 1). Perception of the movement generated by the slip between the visual world and the retina elicits an eye or head movement which acts to cancel the stimulus. The gain of the system with the feedback intact varies but is never more than about 0.9. Unity gain would mean perfect compensation with no slip and this cannot occur if the visual input is the sole driving force.

Different parts of the eyes of various arthropods are known to be differently sensitive to optokinetic stimuli. In mantids and in flies a moving stimulus presented to the anteriorly-facing portions of the eyes releases a greater response than when the same stimulus is presented only at the side (Collett and Land, 1975; Rossel, 1979). Conversely, in crabs, which more often walk sideways, larger eye movements to moving stimuli are released when these are presented at the sides of the eyes (Sandeman,

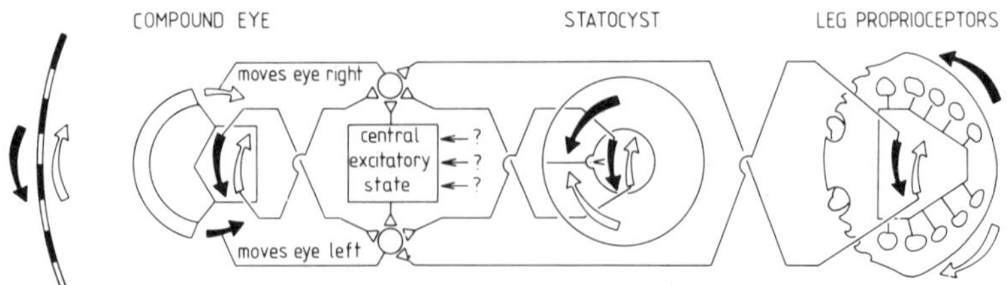

Figure 1 Sensory systems controlling horizontal eye movements in the crab. The movement of a vertically striped visual field either to the left (filled arrow) or to the right (unfilled arrow) is detected by the compound eye. Information about the direction and velocity of the movement is relayed to the eye muscles which move the eye in the same direction as the visual field. The gain of the transfer is affected by the central excitatory state of the animal. Similar directional information about changes in the animal's position are relayed to the same muscle system from the statocyst and from the leg proprioceptors. In every case the eye movements are such that they tend to remain stationary relative to the environment.

1978). The optokinetic response may therefore aid in directing the animal along a straight path by ensuring that the eye area most sensitive to movement across its surface is always pointing to where this is minimal, i.e. in the normal locomotory direction (Reichardt and Poggio, 1976; Poggio and Reichardt, 1976).

Not all optokinetic responses are compensatory in the sense that they form a negative feedback system. In the lobster, movement of a striped visual field from anterior to posterior has a significant effect in maintaining the *forward* walking of the animal (Ayers and Davis, 1977*a*).

The fast phase of the optokinetic response is generated within the central nervous system and does not use proprioceptive cues as a trigger (Horridge and Sandeman, 1964; Sandeman *et al.*, 1975*a*, *b*). The neural mechanism is not known but the appearance of a fast phase in sequential optokinetic responses is invariably preceded by a slow phase. In freely moving animals, saccades, which are the equivalent of fast phases, can occur without the preceding slow phase. The optokinetic system is therefore one which keeps the head or the eyes of the animal "locked" onto the visual environment. Fast saccades break this lock during voluntary turns.

Neurally, the optokinetic systems appear to be relatively simple. In locusts, flies and crabs, directional information is gathered in relatively few wide field motion sensitive interneurones (Kien, 1974*a*, *b*; Dvorak *et al.*, 1975; Sandeman *et al.*, 1975*b*). Where the output of the head or eye muscles has been recorded simultaneously with the optokinetic interneurones, it is found to follow closely the discharges of these interneurones (Kien, 1974*a*, *b*; Sandeman *et al.*, 1975*b*). The evidence points to a direct projection from the interneurones containing the adequately computed directional and velocity information to the appropriate motoneurones.

An aspect of the optokinetic systems, which is well known but has received little attention, is the variability of the gain of the systems, and the dependence of the gain on the overall activity or central excitatory state of the animal (Wiersma and Fiore, 1971). In locusts, the transfer of information from the optomotor neurones to the neck muscle motoneurones will sometimes fail, suggesting the presence of a gate which, if not primed, prevents the passage of the spike and consequently affects the consistency of the compensatory reaction (Kien, 1979).

Ocellar systems

The adults of many insects have ocelli. These are small light-sensitive organs situated at the front and side of the head above the much larger compound eyes, and their possible importance in maintaining stable flight has been reviewed (Kalmus, 1945). In the locust the lens of the ocellus is

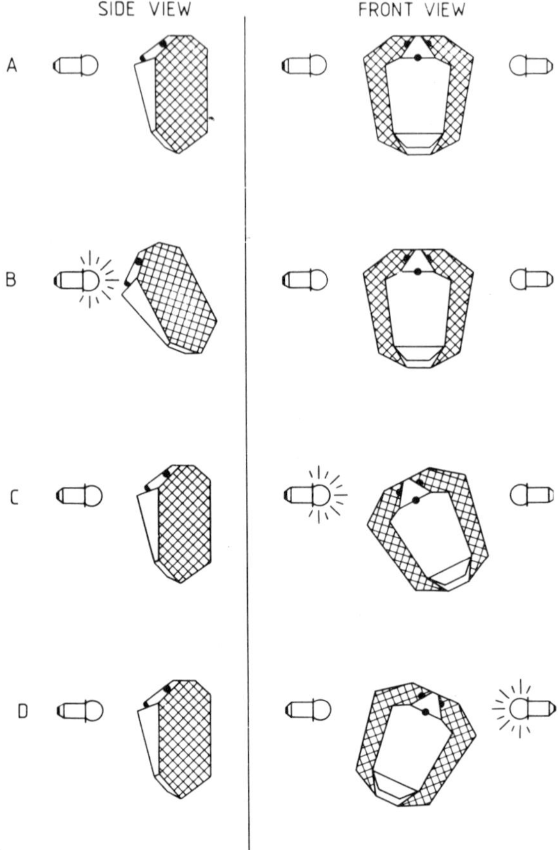

Figure 2 Head movements in dragonflies elicited by increasing the illumination in the receptive field of the individual ocelli. The animal is tethered and made to "fly" by directing a stream of air over it. A: No illumination. B: The anterior ocellus is illuminated and the head pitches forward. C and D: Lateral illumination results in head rolling toward the illuminated side. (From Stange and Howard, 1979.)

underfocused and so optically unsuited for producing a clear image of the environment on the receptor cells (Wilson, 1978). Large second order cells in the ocellar nerve are predominantly sensitive to ultraviolet light and adapt rapidly to illumination. Wilson produced the hypothesis that, among other functions, the ocelli together form a system responsible for maintaining stability about the pitch and roll axes. The ultraviolet-sensitive system of large second order cells divides the visual world into dark and light regions, the ground and the sky. Should the locust roll or pitch in flight, one of the lateral or the anterior ocelli will detect an abrupt decrease in the intensity of light in its visual field. If the output of these second order cells were coupled to appropriate neck muscles to produce a rapid correction of the head attitude, the stability of the animal would be assured, because neck proprioceptors, detecting the resulting misalignment between the head and the body, would act to realign the body behind the head. The optokinetic system is less suited for rapid compensation, concerned as it is always to establish a hold on the visual environment, and restoring systems such as those driven by the ocelli need to act quickly and phasically to override it.

Wilson's hypothesis has received support from behavioural observations on dragonflies (Stange and Howard, 1979), where the ocelli have long been suspected to have a stabilizing effect in flight (Mittelstaedt, 1950). Head movements can be elicited in dragonflies if the insects are first tethered in a windstream and made to "fly", and the ocelli are then individually illuminated. Illumination of the anterior ocellus results in downward tilting of the head; illumination of a lateral ocellus results in head rolling so that the non-illuminated side is rotated upward (Fig. 2). Head movements also follow shading the individual ocelli and in all cases the important parameter is an abrupt change in the level of illumination. Interpreted according to Wilson's hypothesis, the head turns of the dragonfly would serve to keep the lesser source of illumination (i.e. the ground) below the animal.

The latency of the head-turning response in the dragonfly is about 40 ms and the head movement is completed in about 100 ms, suggesting a fairly direct coupling between the receptors and the effectors. Of interest is the observation that dragonfly head movements occur only if the wings are being actively moved by the animal. Animals not in flight show little or no response to ocellar illumination. A direct parallel can be found in the head movements of flies in response to gravity, where orientation of the head occurs only during walking (Horn and Lang, 1978). Locust neck-muscle motoneurones are also controlled by a gating system interposed between them and the sensory hairs on the neck sclerites (Kien, 1979), and compensatory movements of the crayfish uropods to imposed roll, occur only during active extension of the abdomen (Hisada and Takahata, 1979).

Compensatory systems using angular acceleration as an input

A hydrodynamic system

Fluid contained within a hollow toroid can be displaced in relation to the walls of the toroid when angular acceleration is applied about the axis of the toroid, but not by linear acceleration in any direction. This physical phenomenon has been exploited in the evolution of animal sensory systems designed to detect angular acceleration about particular axes. Fluid-filled circular canals are found in the vestibular systems of the vertebrates, and in the statocysts of molluscs and swimming crabs. They form the basis of equilibrium systems which indicate changes in posture or position, as the result of imposed angular accelerations.

In the swimming crab, the normal sac-like statocyst of the crustacean has been elaborated to form a system of two circular canals (one horizontal and one vertical) at right angles to one another. Sensory hairs project across the lumen of the canals and detect the movement of the canal fluid (Sandeman and Okajima, 1972).

Fluid movements in the horizontal canals are known to lead to slow and fast compensatory eye movements (nystagmus) similar to those produced by an optokinetic stimulus (Fig. 1). Direct observation of the sensory hairs through the transparent walls of an isolated but intact statocyst showed that at oscillation frequencies where the eyes of the animal move in antiphase to the body, the hairs are also moving very nearly in antiphase relative to the walls of the statocyst (Janse and Sandeman, 1979*a*, *b*). The position of the hairs therefore directly determines the position of the eyes. Electrical recordings from the individual hairs show that, over a significant part of its physical range of movement, the position of the hair is coded in the discharge frequency of its sensory cell. The hairs can also be displaced by gravity and by fixing the animal in an abnormal position the hairs can be made to operate in a region where the sensory cells code their velocity. The eyes now move with a 90° phase lead relative to the body, confirming that the eye position is directly determined by the discharges in the sensory nerve.

The directness of the connection between the statocyst receptors and the motoneurones of the eye is also known from anatomical and physiological studies. Incoming afferents end in the same area of neuropile occupied by the branching dendrites of the oculomotor neurones, and intracellular recordings from the oculomotor neurones reveal a latency of 3 to 4 ms between volleys in the statocyst afferents and the e.p.s.p.s in the motoneurones (Sandeman and Okajima, 1973*a*, *b*; Silvey and Sandeman, 1976*a*).

Intracellular recordings from the oculomotor neurones of the swimming crabs also reveal a physiological correlate of the behavioural variability in the amplitude of the eye movements seen during maintained oscillation of the animal about its vertical axis. In these experiments the statocyst hairs were stimulated by irrigating the canals, and both the primary afferent discharges and the responses of the individual motoneurones were recorded simultaneously. Motoneurone potentials often fluctuated in phase with the sensory discharges but did not spike. E.p.s.p.s impinging on the motoneurones from other inputs, which were not identified but not related to statocyst stimulation in a phase-dependent way, raised the motoneurone membrane potentials to a level where each cycle from the irrigated statocyst released a burst of motor action potentials (Silvey and Sandeman, 1976*b*). The crab statocyst-eye movement system therefore exhibits the hallmarks of the other compensatory systems: a direct translation of the signal appearing in the nerves of a sensory system, which is tuned by its structure to select certain parameters of an imposed movement, to the motoneurones, and the control of the gain of this transfer by activity not stemming from a specific receptor but from some source measuring or reflecting the overall activity of the animal.

Sensory hairs stimulated by fluid movements around the *vertical* canals in the crab statocyst release a very different but equally interesting compensatory response. If the crab *Scylla serrata* is suspended above the ground and then tilted in a head-up direction, the last walking leg of each side performs circular motions not unlike the movements which accompany swimming. Called the righting reflex, this behaviour is under the direct control of the statocysts. Two large sensory interneurones collect the "head-up" directional information from the statocysts and transfer this in their axons diagonally across the body, i.e. from the left statocyst to the right side of the thoracic ganglion, and from the right statocyst to the left side of the thoracic ganglion. The righting reflex follows activity in these interneurones, whether they are excited by tilting the animal or by directly electrically stimulating the axons of the interneurones (Fraser, 1975). There is, however, an added nicety to the system. The vertical canals are oriented at 45° to the long axis of the body, so that maximum output in one interneurone and minimal output in its contralateral partner is elicited when the animal is tilted diagonally (Fraser and Sandeman, 1975). With diagonal tilting both 5th walking legs beat, but the leg opposite the maximally stimulated statocyst canal beats with a greater frequency and amplitude, and effectively counteracts the diagonally imposed tilt by raising the opposite "corner" of the animal. Thus the intensity of the output from the canals, represented by the frequency of the interneurone discharges, gives a precise indication of the axis, whether orthogonal or not, about which the animal is tilted. The direct transfer of this information into the amplitude and frequency of the beating of the individual 5th legs produces, automatically, the appropriate compensatory reaction. As in the other compensatory reactions, habituation is a feature of this system.

A gyroscopic system

The hind wings of dipterous flies are reduced to small club-shaped organs called *halteres*. Short-bodied, fast-flying flies of the muscid type are often totally dependent on these organs during flight. This can be easily demonstrated by removing or disabling the halteres and throwing the otherwise unharmed insect into the air. It typically executes a few, apparently uncontrolled turns and falls to the ground. A now classical experiment, in which a thread was glued to the back of an animal without halteres, showed that the animal could again fly if stability was returned to it by way of the trailing thread (Pringle, 1948).

The most important function of the halteres in stabilizing the flight of flies is probably in the detection of angular accelerations experienced during rapid turns and the subsequent release of compensatory head and wing movements. The way in which the halteres achieve this is as follows. During flight or walking the halteres beat up and down through an angle of about 170° and at a frequency of between 100 and 200 Hz. They can be compared to two rapidly beating pendula. At the bottom and at the top of their swing, the club-shaped ends of the halteres are for a short time stationary. Their distance from the vertical axis of the fly is also at a minimum. In the middle of their swing, however, the ends of the halteres reach a maximum velocity, are at their maximum distance from the vertical axis of the fly, and have therefore a certain inertia to any force acting about the vertical axis of the fly. It is not certain whether this in itself exerts a stabilizing effect on the fly, but it is known that the rows of campaniform sensilla around the base of the halteres are sensitive to their displacement.

Compensatory head movements in resting flies can be produced by twitching the haltere of one side forwards (Sandeman and Markl, 1980). The head movement is always away from the side on which the haltere is moved. Displacing the haltere backward or up and down released no head movement (Fig. 3). From these results it was speculated that should the fly experience a sudden yaw to the left, for example, when the halteres are oscillating, the haltere on the left will be displaced forwards and release a head turn to the right to compensate for the displacement (Sandeman and Markl, 1980). This hypothesis was tested by rapidly accelerating tethered, flying animals about their vertical axes and photographing them during the applied acceleration. The photographs show that with the halteres intact, the animals compensate for the imposed acceleration by turning their heads against the rotation, and by altering the angle of attack of the individual wings in ways which would resist the imposed movement; with the halteres removed these compensatory movements are absent (Sandeman, 1980).

The sensitivity of the halteres to angular acceleration can be demonstrated by subjecting tethered, walking animals to a rapid oscillation about their vertical axis and photographing them at different positions in the cycle. The results show that the head is in antiphase with the body at angular accelerations which the fly normally experiences during flight. The largest head deflections occur therefore when the maximum acceleratory force is exerted on the halteres.

Physiological studies of the haltere system reveal that moving the

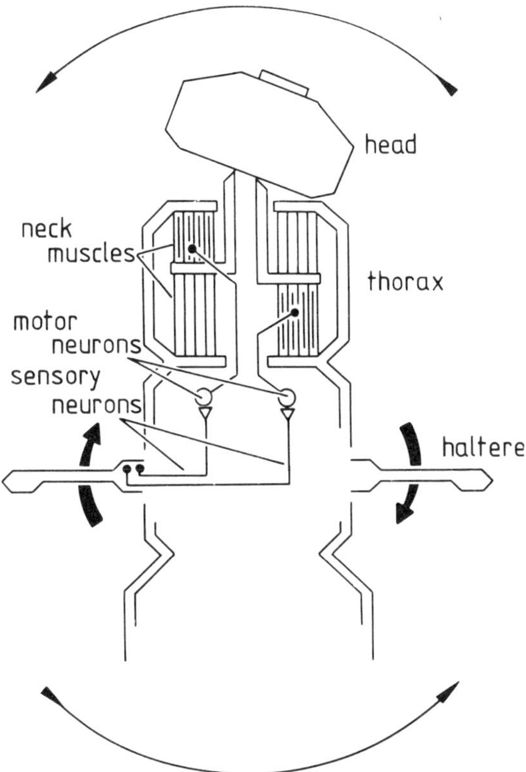

Figure 3 Halteres and the head movement of flies. Forward movement of the left haltere, brought about by a counterclockwise acceleration of the fly, excites receptors at the base of the haltere. This produces contractions in neck muscles which, through the action of neck sclerites, pull the head of the fly to the right. (From Sandeman and Markl, 1980.)

haltere forwards results in a single phasic discharge in the motoneurones of the neck muscles which bring about the head movements. The motoneurone discharges follow, one to one, a stimulus rate of up to 200 Hz, and do not adapt readily. Latencies are in the order of 2 to 3 ms, and cobalt back-filling of the sensory pathways from the haltere nerve shows them to branch widely but, significantly, to send processes into those neuropiles occupied by the endings of the neck and wing motoneurones. Thus, in the fly haltere system, directional receptors, tuned by the remarkable physical structure of the organ, project directly to the muscle systems and automatically produce exactly the appropriate compensatory motions of the head and wings (Fig. 3).

Gating in this system has not yet been directly demonstrated. Stationary flies twitch their heads through only 3 to 4 degrees after comparatively large displacements of the halteres. Walking animals, however, turn their heads through angles of up to 12° in response to deflections of the halteres which must be very small (Sandeman, 1980). This difference could be accounted for by the relatively gross method of moving the haltere in the stationary animal, and the higher rate of repetition of the forward force in the naturally beating haltere. It is also possible that the activity of the halteres itself raises the excitability of the motoneurones in a non-specific manner. The possibility exists that, as earlier suggested by von Buddenbrock (1919), the halteres are also "stimulation" organs signalling a general state of activity of the animal.

Compensatory systems with proprioceptive inputs

The task presented to the crustacean central nervous system of monitoring and controlling the actions of the walking legs is a complex one. Crustacean legs are typically jointed in six or seven places and at each joint there are several proprioceptive devices monitoring its acceleration, velocity and position (Fig. 4). The limb has degrees of freedom in every plane and a sensory input from 14 to 16 complete receptor systems (Wales *et al.*, 1970; Clarac, 1977). That this information is somehow and somewhere combined in a rapid and effective way can be concluded from watching the agility with which shore crabs run over uneven ground without stumbling, or witnessing the immediate implementation of alternative stepping sequences which act to maintain stability if one or more legs are lost. Also included in the repertoire are the necessary refinements

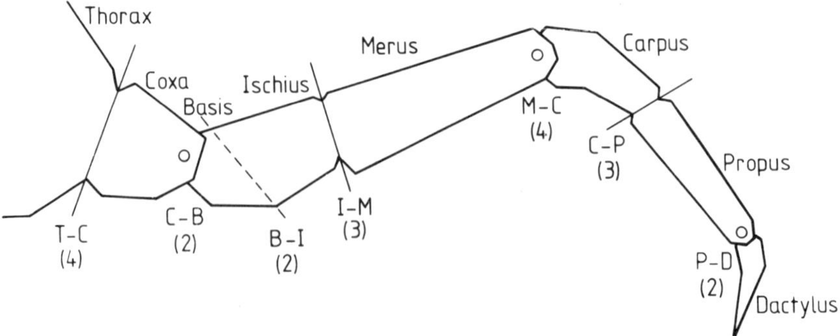

Figure 4 The leg of a decapod crustacean. Lines through the joints indicate that the joint moves about an axis which is parallel to the plane of the page. Circles indicate that the joint axis is at right angles to the page. In the animal this corresponds respectively to an anterior/posterior, and dorso/ventral movement of the limb. The B–I joint is indicated with a dotted line because in the Astacura this is not movable. The numbers in parentheses below each joint represent the numbers of identified sensory systems associated with each joint (Clarac, 1977).

for stopping, turning, backward walking, climbing, and rapid and slow movement.

Compensatory movements associated with the legs can be regarded as either static, or postural changes, or dynamic (locomotory) reactions. These are treated separately below.

Static compensation

The maintenance of stability when standing still is as critical to the animal as when walking, since it needs to compensate for the forces caused by gravity and by movements of the surrounding medium, i.e. air or water, which can be sudden. It is therefore to the animal's advantage to be able to react rapidly and directionally. Insects on trees in gusty weather, crayfish in tidal pools and crabs on wave-exposed rocks are all subjected to quite considerable and sudden forces, and rely upon the rapid detection of the strength and direction of these forces to counteract them with reflexive muscle actions.

Such reactions must be quickly co-ordinated and be appropriate not only to the direction from which the disturbance comes, but also for the particular posture the animal happens to hold at the time. Two animals, both subjected to the same lateral force may have to make very different compensatory adjustments depending on the respective positions of the limbs of each.

If, in an experimental situation, a force is brought to bear on a standing animal, from above or laterally, the animal immediately resists (MacMillan, 1975). These so called "resistance reflexes" are an important part of the stability system, and various interactions between many receptors can be investigated by measuring the force the animal exerts against the imposed disturbance and by observing the compensatory reactions of the eyes, for example, when the legs are displaced (Schöne *et al.*, 1976).

In this way inter-receptor actions in the spiny lobster have been demonstrated. When the animal is firmly held by the body, and the legs are displaced by tilting a board on which the animal stands, the eyes move in a way which can be related to the intensity of the combined compensatory activity of the legs, and to the statocyst as well if the body of the animal is tilted (Neil and Schöne, 1979). If the leg-to-body geometry is altered, for example by fixing the mero-carpopodite joint in particular positions, the gain of the leg-produced eye movements is also altered (Scapini *et al.*, 1978). Similar interactions and weighting of the inputs from various receptor systems can be demonstrated. The compensation brought about by gravity (monitored through the statocyst) is lessened when the animal has contact with the substrate (Schöne *et al.*, 1978). The gain of the eyestalk movements driven by leg proprioceptors is related to the force exerted by the legs and not by the movement. This can be shown by allowing very small leg movements and applying considerable force, in comparison with allowing larger leg movements to occur in the presence of a smaller force (Neil *et al.*, 1979).

Postural compensatory reactions also habituate if they are repeatedly evoked. They rapidly dishabituate if the animal is aroused.

Some indication of the rapidity and directness of the receptor-to-effector connectivity in the leg proprioceptor systems is given by the studies of Bush and colleagues on the thoracic coxal joint. Receptors here have axons which are short and thick and do not conduct action potentials. Instead the electrotonically-conducted receptor potentials are converted directly into motoneurone action potentials which reflect by their frequency the depolarization of the receptor. Behaviourally, this system is responsible for a strong resistance reflex of the thoracic coxal joint, and by feeding back upon itself and its receptor muscles, the receptor system is probably able to set the gain of the system and so adjust for the different postures taken up by the leg (Bush, 1976). The extent to which this device is used elsewhere in the limb is not known, but such adjustments require the receptor to be associated with a receptor muscle system.

Dynamic stability

Walking is a continuing and dynamic process of orientation. Resistance reflexes are less evident during walking in the crustaceans and may be important to compensate rapidly for unexpected movements occurring when the animal walks over slippery or uneven ground (Barnes *et al.*, 1972). In stick insects, however, resistance reflexes do play an active role during walking (Cruse and Pfluger, 1978), and there is evidence to suggest that in the lobster resistance reflexes may be important at the end of the trailing stroke and the beginning of the forward movement of the limb (Davis, 1969; Ayers and Davis, 1977*b*).

Several kinds of reflexive systems important in the control of walking have been discovered in the lobster *Homarus americanus*. If these animals are held by the carapace and forced to stand on a motor-driven treadmill, many will actively walk at the velocity and in the direction determined by the treadmill (Ayers and Davis, 1977*a*). Recording from known muscles in the legs of these animals allowed the identification of four types of reflexes. These are:

1. Resistance or negative feedback reflexes which occur in relation to every joint of the leg (Bush, 1965).
2. Co-operative or positive feedback reflexes which act to move the limb in the direction it is displaced. Three of these systems have been identified, all concerned with movement of the thoracic coxal joint.

3. Distributed reflexes, in which movement at one joint in a limb evokes an output to the motoneurones in another joint of the same limb. Nineteen of these are described. Characteristically the interaction is always between joints which move in the same plane.

4. Intersegmental reflexes in which movements in the joints of one limb affect the motoneurones to the muscles of the other limbs. These are known from relatively few examples and their role is not clear except perhaps for the maintenance of limb co-ordination (Ayers and Davis, 1978).

A remarkable finding in the lobster is that "appropriate" reflexes, i.e. those seen to occur at a particular time in the leg movement cycle during walking, are tuned to a specific velocity of leg movement, and that these velocities occur during normal walking. Movement of the limbs at abnormal velocities resulted in phase shifts of the reflex in relation to the leg movement-cycle and the firing of the reflex at an "inappropriate" time. This is mirrored in the behaviour of the animals —lobsters can be made to walk on the treadmill only within a limited velocity range.

The reflexive systems controlling the limb movements during walking in crustaceans are not sufficient to maintain walking in the absence of central nervous activity. The subsystem of specialized and tuned receptors, their direct connections with the muscle systems, and the constraints imposed by tuning and hard-wiring the entire reflex system may nevertheless be responsible for much of the fine tuning seen during walking. The central commands may be much less precise in their nature than was previously thought, and may act largely by supplying a general activity to the subsystem.

Discussion and conclusions

In spite of their diversity in anatomy and function, the sensory-motor systems described here share several common features.

1. The receptor systems are specialized in their structure and thus often dictate the specific physical parameter to which the sensory cells respond.

2. The connections between the sensory cells and their motoneurones are often very direct.

3. There is evidence of a divergence of the sensory input parallel to the direct addressing of the labelled-line sensory-to-motor system.

4. The built-in anatomical rigidity of the systems does not prevent variability of behaviour, and the gains of the reflexes are often controlled either by some ongoing activity or by the state of arousal of the animal.

These features, although drawn specifically from compensatory systems, in fact represent some of the more typical characteristics of arthropod nervous systems and lead to some generalizations about their overall organization.

The close association between the central terminals of sensory neurones and the branches of motoneurones in the central neuropile is now known from both insects and crustaceans, and there is good evidence that in some systems there are no interneurones interposed between the sensory and motor neurones. This does not mean that interneurones have no part to play, or have not been implicated in arthropod behaviour. It is now possible, however, to recognize two basic classes of interneurones. These are, first, the "in-line" type where the input from a particular set of sensory cells is combined, of which the optokinetic interneurones are a typical example. Termed "sensory" interneurones, they carry the information regarding the direction and velocity of movement in the visual field of the receptors to the motor systems which move the head or the eyes. The giant statocyst interneurones in the crab are another example, although the term "sensory interneurone" is less satisfactory here, because if they are stimulated they will drive the motor system releasing the righting behaviour. Other interneurones in the Crustacea which similarly produce complete behavioural actions when stimulated have been called "command" interneurones. Both sensory and command interneurones are "in line" between the receptor and effector.

The second class of interneurones which have recently received more attention are not "in line" between the sensory and motor systems but converge on the sensory-motor junctions of the more direct systems and modulate them. An interesting example of such a "modulator" interneurone is provided by the DUM cells in the locust thoracic ganglion (Evans and O'Shea, 1977; Hoyle and Dagan, 1978). These interneurones are responsive to a large number of sensory inputs but adapt so rapidly that it is hard to characterize them in terms of their sensory input. They function in this sense as novelty detectors. Their output controls the gain of the motor system driving the fast extensor muscle of the tibia, important for jumping.

That "in line" interneurones can also act as modulators has been elegantly demonstrated in crayfish (*Procambarus clarkii*) where uropod movements under the control of the statocyst are gated by activity in interneurones, bringing about extension of the tail (Hisada and Takahata, 1979).

The multimodality of modulator interneurones is a point of particular interest when considering the overall organization of the central nervous system and behaviour. The unimodal specificity of the sensory cells is lost when their inputs are combined in these multimodal cells. The interneurones contain information which represents a particular mixture of sensations. Characterization of these interneurones could depend on the mixture, or "colour", produced by the combination of specific receptor modalities, and, importantly, by their outputs. So far no real attempt has been made to describe identified interneurones in this way, or to show that the mixtures found within the identified interneurones are always the same in a particular cell, and have an effect on the same specific set of motor systems. An intriguing finding is that in some multimodal interneurones in the bee brain, relative sensitivity to different sensory modalities changes during conditioning (Erber, 1980).

A concept emerging from several studies on compensatory systems is that the sensory information gathered into multimodal interneurones parallels the activity of the hard-wired, directly addressed systems and is used to control their gains (Silvey and Sandeman, 1976*b*; Kien, 1979). Such a system is illustrated in Fig. 5. In compensatory systems the causal

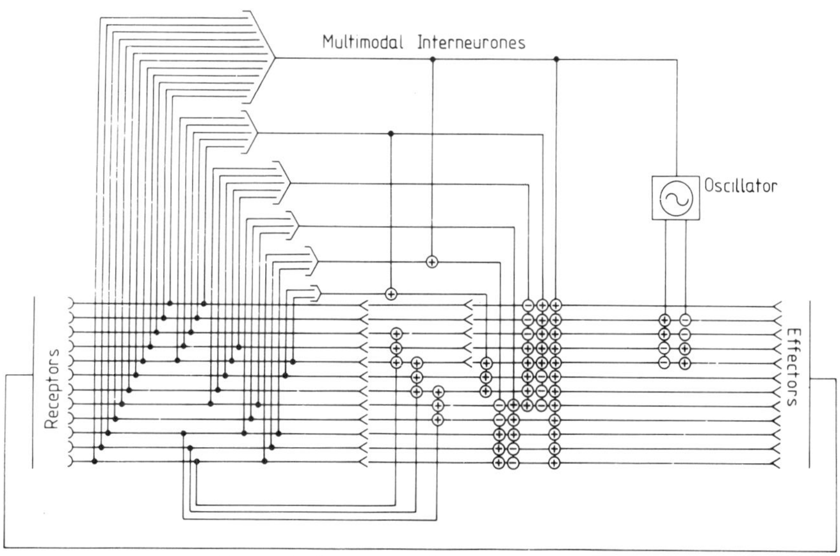

Figure 5 A model of the organization of the neurones in the central nervous system of arthropods. The scheme is derived from studies of sensory systems and their related compensatory reactions. Information from receptors at the left of the diagram is highly selected by the receptors and the receptor systems. This information can be addressed directly to the effector motoneurones, or to the motoneurones via sensory "in line" interneurones. Information from two or many tuned receptors is also collected by multimodal "modulator" interneurones which are graded according to the complexity of their input. The output of the multimodal neurones either increases or decreases the gain of the directly addressed motor systems, and also acts through central oscillators which in turn activate the sensory-motor subsystems. Modulation of the motor systems can also be achieved directly by diverging sensory inputs or by the action of one "in line" system on another (Hisada and Takahata, 1979). A physical feedback is created by the action of the motoneurones on the receptor inputs, which in the compensatory systems are usually sensitive to the motion produced by the effectors.

and dominating factor in the movement made by the animal lies in the sensory input, but in walking animals (though not necessarily in all flying insects, Heide, 1979) the dominant influence which sets the cyclical pattern of the appendages stems from the central oscillators (Davis, 1976), although peripheral reflexes act to tune the output of the oscillator to prevailing conditions.

The model in Fig. 5 may be applied to more than just the compensatory actions, and implies that all observed behaviour is the direct result of the careful combination of sensory inputs to form specific, complex mixtures which modulate the gains of the simpler hard-wired subsystems. What the animal *will* do at any stage depends on the titration of the various modulators, one against the other. What the animal *can* do is restricted by the bandwidths of the reflexive subsystems.

REFERENCES

Ayers, J. L. and Davis, W. J. (1977*a*) Neuronal control of locomotion in the lobster. I. Motor programs for forward and backward walking *J. comp. Physiol.*, **115**, 1–27.

Ayers, J. L. and Davis, W. J. (1977*b*) Neuronal control of locomotion in the lobster. II. Types of walking reflexes *J. comp. Physiol.*, **115**, 29–46.

Ayers, J. L. and Davis, W. J. (1978) Neuronal control of locomotion in the lobster. III. Dynamic organization of walking reflexes *J. comp. Physiol.*, **123**, 289–298.

Barnes, W. J. P., Spirito, C. P. and Evoy, W. H. (1972) Nervous control of walking in the crab *Cardisoma guanhumi*. II. Role of reflexes in walking *Z. vergl. Physiol.*, **76**, 16–31.

Buddenbrock, W. von (1919) Die vermutliche Lösung der Halterenfrage *Pflügers Archiv.*, **175**, 125–164.

Bush, B. M. H. (1965) Leg reflexes from chordotonal organs in the crab, *Carcinus maenas Comp. Biochem. Physiol.*, **15**, 567–587.

Bush, B. M. H. (1976) "Non-impulsive thoracic coxal receptors in crustaceans" in *Structure and Function of Proprioceptors in the Invertebrates* (ed. Mill, P.) Chapman and Hall, London.

Clarac, F. (1977) "Motor co-ordination in crustacean limbs" in *Identified Neurons and Behaviour of Arthropods* (ed. Hoyle, G.) Plenum Press, New York.

Collett, J. S. and Land, M. F. (1975) Visual control of flight behaviour in the hoverfly *Syritta pipiens* L *J. comp. Physiol.*, **99**, 1–66.

Cruse, H. and Pflüger, H-J. (1978) Wird die Stellung des Kniegelenkes auch beim laufenden Insekt geregelt? *Verh. Dtsch. Zool. Ges.*, **260**.

Davis, W. J. (1969) Reflex organization in the swimmeret system of the lobster. I. Intrasegmental reflexes *J. exp. Biol.*, **51**, 547–563.

Davis, W. J. (1976) "Organizational concepts in the central motor networks of invertebrates" in *Neural Control of Locomotion* (eds. Herman, R., Grillner, S., Stein, P. S. G., Stuart, D.) Plenum Press, New York.

Dvorak, D. R., Bishop, L. G. and Eckert, H. E. (1975) On the identification of movement detectors in the fly optic lobe *J. comp. Physiol.*, **100**, 5–23.

Erber, J. (1980) Neural correlates of non-associative learning in the honeybee *Verh. Dtsch. Zool. Ges.* (in press).

Evans, P. D. and O'Shea, M. (1977) An octopamine neurone modulates neuromuscular transmission in the locust *Nature*, **270**, 257–259.

Fraser, P. (1975) Three classes of inputs to a semicircular canal interneuron in the crab *Scylla serrata*, and a possible output *J. comp. Physiol.*, **104**, 261–271.

Fraser, P. and Sandeman, D. C. (1975) Effects of angular and linear accelerations on semicircular canal interneurons of the crab *Scylla serrata J. comp. Physiol.*, **96**, 205–221.

Heide, G. (1979) Proprioceptive feedback dominates the central oscillator in the patterning of the flight motoneuron output in *Tipula* (Diptera) *J. comp. Physiol.*, **134**, 177–189.

Hisada, M. and Takahata, M. (1979) "Control of uropod position by descending statocyst-driven interneurons in the crayfish" in *Integrative Control Functions of the Brain*, Vol. II (eds. Ito, M., Tsukahara, N., Kubota, K., Yagi, K.) Kodansha, Tokyo; Elsevier, Amsterdam.

Horn, E. and Lang, H. G. (1978) Positional head reflexes and the role of the prosternal organ in the walking fly *Calliphora erythrocephala J. comp. Physiol.*, **126**, 137–146.

Horridge, G. A. and Sandeman, D. C. (1964) Nervous control of optokinetic responses in the crab *Carcinus Proc. Roy. Soc.* (*B*), **161**, 216–246.

Hoyle, G. and Dagan, D. (1978) Physiological characteristics and reflex activation of DUM (octopaminergic) neurons of locust metathoracic ganglion *J. Neurobiol.*, **9**, 59–79.

Janse, C. and Sandeman, D. C. (1979*a*) The role of the balance organs in the induction of phase and gain in the vestibulo-ocular reflex of the crab *Scylla serrata J. comp. Physiol.*, **130**, 95–100.

Janse, C. and Sandeman, D. C. (1979*b*) The significance of canal receptor properties for the phase and gain of the vestibulo-ocular reflex in the crab *Scylla serrata J. comp. Physiol.*, **130**, 101–111.

Kalmus, H. (1945) Correlations between flight and vision, and particularly between wings and ocelli in insects *Proc. Roy. Ent. Soc. Lond.*, **A20**, 84–96.

Kien, J. (1974*a*) Sensory integration in the locust optomotor system. I. Behavioural analysis *Vision Res.*, **14**, 1245–1254.

Kien, J. (1974*b*) Sensory integration in the locust optomotor system. II. Direction selective neurons in the circumoesophageal connectives and optic lobe *Vision Res.*, **14**, 1255–1268.

Kien, J. (1979) Variability of locust motoneuron responses to sensory stimulation: a possible substrate for motor flexibility *J. comp. Physiol.*, **134**, 55–68.

MacMillan, D. L. (1975) A physiological analysis of walking in the American lobster *Homarus americanus Phil. Trans. Roy. Soc. B*, **270**, 1–59.

Mittelstaedt, H. (1950) Physiologie des Gleichtgewichtsinnes bei fliegenden Libellen *Z. vergl. Physiol.*, **32**, 422–463.

Neil, D. M. and Schöne,. H. (1979) Reactions of the spiny lobster *Palinurus vulgaris* to substrate tilt. II. Input–output analysis of eyestalk responses *J. exp. Biol.*, **79**, 59–68.

Neil, D. M., Schöne, H. and Scapini, F. (1979) Leg resistance reaction as an output and an input. Reactions of the spiny lobster, *Palinurus vulgaris* to substrate tilt. VI *J. comp. Physiol.*, **129**, 217–221.

Poggio, T. and Reichardt, W. (1976) Visual control of orientation behaviour in the fly. II *Quart. Rev. Biophys.*, **9**, 377–438.

Pringle, J. W. S. (1948) The gyroscopic mechanism of the halteres of *Diptera Phil. Trans. R. Soc. B*, **233**, 347–384.

Reichardt, W. and Poggio, T. (1976) Visual control of orientation behaviour in the fly. I. A quantitative analysis *Quart. Rev. Biophys.*, **9**, 311–375.

Rossel, S. (1979) Regional differences in photoreceptor performance in the eye of the praying mantis *J. comp. Physiol.*, **131**, 95–112.

Sandeman, D. C. (1978) Regionalization in the eye of the crab *Leptograpsus variegatus*: Eye movements evoked by a target moving in different parts of the visual field *J. comp. Physiol.*, **123**, 299–306.

Sandeman, D. C. (1980) Angular acceleration, compensatory head movements and the halteres of flies (*Lucilia serricata*) *J. comp. Physiol.*, **136**, 361–367.

Sandeman, D. C. and Okajima, A. (1972) Statocyst induced eye movements in the crab *Scylla serrata* I. The sensory input from the statocysts *J. exp. Biol.*, **57**, 187–204.

Sandeman, D. C. and Okajima, A. (1973*a*) Statocyst induced eye movements in the crab *Scylla serrata*. II. Response of the eye muscles *J. exp. Biol.*, **58**, 197–212.

Sandeman, D. C. and Okajima, A. (1973*b*) Statocyst induced eye movements in the crab *Scylla serrata*. III. The anatomical projections of the sensory and motor neurons and the responses of the motor neurons *J. exp. Biol.*, **59**, 17–38.

Sandeman, D. C., Erber, J. and Kien, J. (1975*a*) Optokinetic eye movements in the crab *Carcinus maenas* I. Eye torque *J. comp. Physiol.*, **101**, 243–258.

Sandeman, D. C., Kien, J. and Erber, J. (1975*b*) Optokinetic eye movements in the crab *Carcinus maenas*. II. Responses of optokinetic interneurons *J. comp. Physiol.*, **101**, 259–274.

Sandeman, D. C. and Markl, H. (1980) Head movements in flies (Calliphora) produced by deflection of the halteres *J. exp. Biol.*, **85**, 43–60.

Scapini, F., Neil, D. M. and Schöne, H. (1978) Leg to body geometry determines eyestalk reactions to substrate tilt. Substrate orientation in spiny lobsters. IV *J. comp. Physiol.*, **126**, 287–291.

Schöne, H., Neil, D. M. and Scapini, F. (1978) The influence of substrate contact on the gravity orientation. Substrate orientation in spiny lobsters. V *J. comp. Physiol.*, **126**, 293–295.

Schöne, H., Neil, D. M., Stein, A. and Carlstead, M. K. (1976) Reactions of the spiny lobster, *Palinurus vulgaris*, to substrate tilt. I *J. comp. Physiol.*, **107**, 113–128.

Silvey, G. E. and Sandeman, D. C. (1976*a*) Integration between statocyst sensory neurons and oculomotor neurons in the crab *Scylla serrata*. III. The sensory to motor synapse *J. comp. Physiol.*, **108**, 53–65.

Silvey, G. E. and Sandeman, D. C. (1976*b*) Integration between statocyst sensory neurons and oculomotor neurons in the crab *Scylla serrata*. IV. Integration phase lags and conjugate eye movements *J. comp. Physiol.*, **108**, 67–73.

Stange, G. and Howard, J. (1979) An ocellar dorsal light response in a dragonfly *J. exp. Biol.*, **83**, 351–355.

Wales, W., Clarac, F., Dando, M. R. and Laverack, M. S. (1970) Innervation of the receptors present at the various joints of the pereiopods and third maxillipede of *Homarus gammarus* (L.) and other macruran decapods (Crustacea) *Z. vergl. Physiol.*, **68**, 345–384.

Wiersma, C. A. G. and Fiore, L. (1971) Factors regulating the discharge frequency in optomotor fibres of *Carcinus maenas J. exp. Biol.*, **54**, 497–505.

Wilson, M. (1978) The functional organization of locust ocelli *J. comp. Physiol.*, **124**, 297–316.

CHAPTER SIXTEEN
SOME ASPECTS OF ELECTRORECEPTION IN WEAKLY ELECTRIC FISH

T. SZABO

Introduction

Although the existence of electroreception was discovered only three decades ago, knowledge in this area has increased to such an extent in the past thirty years (Bennett, 1971; Fessard, 1974) that it is no longer possible to give a short review of this particular field of sensory physiology. This presentation has therefore been restricted to a relatively small area which concerns some aspects of electroreception in weakly electric fish. A brief look at the state of our knowledge in this area, especially at recently acquired data, may indicate new directions for further research.

Weakly electric fish possess, on the one hand, electrogenic organs which emit low voltage signals (electric organ discharge, EOD) into the highly

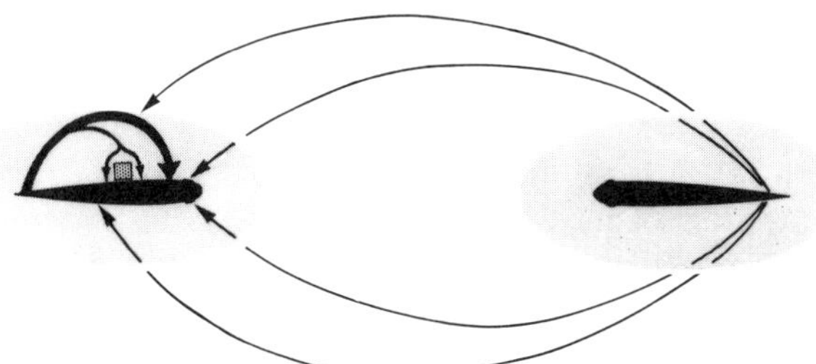

Figure 1 Schematic representation of the two kinds of electrical stimulation received by a weakly electric fish (*left*). Thick arrow indicates self-stimulation by the fish's own discharge; an object (dark square) of a conductivity different from that of the water distorts the electric field (set up by the discharge) at the level of the cutaneous electroreceptors. The shaded area represents the part of the electric field where an object can still modify the autostimulatory effect of the discharge at the level of the electroreceptors. Four thin arrows indicate exogenous stimulation emitted by a congener (*right*).

conductive environmental medium, and, on the other hand, special sense organs, so-called electroreceptors, specialized in perceiving electric signals. In the natural environment this electrosensory system is stimulated by the fish's own electric discharge and by those emitted by congeners. In our attempt to "make sense of sense organs", a pertinent question arises: how indeed do electroreceptors make sense of the varying information which they receive randomly through congener EODs in addition to that which the fish obtains through its own discharge (Fig. 1)?

The problem presented by this double stimulation is not unique to electric fish. Other animal species, such as bats or dolphins with their radar- and sonar-like systems, encounter similar problems of distinction between information from their own and foreign stimulus signals. However, the case of weakly electric fish is somewhat unusual because the electric signals are not emitted voluntarily but continuously from very early in life. Each individual, from the 8th day of its existence (Kirschbaum and Westby, 1975), lives in its own electric field, which is created by the continuous emission of EOD pulses. The repetition rate of the latter depends on the auto-rhythmically active encephalic centre, the EOD pacemaker nucleus, this being the key to the fish's electrical behaviour.

The electromotor command system

Gymnotidae

The first electrophysiological and morphological experiments on the command system of the EOD of weakly electric fish showed that in Gymnotidae the pacemaker nucleus has a simple structure (Szabo and Enger, 1964). It consists of two kinds of cells: large relay cells, the axons of which compose the descending spinal tract, and small pacemaker cells, whose rhythmical pacemaker activity determines the EOD rate. Evidence from electrophysiological and electronmicroscopical observations has shown that the pacemaker cells (Bennett *et al.*, 1967) are connected to the relay cells through electrotonic coupling, and to each other by way of the prejunctional fibres which may serve to synchronize the activity of all pacemaker elements. The relay cells connect pacemaker cells and electromotoneurones innervating the electrocytes by way of long axons. This relatively simple scheme has been partly confirmed for many gymnotid species (Ellis and Szabo, in press), and the largest elements have been identified by HRP labelling as relay cells. The connections between small pacemaker cells and also between pacemaker and relay cells are made through long and multiply-branched pacemaker axons and club endings (Fig. 2). Surprisingly, in *Sternarchus* and *Eigenmannia* where accurate synchronization of the different elements at high frequency is required,

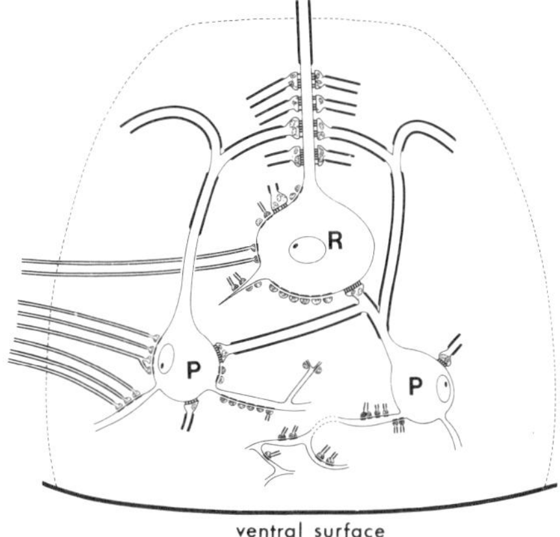

Figure 2 Scheme of the synaptic organization within the pacemaker nucleus in *Sternarchus albifrons*. Two small pacemaker cells send their strongly branching axons to one of the large relay cells, on one hand, and to the neighbouring pacemaker cells, on the other hand. The synaptic contacts are made by gap junctions at both levels. Note the great density of club endings with gap junctions at the relay cell initial segment. Both cell types receive chemical terminal boutons from small myelinated fibres of extranuclear origin (Courtesy of Dr K. Elekes).

neither dendro-dendritic nor somato-somatic junctions were found. Differences have been established at the synaptic level between *Sternarchus* on one hand, and *Eigenmannia* and the low frequency *Hypopomus* on the other: in the former the axosomatic club endings form gap junctions whereas in the latter there are mixed synapses (Elekes and Szabo, 1980*a* and *b*).

Concerning the cellular organization of the pacemaker nucleus, the two cell types, pacemaker and relay cells, are intermingled in the high-frequency *Eigenmannia* and *Sternarchus*, whereas in the low-frequency fish *Sternopygus*, *Gymnotus* and *Hypopomus* they form two separate nuclei embedded in a common network. In *Hypopomus* two ultrastructurally different types of pacemaker cells were found, which suggests greater complexity in this nucleus. A common feature of all gymnotid pacemaker nuclei (Elekes and Szabo, 1980*a*) is their afferences of extranuclear origin, which are thin, myelinated fibres ending in boutons with chemical synapses on the cell bodies and dendrites of the pacemaker and relay cells. It is therefore possible that they modulate the EOD rate at both levels. If the pacemaker structure of different species is compared, it appears that the organization is simpler in the high-frequency *Sternarchus* than in *Eigenmannia*, but much more complex in the low-frequency *Hypopomus*.

These structural differences can be related to the varying electric behaviour of the different species, i.e. to the different degrees of variability in their electric emission (see Hopkins, 1977). *Sternarchus* can raise its discharge rate transiently or shift it progressively; *Eigenmannia* can in addition decrease its discharge frequency and stop its electric emission. All these variations in both fish can be caused only by electrical stimulation. *Hypopomus* and other low-frequency fish can vary their electric emission in the same manner, but the electric behaviour can be influenced by stimulation of several other sensory modalities besides the electric sense.

Mormyridae

That a larger repertoire of types of electric emission is related to a more complex command system is even more distinctly demonstrated by the other family of weakly electric fish, the Mormyridae. One of the differences between the two weakly-electric fish families lies in the functional properties of their medullary centre: in contrast to gymnotids, in mormyrids this centre represents only a *relay* between a higher pacemaker centre—probably in the mesencephalon—and the spinal electromotoneurones. The autorhythmic discharge rate is dependent on the former, the structure of which has still not been identified.

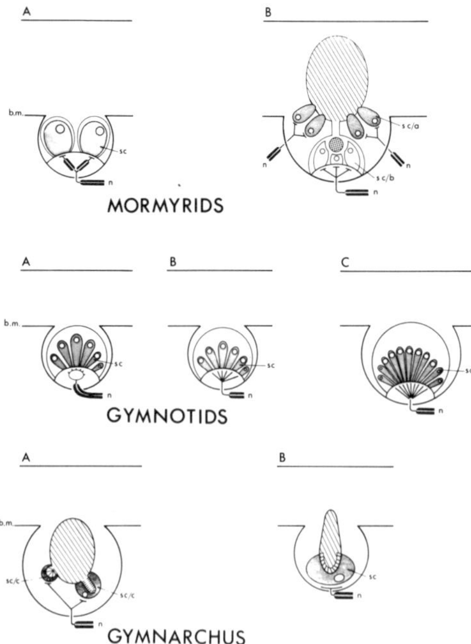

Figure 3 Schematic drawing of the two main types of phasic electroreceptors characteristic for weakly electric fish and *Electrophorus electricus*. A, common tuberous organ with characteristic myelinated pro-terminal fibre (except *Gymnarchus*) functionally identified as pulse marker. B (and C), specific tuberous organ; structurally different in the three families but with similar field intensity coding function.

In mormyrid larvae, a particular structure can be found in the floor of ventricle III; it is already differentiated by 8 days of age when the larvae produce their first electric emission. This structure, which probably corresponds to the pacemaker structure, is located in the same area from which a EOD-associated signal can be recorded in adults (Aljure, 1964). It is a peculiarity, however, that this structure, in contrast to the single medullary pacemaker nucleus in gymnotids, is two-sided.

A third feature of the command system in mormyrids is that it controls incoming electrosensory information by influencing it—positively or negatively—at the rhombencephalic level (see Fig. 11). A second control may exist by means of direct pathways recently established anatomically at the mesencephalic level (unpubl. obs.).

The electric emission pattern of mormyrids is in keeping with the complexity of their command system. Mormyrids do not have a regular basal frequency, and it is probably for this reason that they lack a unique pacemaker nucleus. The autorhythmic, but "irregular" emission pattern almost certainly depends on the interactions within the bilateral mesencephalic control centre.

The electrosensory system

If there are fundamental differences in the electromotor command system between Gymnotidae and Mormyridae, the electrosensory system in both is fundamentally similar and shows strong evolutionary convergence.

Morphological aspects of electroreceptors

In the first description of specialized sense organs belonging to the lateral line system and localized in the skin of weakly electric fish (Szabo, 1965), two classes were distinguished, the ampullary and the tuberous organs. The former have been identified as tonic, the latter as phasic electroreceptors. Only the phasic electroreceptors are adequately stimulated by the fish EOD and only these will be considered here. Fig. 3 gives a schematic illustration of the tuberous receptor structure of mormyrids, gymnotids and *Gymnarchus*. In each of these fish families two kinds of tuberous receptors were distinguished on the basis of the innervation pattern, there being myelinated preterminal fibres and a large axon diameter in the first (A) and unmyelinated preterminal fibres and a small axon diameter in the second (B, C). Subcategories may exist in both groups (Echague and Trujillo-Cenoz, pers. comm.) and functional differences have also been detected (Bastian, 1976; Hopkins, 1976; Scheich *et al.*, 1973). Correlations between morphological and physiological data are still lacking.

The puzzling complexity of the receptors in the category B of mormyrids has never been analysed from a functional point of view and little is known about the functional properties of the two receptor categories in *Gymnarchus* (see Bullock *et al.*, 1975). All in all very little progress has been made since 1965 when a morphological classification of electroreceptors was first established (Szabo, 1965).

Functional aspects of phasic electroreceptors

Although the idea that in weakly electric fish specialized receptors must be responsible for detection of variations in the fish's own electric field was put forward by Lissmann in 1958 (see Lissmann and Machin, 1958), the fact that electric field intensities were analysed by such receptors was first demonstrated by Hagiwara, Kusano and Nagishi (1962), who recorded the sensory messages in the afferent lateral line nerve fibres in gymnotid fish. Several mechanisms have been described since that time: local electric field variation at the level of a receptor can be indicated by the number of sensory impulses and/or by their latency measured from the stimulus onset (Fig. 4); in high-frequency fish this parameter can be defined by the probability of impulse occurrence. Regardless of the method of measuring the different characteristics of the sensory message, the function of these receptors is to quantify the electric stimulus; in other words the electroreceptors encode the intensity of the electric event in the afferent nerve fibre and are therefore called *intensity coders*.

In 1970 a new type of electroreceptor was detected (Szabo, 1970), the activity of which was independent of local field variations (Fig. 4); above threshold this receptor type generates a single spike of constant short

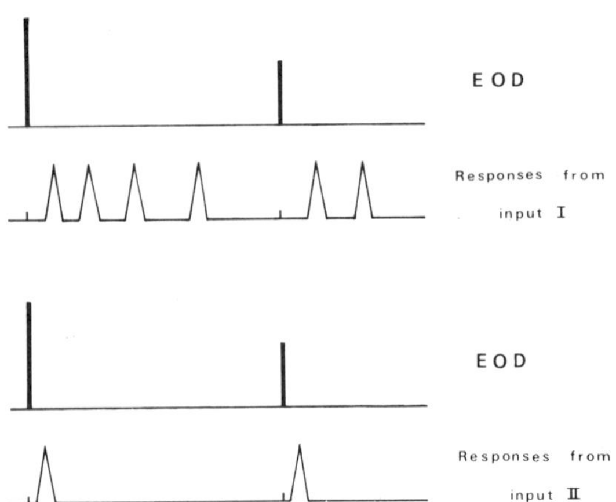

Figure 4 Basic coding mechanisms in the peripheral electrosensory system. Input I codes the intensity of the local electric field; input II yields information on occurrence of electric pulses (pulse marker).

latency carried by fast-conducting, thick nerve fibres. This kind of receptor conveys one kind of information only, namely that of the occurrence of an electric signal (pulse) and was therefore named a *pulse marker* (Bastian, 1976). Curiously, the threshold sensitivity of pulse markers appears different when examined in different fish. In mormyrids they are almost 100 times more sensitive than the intensity coders; these receptors were thought therefore to be active in electrocommunication. In some gymnotids the threshold sensitivity differs less but the pulse markers are still more sensitive than intensity coders (Scheich *et al.*, 1973). In contrast, some other gymnotids possess pulse markers of extremely low sensitivity (Bastian, 1976) which may be involved in active electrolocation mechanisms. Besides these two receptor categories—intensity coders and pulse markers (corresponding to two kinds of sense organs with clearly different morphological characteristics), it has been shown that there are subcategories amongst the intensity coders, and these have been classified according to their frequency response characteristics (wide band, narrow band or low frequency). Several authors (Bastian, 1976; Hopkins, 1976) have found that the frequency sensitivity of the electroreceptors in gymnotids matches the peak power of the fish's own electric signal which would attribute to the latter a high specificity. Similar results have been obtained recently for pulse markers in mormyrid fish (Hopkins, pers. comm.). This specificity, on one hand, would protect the fish electrolocating system against the non-specific EOD pulses of other species, and, on the other hand, would enable the fish to recognize conspecific pulses, allowing communication between congeners.

In spite of these functional differences at the receptor level, we still cannot distinguish more than two categories of receptors in either family of weakly electric fish in view of the kind of sensory message conveyed through the afferent sensory fibres: intensity coders and pulse markers. Although subcategories have been established in the former type according to the maximum number of sensory impulses provoked by maximum stimulus intensity (Kramer-Feil, 1976; Suga, 1967), no functional significance has yet been attributed to them. As it will be seen below, the two types of receptors correspond to peripheral inputs from two distinct sensory systems.

The electrosensory pathways

The electrosensory pathways (see Fig. 5) belong to the acoustico-lateral system in both weakly electric fish families; recent experimental anatomical investigations in mormyrids (Haugedé-Carré, 1980) have allowed determination of two distinct neuronal contingents in the peripheral as well as the central nervous system, carrying on one hand mechanosensitive and on the other hand electrosensitive impulses. The mechanosensitive contingent peripherally unites the afferent and efferent fibres of the lateral line neuromasts, labyrinth and canal organs, whereas the electrosensitive contingent combines those of tonic (ampullary) and phasic (tuberous or mormyromast) electroreceptors (Bell and Russell, 1978; Bell, pers. comm.).

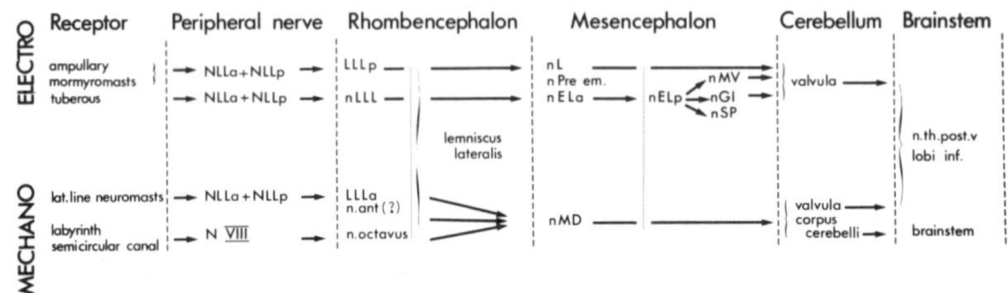

Figure 5 Anatomically identified connections of the acoustico-lateral system in mormyrids carrying mechano- and electrosensory information. It appears that this information may converge first only at the output of the valvula cerebelli. NLLa and NLLp, anterior and posterior lateral line nerves; N VIII acoustic nerve; LLLa and LLLp, anterior and posterior lateral line lobe; nLLL, lateral line lobe nucleus; n ant. and octavus, anterior and octavus nuclei; nL, nucleus lateralis; n Pre em, nucleus preeminentialis; nELa and nELp, anterior and posterior exterolateral nucleus; n MD and n MV, mediodorsal and medioventral nucleus; GI, ganglion isthmi; n SP, nucleus subpreeminentialis; n th post v, postero-ventral thalamic nucleus; lobi inf., inferior lobe.

The mechanosensitive fibres which constitute nerve VIII project on to the VIII nuclei, whereas those from the lateral line nerves project on to the anterior lateral line lobe. At the rhombencephalic level there is also a convergence of primary mechanosensitive fibres at the *eminentia granularis* (not illustrated in Fig. 5).

Mechanosensitive impulses of acoustic and lateral line origin converge upon the medio-dorsal nucleus of the mesencephalon and from there to the corpus and valvula of the cerebellum. The projection area of the electrosensory fibres which constitute the larger part of both lateral line nerves is quite different, this terminates in the posterior lateral line lobe (LLLp) and lateral line lobe nucleus (nLLL) with a somatotopic distribution. Furthermore, tuberous afferent fibres end in the nLLL whereas those of the two other receptor types end in the LLLp. The rhombo-mesencephalic projections of the electrosensitive fibres traversing the *lemniscus lateralis* are still grouped according to their peripheral origin: the lateral line lobe nucleus projects to the anterior exterolateral nucleus while the posterior lateral line lobe projects to the lateral mesencephalic nucleus. A relative small fibre bundle emerging from the posterior part of the LLLp ends in the *nucleus preeminentialis* at the base of the mesencephalon. Electrosensory inputs from mormyromasts (and from ampullary receptors, see Russell and Bell, 1978) are transmitted from the lateral mesencephalic nucleus directly at the valvula cerebelli. The information

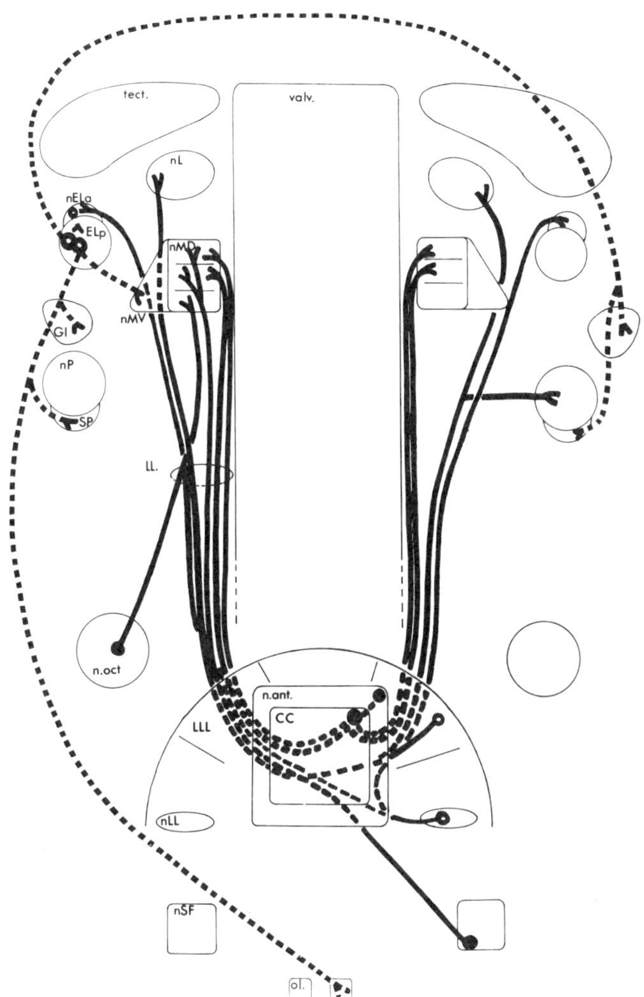

Figure 6 Mapping of structures connected to the acoustico-lateral area in the mormyrid brain. LLL, posterior lateral line lobe; CC, crista cerebelli, i.e. anterior lateral line lobe; n ant, anterior nucleus; nLLL, lateral line lobe nucleus; ol., olive; n SF, nucleus subfunicularis; n oct, nucleus octavus; LL, lateral lemniscus; sP, nucleus subpreeminentialis; nP, nucleus preeminentialis; GI, ganglion isthmi; n MV and n MD, nucleus medioventralis and mediodorsalis; n ELa and n ELp, nucleus exterolateralis anterior and posterior; nL, nucleus lateralis; valv, valvula cerebelli; tect.. optic tectum. (By courtesy of Dr F. Haugedé-Carré.)

from tuberous receptors also arrives at the valvula but this takes place by a complicated pathway having several intramesencephalic relays (Fig. 5). Therefore, mechanosensitive and electrosensitive impulses are conveyed in parallel, but distant pathways from the receptor to the mesencephalic level whilst acoustic and lateral line impulses converge at several levels in the rhombencephalon (Fig. 6) as well as in the mesencephalon. In contrast, electrosensory impulses coming from the different types of electroreceptors do not converge until the cerebellar cortical level.

The lack of convergence in the electrosensory pathways is not surprising if one considers on the one hand the functional differences among the categories of electroreceptors and on the other hand the different kinds of processing of the sensory messages. Indeed, the sensory information arising in the intensity coders is integrated once (or twice) at the rhombencephalic, a second time at the mesencephalic level and a third time in the cerebellum. In contrast, the pulse marker messages are only relayed at the different encephalic levels: in the lateral line nucleus and then in the mesencephalic extero-lateral nucleus. The relays provided with electrotonic junctions allow rapid transmission of the sensory message which arrives at the mesencephalon within a few milliseconds. A surprising development is the sudden slowdown of conduction and transmission from this point onwards, which results in a delay of 20 ms at the cerebellum (Russell and Bell, 1978).

While functional and anatomical pathways have been well established for electrosensory impulses, little functional analysis has yet been undertaken to elucidate the integration processes of primary or secondary sensory messages. We know somewhat more about the pathways which control the sensory messages at different encephalic levels. It is well known that the activity of mechanoreceptors (i.e. sense organs with ciliated sensory cells) can be regulated at the level of the sense organ by efferent peripheral nerves originating in the medullary brainstem (Roberts, 1978). No such efferences occur at the electroreceptors and the peripheral electrosensory message enters the brain without modulation. In contrast, there is a possibility of controlling the electrosensory message in the brain. Although there is a great similarity between the mormyrid and gymnotid electrosensory systems (Szabo and Fessard, 1974), there is an essential difference in their efferent motor control; only mormyrids possess such a control system, while gymnotids seem to lack it altogether. The electrosensory system of mormyrids is under the influence of several efferent pathways, the signals in which are associated with those of the EOD pacemaker activity. Three efferent pathways have been described to date, two towards the pulse marker and one towards the intensity coding system. The first (Fig. 7), the only pathway to have been physiologically demonstrated, is inhibitory, blocking at the rhombencephalic level the afferent impulses provoked by the fish's own discharge. The second is an anatomically established pathway which projects to the mesencephalic exterolateral nucleus, but its function is not yet known. The mesencephalic control has a facilitatory action on the intensity coder system at the rhombencephalon. The timing of this facilitation is the same as that of the inhibition in the pulse marker system, i.e. it occurs exactly when the

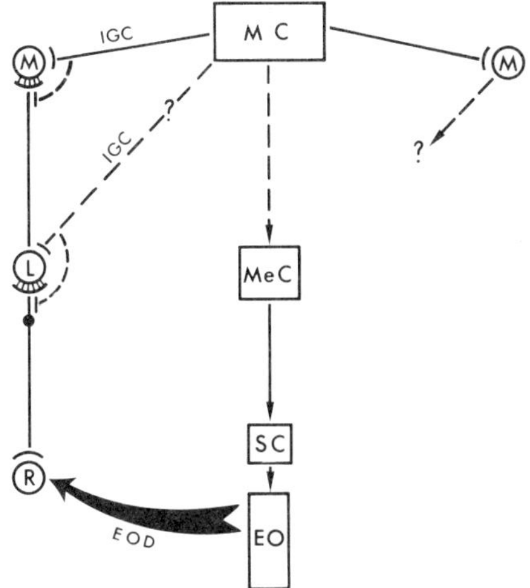

Figure 7 Scheme of intrinsic gating controls (IGC) by the mesencephalic "command" centre (MC) at the rhombencephalic (L) and mesencephalic (M) level of the pulse marker system. Sensory afferent impulses elicited in the common tuberous organs (R) by the fish's own electric organ discharge (EOD) and conveyed through electrotonic junctions at L and M, can be modified by the IGC. The IGC at L has an inhibitory effect probably at the presynaptic level. The function of established anatomical connections between MC and M is unknown. Anatomical pathways from MC to the medullary command (MeC) remain to be identified. Dashed lines indicate connections not identified anatomically. EO, electric organ; SC, spinal electromotoneurones; MeC, medullary relay.

sensory information set up by the fish's own EOD arrives at the rhombencephalon. These rhombencephalic units have a high threshold and only transfer messages towards higher encephalic levels when their threshold has been lowered by the facilitatory effects of the mesencephalic control. This means that the fish's intensity coding system, for which the fish uses the self-stimulating effects of this EOD, is protected twice by high threshold sensitivity against stimulations of congeners.

Behavioural aspects of the electromotor-sensory system

One can speculate about the advantages to the fish of this particular sensory system. As mentioned in the introduction, the problem confronting a weakly electric fish is to distinguish between its own (SI) and congener (SE) EODs, which in certain behavioural situations stimulate the fish's electrosensory system at the same time (Szabo, 1977; Szabo *et al.*, 1979).

Since we know the characteristics of this electrosensory system we shall consider two behavioural situations (Fig. 8): one in which fish A approaches fish B from a relatively great distance (Fig. 8a) and another in

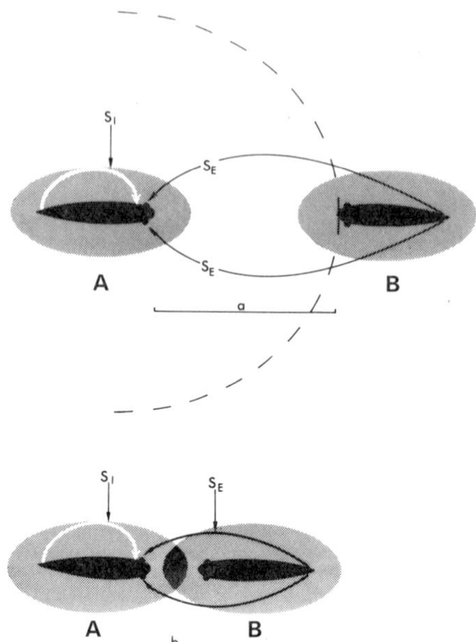

Figure 8 Electrical stimulation of fish A (S_I intrinsic stimulus) by a congener B (S_E extrinsic stimulus). Above: at large interfish distance (a) the stimulatory effect of fish B intervenes only at the level of the pulse marker (fast) channel of fish A. Below: at short interfish distance both electrosensory channels are stimulated by the congener's discharge. Shaded area, spatial limits of electrolocation by the fish's own EOD (white arrow). Dashed line, limits of the stimulatory effect of fish B on fish A.

which the two fish are close together (Fig. 8, distance b). Let us consider the functioning of the sensory system in fish A.

At a large interfish distance (a) the stimulation intensity of fish B's EOD is just sufficient to excite the pulse marker receptors of fish A, which in mormyrids have a much lower threshold than the intensity coders. Thus fish B's signals are already selected at the receptor level. It remains, however, to distinguish between SI and SE on the pulse marker channel. In order to keep the signal sequence of fish B undisturbed, fish A has two alternatives. Firstly, it can cease its electric emission, thus allowing only extrinsic information (Inf SE) to reach fish A's higher encephalic centres (Fig. 9). The disadvantage of this solution is that fish A must renounce the use of the second channel for electrolocation. The second alternative is that fish A continues to discharge (Fig. 10). Its own EOD will not interfere with the EOD of the congener on the pulse marker channel, as the information set up by its own EOD will be blocked by inhibitory internal feedback. Thus information SE remains undisturbed while the electrolocating system can still operate.

Figures 9 and 10 Functioning of SI fish's double electrosensory system at large interfish distance shown in Fig. 8(a).

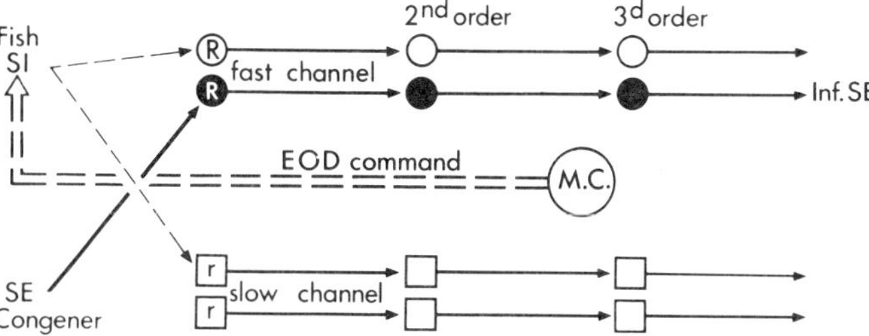

Figure 9 Activation of pulse marker (fast) channel only by congener SE while SI fish is electrically silent, i.e. mesencephalic command (M.C.) non active.

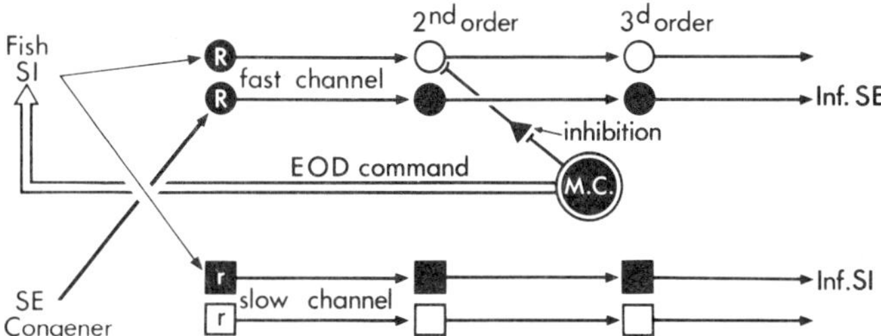

Figure 10 Simultaneous stimulation of pulse marker channel by SE and SI. SI and SE are selected by the M.C. controlled inhibitory intrinsic feedback at the rhombencephalic level (see Fig. 7). SI also stimulates the intensity coding (slow) channel (see also Fig. 10) while SE is insufficient because of large interfish distance. SI, fish's self-stimulation; SE, stimulation by congener; Inf E, information from congener; Inf SI, information through self-stimulation.

In the case of a short interfish distance (Fig. 8, bottom) the intensity of fish B's EOD is strong enough to stimulate both sensory channels of fish A. In other words, both channels will be stimulated by SI and SE (Fig. 11). For the pulse marker system this situation brings no new problem; the inhibitory feedback control takes care of interference between the effects of SI and SE by suppression of SI; only Inf SE penetrates to higher centres. The receptors of the intensity coding system will be excited by fish B's as well as by fish A's own discharge; however, information from the congener (SE) will not reach higher centres because of the high threshold of the second order neurones. On the contrary, information from fish A's own discharge (Inf SI) will be transmitted thanks to the facilitatory mechanism of the mesencephalic control at the same site.

In conclusion, it can be stated that the efferent mesencephalic control which operates in phase with the pacemaker represents a double gate system displaying opposite effects on the two sensory channels. It allows

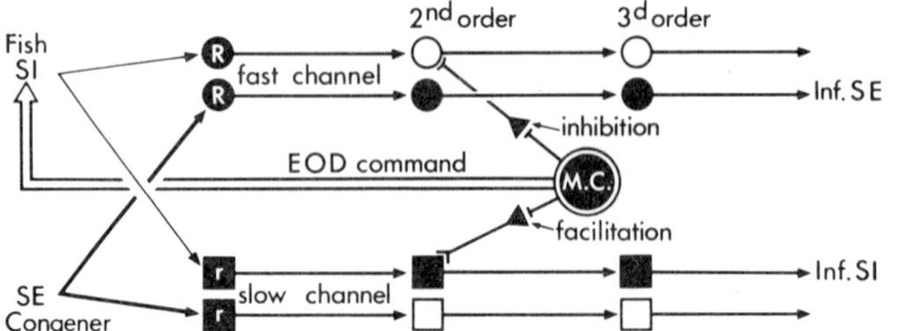

Figure 11 Functioning of SI fish's double electrosensory system at small interfish distance shown in Fig. 8(b). Selection of SI and SE on pulse marker (fast) channel as explained in Fig. 9. Protection of intensity coding (slow) channel at strong SE stimulation is by high threshold block at the 2nd level; it is released by M.C. facilitation for SI occurrence.

the fish to receive information from congeners without disturbing its own electrolocating system; electro-orientation and electrocommunication are simultaneously possible.

This mechanism seems to be native to mormyrids. No such control has been detected at the level of the double electrosensory system of gymnotids (Heiligenberg, 1977), and the neuronal basis of the mechanism permitting these fish to resolve the same problem which they encounter during their social behaviour remains to be found.

REFERENCES

Aljure, E. (1964) *Neuronal control system of electric organ discharges in Mormyridae* Ph.D. Thesis, Columbia Univ., New York.

Bastian, J. (1976) Frequency response characteristics of electroreceptors in weakly electric fish (Gymnotoidei) with a pulse discharge *J. Comp. Physiol.*, **112**, 165–180.

Bell, C. C. and Russell, C. J. (1978) Termination of electroreceptor and mechanical lateral line afferents in the mormyrid acousticolateral area *J. Comp. Neurol.*, **182**, 367–382.

Bennett, M. L. V., Pappas, G. D., Aljure, E. and Nakajima, Y. (1967) Physiology and ultrastructure of electrotonic junctions. IV. Medullary electromotor nuclei in gymnotid fish *J. Neurophysiol.*, **30**, 180–203.

Bennett, M. V. L. (1971) "Electric organs—Electroreceptors" in *Fish Physiology* (eds. Hoar, W. S., Randall, D. J.) Academic Press, New York, Vol. V, 347–574.

Bullock, T. H., Behrend, K. and Heiligenberg, W. (1975) Comparison of the jamming avoidance response in gymnotoid and gymnarchid electric fish: A case of convergent evolution of behavior and its sensory basis *J. Comp. Physiol.*, **103**, 97–121.

Elekes, K. and Szabo, T. (1980*a*) Synaptology of the command (pacemaker) nucleus in the brain of the weakly electric fish, *Sternarchus* (*Apteronotus*) *albifrons Neuroscience* (in press).

Elekes, K. and Szabo, T. (1980*b*) Comparative synaptology of the pacemaker (command) nucleus of the brain of weakly electric fish (Gymnotidae) (in press).

Ellis, D. B. and Szabo, T. (1980) HRP identification of different cell types in the command (pacemaker) nucleus of several gymnotid species *Neuroscience* (in press).

Fessard, A. (ed.) (1974) *Handbook of Sensory Physiology*, Vol. III/3, Springer Verlag, Berlin.

Hagiwara, S., Kusano, K. and Nagishi, K. (1962) Physiological properties of electroreceptors of some gymnotids *J. Neurophysiol.*, **25**, 430–449.

Haugedé-Carré, F. (1980) *Contribution à l'étude des connexions du torus semicircularis et du cervelet chez certains mormyrides.* Thesis, Université de Paris VII.

Heiligenberg, W. (1977) *Principles of electrolocation and jamming avoidance in electric fish. A neuroethological approach. Studies of brain function,* Vol. I, Springer Verlag, Berlin-Heidelberg-New York.

Hopkins, C. (1976) Stimulus filtering and electroreception: Tuberous electroreceptors in three species of gymnotoid fish *J. Comp. Physiol.*, **111**, 171–208.

Hopkins, C. D. (1977) "Electric communication" in *How Animals Communicate* (ed. Sebeok, T. A.) Indiana Univ. Press, Bloomington, 263–289.

Kirschbaum, F. and Westby, G. W. M. (1975) Development of the electric discharge in Mormyrid and Gymnotid fish (*Marcusenius* sp. and *Eigenmannia virescens*) *Experientia*, **31**, 1290.

Kramer-Feil, U. (1976) Analyse des sinnesphysiologischen Eigenschaften der Einheit Elektrorezeptor (Mormyromast) -sensible Faser des schwachelektrischen Fisches *Gnathonemus petersii* (Mormyridae, Teleostei) Thesis, University of Frankfurt.

Lissmann, H. W. and Machin, K. E. (1958) The mechanism of object location in *Gymnarchus niloticus* and similar fish *J. Exp. Biol.*, **35**, 451–486.

Roberts, B. L. (1978) "Mechanoreceptors and the behaviour of elasmobranch fishes with special reference to the acoustico-lateralis system" in *Sensory Biology of Sharks, Skates and Rays* (eds. Hodgson, E. S., Mathewson, F.) Office of Naval Research, Dept. of the Navy, Arlington, VA.

Russell, C. J. and Bell, C. C. (1978) Neuronal responses to electrosensory input in the mormyrid valvula cerebelli *J. Neurophysiol.*, **41**, 1495–1510.

Scheich, H., Bullock, T. H. and Hamstra, R. H. Jr. (1973) Coding properties of two classes of afferent nerve fibers: High frequency electroreceptors in the electric fish, *Eigenmannia J. Neurophysiol.*, **36**, 39–60.

Suga, N. (1967) Coding in tuberous and ampullary organs of a gymnotid electric fish *J. Comp. Neurol.*, **131**, 437–451.

Szabo, T. (1965) Sense organs of the lateral line system in some electric fish of the Gymnotidae, Mormyridae and Gymnarchidae *J. Morph.*, **117**, 229–250.

Szabo, T. (1970) Morphologische und funktionelle Aspekte bei Elektrorezeptoren *Verh. Deutsch. Zool. Ges.*, **64**, 141–148.

Szabo, T. (1977) Le problème du poisson électrique: comment distinguer ses propres signaux de ceux émis par ses congénères? *La Recherche*, Vol. 8 (**78**), 484–485.

Szabo, T. and Enger, P. S. (1964) Pacemaker activity of the medullary nucleus controlling electric organs in high-frequency Gymnotid fish *Z. vergl. Physiol.*, **49**, 285–300.

Szabo, T., Enger, P. S. and Libouban, S. (1979) Electrosensory systems in the mormyrid fish, *Gnathonemus petersii*: special emphasis on the fast conducting pathway? *J. Physiol.* (Paris), **75**, 409–420.

Szabo, T. and Fessard, A. (1974) "Physiology of electroreceptors" in *Handbook of Sensory Physiology*, Vol. III/3 (ed. Fessard, A.) Springer Verlag, Berlin-Heidelberg-New York.

CHAPTER SEVENTEEN

CUTANEOUS SENSORY SYSTEMS

A. IGGO

Introduction

The skin provides a major sensory input, and adopting the general line of attack suggested by Laverack (this volume) it can be analysed in terms of the kinds of environmental and intrinsic forms of energy that impinge on it. These are *mechanical* (physical changes in the static and dynamic mechanical forces that can be envisaged as acting on the surface and causing displacement, pressure, shear stresses etc.); *thermal* changes due to radiant energy exchange or by conduction; *electromagnetic fluxes*; and finally, a host of *chemicals*, some produced in the skin by injury and local inflammation, others used in aggression or defence.

Analysis of the cutaneous senses can use behavioural techniques yielding results that offer a valuable guide to the kinds of stimulus parameters to be explored in detailed analytical investigations. In the work described below, morphological and electrophysiological techniques in combination with quantitatively controlled mechanical, thermal and some chemical stimuli have been used to analyse the neurophysiological mechanisms. The results can broadly be seen as establishing that the skin contains a variety of specialized receptors that encode, in a highly specific manner, various parameters of the whole gamut of actual or possible environmental changes. For example, there are mechanoreceptors that respond only to vibratory changes in the position of hairs and which are indifferent to steadily maintained deflection of the hair or to the temperature of the skin. Conversely, there are other receptors that are excited only by skin temperatures in a particular range and by changes in temperature in a particular direction, but which are quite unaffected by any mechanical stimuli, short of those which are potentially destructive. Thus the peripheral receptors have the remarkable capacity to sample given parameters of the environment. The mechanism of this transduction continues to be one of the major challenges in sensory physiology, although it is quite clear that the overall mechanism converts one or another of the environmental parameters into a change in membrane permeability. This is expressed as a generator potential that leads to the setting up of action potentials that travel into the central nervous system and are the actual sensory messages in most sensory systems. Once these messages enter the mammalian nervous system they become an element in a complex interacting neuronal network, which both separates and combines them in varying degree, first in the spinal cord and later in ascending sensory pathways that pass through several "relay stations" on their way to the sensory cortex. At each of these relay nuclei, the onward transmission of the sensory information can be modified by interaction with other incoming signals, as well as by powerful descending controls that emanate from higher centres in the brain.

The outcome of all this activity is, in man, a sensory experience which can be expressed verbally. In other animals we can only infer the existence of the sensory experience and attempt to judge its character by the study of behaviour.

Cutaneous receptor mechanisms

Single unit electrophysiological methods (Brown and Iggo, 1967) provide a convenient method for tapping off the sensory impulses. Two main variants are used, either microdissection of peripheral nerves and extracellular recording of the action potentials, or insertion of microelectrodes into the receptor, a peripheral nerve fibre or the dorsal root ganglion cell itself. In combination with quantitatively controlled natural stimulation of the receptors in the skin, these methods can yield a precise analysis of the skin receptors and as a result several well-defined kinds of cutaneous sensory receptor have now been described. The further combination of these techniques with exact marking of the location of the receptor, during electrophysiological recording, and its subsequent histological examination, has provided evidence for the correlation of morphological and functional characteristics of the receptors.

Three main categories of receptors are recognized on the basis of functional studies—mechanoreceptors, thermoreceptors and nociceptors. Within each group, there is further subdivision based on various parameters of the responses and characteristics of the receptive fields and afferent fibres. This functional classification has only slowly emerged from the experimental work, and has required the use of exact quantitative analytical methods. The validity of the classification has been greatly enhanced by the results of combined functional and morphological studies (e.g. Iggo and Muir, 1969) and further strengthened by analysis of the central pathways which are referred to later.

Cutaneous mechanoreceptors

The major characteristics of the responses of mechanoreceptors are illustrated in Fig. 1. This diagram shows that there are several significant parameters of the stimulus that can be encoded. These are its presence, amplitude, dynamic and static elements, duration and direction. For each receptor illustrated in Fig. 1, the stimulus is the same—namely indentation of the skin with a small, smooth-tipped mechanical probe, initially placed just above the skin, then advanced at a constant velocity to a maintained indentation, after which it is vibrated at three different frequencies (20, 100 and 300 Hz) and finally is withdrawn at constant velocity from the skin. As is shown, there are some receptors (P.C.) that respond only to very high rates of change of position of the probe, others (R.A.) that respond to lower velocities of stimulation, but not to steady deformation, and still others (S.A.) that can encode static and slowly moving stimuli but not the high frequencies. Each of these illustrated examples is innervated by myelinated afferent fibres in mammals. In addition, there are other quite sensitive mechanoreceptors with non-myelinated afferent fibres that are excited, but to a low frequency only, by slowly moving stimuli (C–mech.). Each kind of receptor is able to extract and encode certain parameters of the mechanical stimulus.

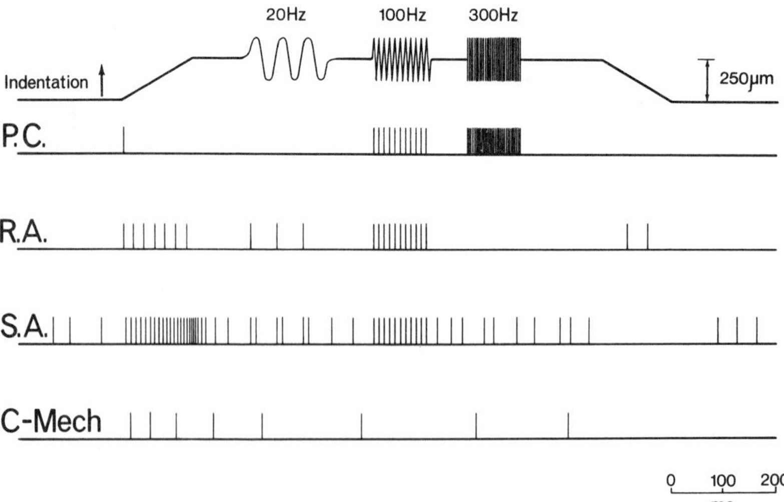

Figure 1 Diagrammatic illustration of the responses of four kinds of cutaneous mechanoreceptor to mechanical indentation of the skin, showing their differential sensitivity at various frequencies. The upper tracing shows the wave form of the stimuli, and the receptors are: P.C.—Pacinian corpuscle; R.A.—rapidly adapting receptor such as a hair follicle Type G unit; S.A.—slowly adapting receptor such as an SAII unit; C–mech—sensitive mechanoreceptor with a non-myelinated (C) afferent fibre (from Iggo, 1977).

The correlative morphological and functional studies began with the Pacinian corpuscle (Gray and Matthews, 1951) which because of its size (up to 2 mm × 1 mm) is visible to the naked eye and can be dissected out of the animal for recording *in vitro*. It quickly became evident that this receptor detects vibratory stimuli, with maximum sensitivity to frequencies about 300–400 Hz and that it is indifferent to, or at least not excited by, thermal stimuli, apart from the inevitable Q_{10} effects (Hunt, 1974). The Pacinian corpuscle was also an early candidate in electron-microscopical studies (Pease and Quilliam, 1957) which pioneered the subsequent detailed ultrastructural analysis of cutaneous receptors.

Other cutaneous receptors proved more resistant to correlative studies. The fortunate chance that the cat is a favoured neurophysiological subject, and that in its skin there are receptors with a visible epidermal location, led to the discovery of another now well-known afferent unit (defined as including the sensory receptor, its afferent axon, dorsal root ganglion cell and centrally directed axon and terminations). As early as 1875 Merkel, in histological studies, had described a touch cell (*Tastzell*) in the skin. Almost a century later it was established as the associated cell for the slowly-adapting Type I (SAI) cutaneous mechanoreceptor in correlative functional and morphological studies. It is illustrated in Fig. 2, which is based on a full description in Iggo and Muir (1969). The Merkel cell (Fig. 2B) is intimately associated with an expanded terminal of the myelinated afferent nerve fibre. This subdivides freely as it enters the receptor, and there are 50–70 nerve terminal discs in a single spot-like receptor, shown in cross section in Fig. 2A. The typical response to mechanical stimulation is shown in Fig. 2C, and is a slowly-adapting discharge of impulses that starts when the stimulus probe begins to indent the receptor's surface. The interspike interval (ISI) histogram (Fig. 2E) illustrates a conspicuous feature of the afferent discharge during sustained mechanical indentation of a receptor. The distribution is semi-Poisson, probably best described by a gamma-function where gamma has a value greater than one (which it would have in the case of a Poisson distribution) and is typical of a distribution generated by a random distribution of interspike interval lengths. The nature of the ISI distribution gives some clue as to the characteristics of the spike-generating mechanism in the receptor (Chambers *et al.*, 1972). The slowly-adapting mechanoreceptors also display a thermal sensitivity, which is expressed as a modulation of the response to a mechanical stimulus (Fig. 2D). Because the response is superficially similar to that of specific thermoreceptors (see below) I have called them "spurious thermoreceptors" (Iggo, 1969) and analysed in some detail their possible contribution to thermal sensory input. The normal functional properties of the afferent unit are disrupted by denervation and subsequent re-innervation of the skin (Brown and Iggo, 1963; Burgess *et al.*, 1974) and clearly the Merkel cell is an integral

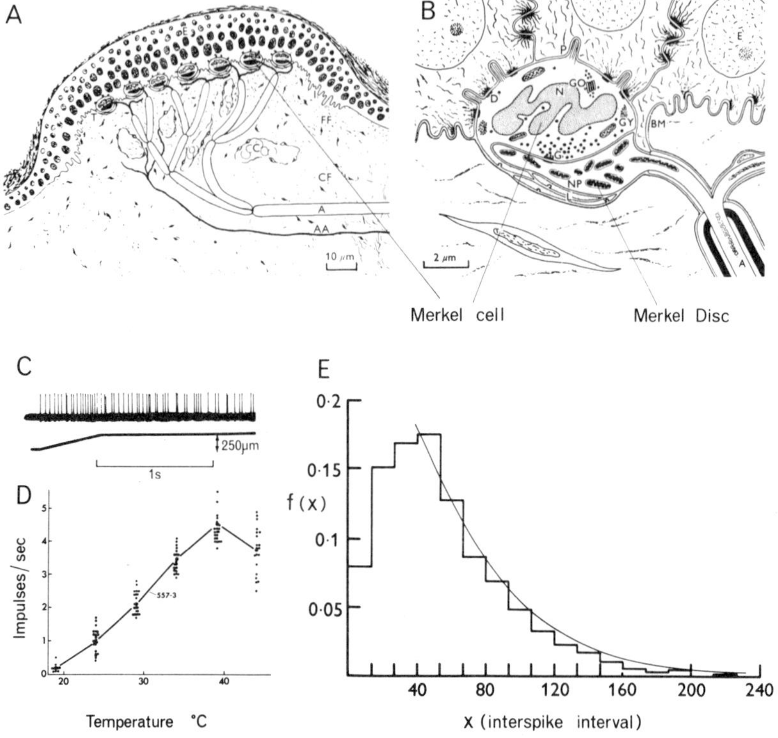

Figure 2 SAI (slowly adapting Type I) cutaneous mechanoreceptor, in hairy skin of the cat. A, diagram of a cross section of the touch dome. B, diagram of a component Merkel cell and associated nerve-ending (Merkel disc) lying at the base of the epidermis. C, discharge of impulses in the myelinated afferent fibre (upper) when surface of a touch dome is indented (lower). E, interspike interval histogram and fitted exponential curve of the adapted discharge of an SAI unit. D, effect of different steady temperatures (abscissa) on the adapted discharge (ordinate) of an SAI unit (based on Iggo and Muir, 1969).

component of the normal receptor, although whether it is actually the transducer cell is still debated (Gottschaldt and Kräft, 1978).

Studies of the kind just described have been extended to other cutaneous mechanoreceptors (SAII, Ruffini ending, Chambers *et al.*, 1972; R. A. Krause *cylindrische endkolben*, Jänig, 1971; Iggo and Ogawa, 1977) and these and similar investigations lead to the conclusion that the various functional categories have a morphological basis (Iggo, 1976; Iggo and Gottschaldt, 1974) and make it possible to tabulate the mechanoreceptors in a systematic manner (e.g. Burgess and Perl, 1973).

In various situations, particularly in the head, there may be a further elaboration of the mechanoreceptors. So far, the various kinds of mechanoreceptor have been considered as separate and independent categories. However, several specialized aggregations that form complex sense organs are known, such as Eimer's organ in the snout of the mole (Quilliam, 1966), the bill-tip organ in ducks (Gottschaldt and Lausmann, 1974; Berkhoudt, 1976) and sinus hairs (e.g. vibrissae in many mammals). These last structures have been analysed in detail, both morphologically (Fig. 3A) (Andres, 1966) and functionally (Fig. 3A, B, E) (Gottschaldt *et al.*, 1973). They are richly innervated (up to 250 myelinated afferent fibres to a sinus hair follicle) and contain at least four well-defined types of organized receptor (Merkel cells, lanceolate endings of two kinds, and lamellated receptors). The electrophysiological analysis by Gottschaldt *et al.* (1973) concluded that it was possible to correlate the several kinds of functional unit with these receptors. Thus the sinus hairs are mechanosensory organs, able to analyse the movements of the vibrissae in terms of direction, velocity, amplitude and duration of displacement, and to do this call on the specialized functional aspects of several kinds of mechanoreceptor. These sinus hairs are particularly numerous in the snout and tail of the mole (*Talpa europea* L.) an animal that is peculiarly dependent on its cutaneous mechanoreceptors, since it is sightless. Sighted animals,

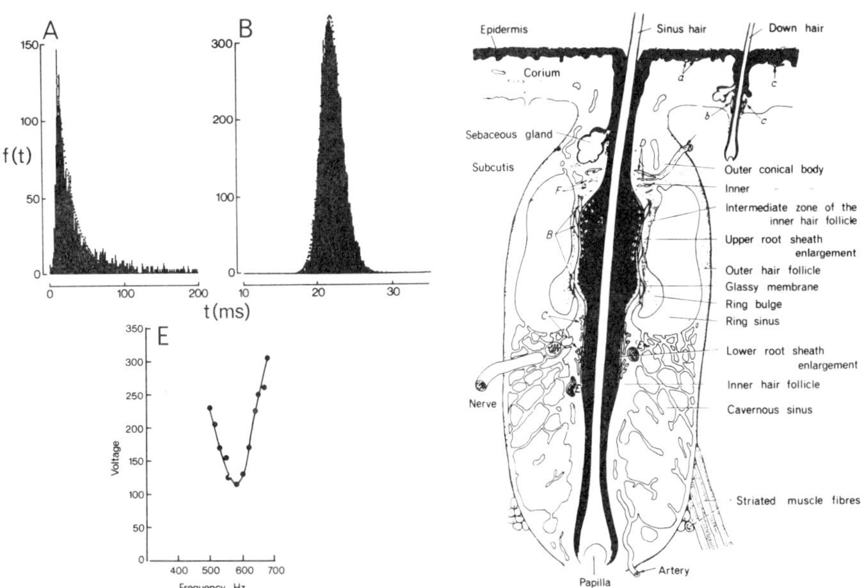

Figure 3 Sinus hair follicle (vibrissa of rat) showing the complex structure of a follicle, with its sensory nerve endings; A—Merkel cells; B—straight lanceolate ending; C—branched lanceolate endings; D—circular lanceolate endings and E—lamellated corpuscles (after Andres, 1966). The left-hand figures A, B and E show (A and B) inter-impulse-interval histograms recorded during steady deflection of a hair and purporting to come from Merkel receptors and lanceolate ending respectively; and (E) a threshold sensitivity curve for a vibration sensitive receptor, presumably a lamellated corpuscle (from Gottschaldt *et al.*, 1973).

however, also show a considerable dependence on their vibrissae. Rats (Vincent, 1913) and cats in the dark (Schmidberger, 1932) use their vibrissae for orientation, locomotion and equilibration.

Cutaneous thermoreceptors

Single unit electrophysiological studies have now convincingly established the existence in the skin of specific thermosensory afferent units. Sensory evidence for their existence came from the studies of Blix (1884) and Thunberg (1902) who first described cold and warm spots in human skin. Electrophysiological validation had to await refinement of techniques and only in 1951 were single unit results published for thermal receptors in the tongue (Hensel and Zotterman, 1951) and then in the facial skin (Boman, 1958). Cutaneous thermoreceptors of the general body surface were described later, because the small size of the afferent fibres proved to be a severe technical challenge. The afferent fibres in cats and rats are non-myelinated, with conduction velocities of about $1\ \mathrm{m\,sec^{-1}}$. Typical thermoreceptor responses are illustrated in Fig. 4. These are for cold and warm receptors in scrotal skin of the rat (Fig. 4A, B) and for cold receptors of forearm skin in the monkey (Fig. 4C). A characteristic feature

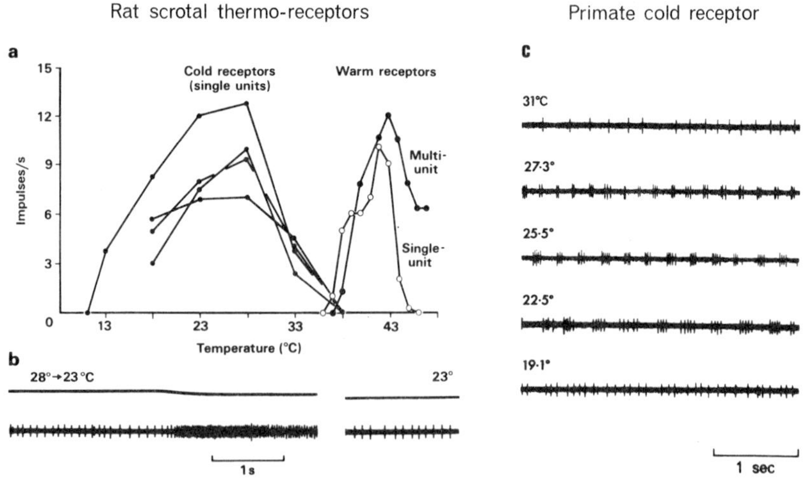

Figure 4 Typical specific cutaneous thermoreceptor responses. (a) and (b) are from single unit electrophysiological studies in the rat. In (a) static thermal sensitivity curves for cold and warm receptors are shown, with the characteristic maximum responses of cold receptors at 23 to 30°C and of warm receptors 41 to 42°C. (b) shows a typical non-primate cold receptor response to cooling the skin from 28 to 23°C and the sustained discharge at a steady 23°C which is at a lower frequency than at a steady 28°C. (c) shows a typical primate cold receptor response during progressive cooling of the skin; there is a distinct patterning of the discharge (based on Iggo, 1969).

of the thermoreceptors is that they are able to sustain a continuous discharge at constant skin temperatures (Fig. 4B), at a rate that is dependent on skin temperature (Fig. 4A), so that the receptors are able to provide continuous information. The cold receptors have maximal sensitivity about 25–30°C (Fig. 4A) in a variety of species, in contrast to the warm receptors that are maximally excited about 40–42°C. The other significant difference is that the cold receptors are excited by a fall in temperature and inhibited by a rise, whereas the warm receptors show the opposite behaviour.

In many reports the thermoreceptors are described as firing with relatively uniform interspike intervals, and, as shown in Fig. 4A, the thermal sensitivity curve is bell-shaped. It is evident that, at static temperatures, the receptors provide ambiguous information, since except at peak discharge rates, there are always two temperatures for any given rate of discharge. Some cold receptors, particularly those in primate skin (Iggo, 1969) have an added feature in the afferent discharge, which, at least theoretically, can provide unambiguous information over a given temperature range. Fig. 4C shows the characteristic pattern of discharge of a monkey cold receptor during dynamic cooling of the skin. On first appearance at 31°C and above, the impulses are regularly spaced and single, below 27°C they are in pairs, and then at lower temperatures successively in triplets and quadruplets, before finally at 20°C and below they appear in an irregular stream. Thus over a range of temperatures between about 31.5–20°C there is a distinctive pattern of discharge, and the number of impulses in each burst is in negative linear relation to skin temperature. Here then is a possible method of encoding skin temperature in an unambiguous manner (Iggo, 1969).

The morphology of specific thermoreceptors is largely undecided. A single successful attempt at a morpho-functional correlation has been reported by Hensel *et al.* (1974). In electrophysiological experiments these workers marked the receptive fields of cold receptors on the nose of cats, and on subsequent electron-microscopical examination found distinctive nerve terminals of myelinated fibres at the base of the epidermis. The receptors were not encapsulated and their structure was relatively simple. It is clear from these results, and from the previously described properties of Ruffini (Chambers *et al.*, 1972) and Krause endings (Iggo and Ogawa, 1977) that neither of these are thermoreceptors as was suggested by von Frey (1895).

Cutaneous nociceptors

The third category of cutaneous receptors are the nociceptors. These were first predicted on the basis of Müller's "Doctrine of Specific Nerve Energies" (1844) and von Frey and Goldscheider's anatomo-sensory correlations. Electrophysiological studies have established the existence of afferent units with a high threshold to natural stimuli, such as pressure and deformation of the skin, and temperature changes (Zotterman, 1939). Detailed single unit studies revealed that many have non-myelinated afferent fibres (Iggo, 1959, 1960; Bessou *et al.*, 1971; Burgess and Perl, 1973 for review). Within this group of afferent units there are some that are excited only by severe or potentially damaging mechanical stimuli, such as squeezing the skin with toothed forceps, others that are excited at skin temperatures greater than 43°C and others excited by both. Among the smaller myelinated axons there are units excited by severe mechanical stimuli (Perl, 1968), but not by temperature changes. An important feature of these various kinds of nociceptor is that their thresholds for excitation are at intensities of stimulation that have already saturated the impulse-carrying capacity of the sensitive mechanoreceptors, or are at, or beyond, the limits of the response range of the sensitive thermoreceptors (Burgess and Perl, 1973).

It is evident that the skin senses include a group of receptors that are well-placed to provide the central nervous system with an effective warning mechanism that can alert it to potentially or actually damaging conditions. It not only detects external stimuli, but can also signal local changes in the tissues. A characteristic feature of damaged tissues is the development of inflammation, associated with the formation and release of several chemical compounds, including histamine, 5-hydroxytryptamine, bradykinin and prostaglandin E_1 and E_2. These substances can excite and/or modulate activity in the cutaneous nociceptors. In this way the central nervous system can be informed about the local tissues' response to injury. At present the full range of chemical substances involved is a matter of conjecture, but even so enough is known to establish that thermal nociceptors can have their response to thermal stimuli enhanced by bradykinin and prostaglandin E (Beck and Handwerker, 1974). Furthermore the action of non-steroidal anti-pyretic analgesics such as aspirin (acetyl salicylic acid) is explicable in terms of its ability to inhibit prostaglandin synthetase. This reduces the tissue concentration of prostaglandin E, thereby removing its potentiating action on bradykinin so that the latter has a weaker excitatory action on the nociceptors.

In summary, the evidence points to the existence in the skin of a set of morphologically distinctive receptors that encode external and internal environmental changes as trains of nerve impulses. The variety of receptors enables various parameters of these stimuli to be extracted and encoded by different afferent units so that the central nervous system is supplied with pre-packed information along private lines.

The next question that arises is whether this information is preserved in the central nervous system, and, if so, how this is done.

Cutaneous sensory mechanisms in the spinal cord

Afferent fibre distribution

The afferent fibres from the skin nearly all enter the spinal cord via the dorsal spinal roots (Bell–Magendie law), although attention has recently been drawn to the neglected small number that enter via the ventral spinal roots (Clifton *et al.*, 1974).

New techniques are revealing hitherto unsuspected features of the distribution of the sensory fibres in the spinal cord. The broad separation of large myelinated fibres (now known to come from sensitive mechanoreceptors in the skin) which send collaterals up the dorsal columns and, at segmental levels, into the deeper levels of the dorsal horn, from the smaller myelinated and non-myelinated fibres that end superficially in the dorsal horn, is well known. New information has come from the use of intracellular ionophoresis of horseradish peroxidase (HRP) (Snow *et al.*, 1976) into identified cutaneous afferent fibres (Brown *et al.*, 1977; Light and Perl, 1979) and the reconstruction in serial section of the distribution of the fibre collaterals and their terminals. On one hand this new work has re-affirmed the earlier known separation of large and small fibres, and on the other has established that the morphology of the fibre terminations is correlated with the functional characteristics of the cutaneous receptors. For example, the hair follicle afferents form flame-shaped arbors distributed in long fillets in laminae III and IV of the dorsal horn, whereas the myelinated mechanical nociceptors have terminals in laminae I and II.

These new results further reinforce the hypothesis that the cutaneous afferent units form distinctive highly specified elements with both the peripheral and central terminals possessing distinctive characteristics. Müller's ancient Doctrine of Specific Nerve Energies is re-emerging in modern dress.

Second-order neurones

All the afferent fibres terminate synaptically in the spinal cord and the onward flow of sensory information is therefore carried by the neurones with which they synapse or by others still further along the chain. These are two main streams of information, either along the collaterals in the dorsal columns to cuneate and gracile nuclei at the rostral end of the spinal cord, or into the ipsilateral dorsal horn and thence via ascending pathways to the brain.

The kind of sensory processing that can occur is illustrated by some examples of neuronal activity in the dorsal horn. In general the incoming sensory information excites the second-order neurones, and the effectiveness of the input depends on the excitability of these neurones. This can be enhanced or reduced by excitatory or inhibitory synaptic action of either local (segmental) or remote (descending) origin. In addition, there are presynaptic actions (Schmidt, 1973) that can reduce the effectiveness of a sensory impulse by lowering its synaptic potency. The outcome of the various interactions may significantly modify the sensory input so that the onflow in the ascending sensory pathways may be transformed. The analysis of such transformations in the cutaneous sensory system is at an early stage, and it is too soon to say whether it has characteristics similar to those found in visual systems. In one respect it is very different, because of the great diversity of cutaneous sensory receptors in contrast to the rather limited variety of receptors that are present in the retina.

Dorsal horn neurones

The basic recording technique makes use of microelectrodes to extract single-unit responses, either metal electrodes which are robust and very effective for recording from axons (Brown, 1968), or glass micropipette electrodes that are necessary for intracellular recordings from cell bodies or large axons. The latter technique has two advantages: exact identification of neurones by Procion yellow or HRP marking (Brown *et al.*, 1980) is possible, and synaptic potentials can be analysed. The latter information is particularly valuable for analysis of intercellular interactions, but the technique is challenging and information is only slowly accruing from its use.

Several classificatory systems are used to introduce order into the variety of neuronal responses that can be recovered electrophysiologically from the dorsal horn. One system (Iggo, 1974) uses the characteristic afferent input and distinguishes classes based on the excitation of the dorsal horn neurones by mechanoreceptors, nociceptors and thermoreceptors as follows: *Class 1* are excited by mechanoreceptors only; *Class 2* are excited by both mechanoreceptors and nociceptors; *Class 3* are excited by nociceptors only and *Class 4* are excited by specific thermoreceptors. Within each class further sub-division is possible, but the general conclusion to be drawn is that the specialization of the sensory units is, at least to some degree, preserved in the organization of the second-order neurones.

The changes evoked in the relatively specific Class 3 nociceptor neurones are illustrated, as is their location, in Fig. 5. A noxious stimulus such as squeezing or heating the skin to above 45°C, evokes a high-frequency discharge. This, as seen in Fig. 5B, may long outlast the stimulus, and the persistence of the discharge is an indication of the added influence of the dorsal horn interneuronal network. In sensation it is paralleled by the prolonged sense of discomfort or pain that may be conjured up by such a stimulus. These Class 3 neurones are particularly concentrated in the superficial dorsal horn, where the nociceptive afferent

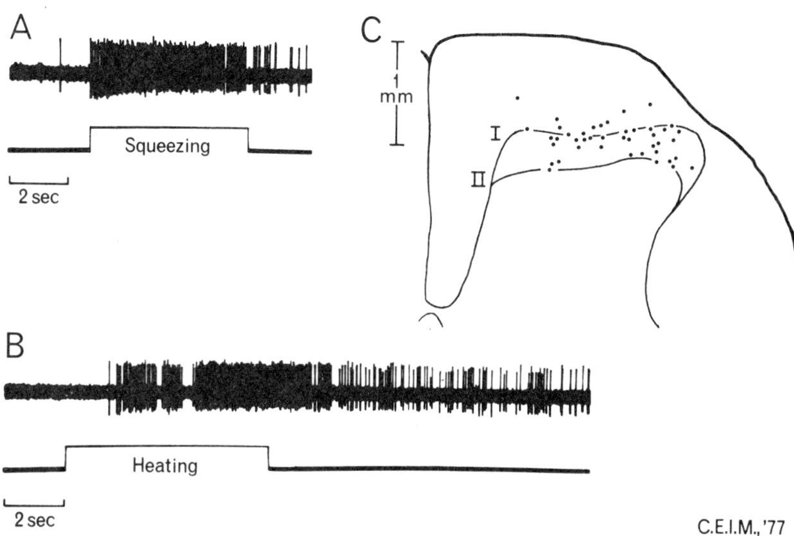

Figure 5 A nociceptor-driven (Class 3) dorsal horn neurone in the lumbar spinal cord of an anaesthetized cat, showing the vigorous discharges, in an otherwise silent neurone, caused by (A) squeezing and (B) nocuous heating (to 45°C) of the skin of the hind foot. Note the persistence of the discharge after the heat is withdrawn; this is a central phenomenon. The locations of recording sites in the superficial dorsal horn for this and similar neurones is shown in C (from Cervero *et al.*, 1976).

units are now known to end (Christensen and Perl, 1970; Cervero *et al.*, 1976; Light and Perl, 1979).

These particular dorsal horn neurones are not excited by sensitive mechanoreceptor afferents, but their activity can be inhibited from that source (Cervero *et al.*, 1976) so that the actual sensory outflow from them depends on the balance of mechanoreceptor and nociceptor activity, as postulated in the "reciprocal sensory interaction" model of Cervero and Iggo (1978).

Another example is provided by the thermosensory (or Class 4) dorsal horn neurones, illustrated in Fig. 6. Once again the neurones are in the superficial dorsal horn (Iggo and Ramsay, 1976), where the small afferent fibres from the specific thermoreceptors end. These dorsal horn neurones are unaffected by an afferent inflow from the mechanoreceptors or nociceptors, but, as shown, are responsive to an input from the thermoreceptors. Their behaviour is consistent with the view that they are excited by the specific cold receptors. They have a sustained discharge when the skin is held at 27°C, a temperature at which cold receptors are tonically very active (Fig. 4A); this discharge stops when the skin is warmed to

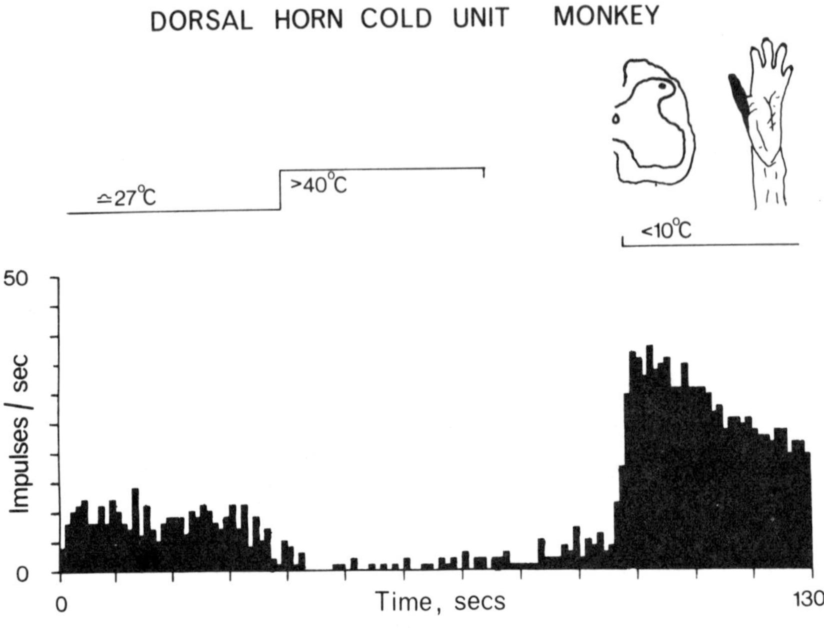

Figure 6 A thermosensory neurone in the dorsal horn of an anaesthetized monkey showing the responses at different steady skin temperatures. The upper right-hand inset shows the recording site in the lumbo-sacral spinal cord and the excitatory receptive field in the skin (from Iggo and Ramsey, 1976).

40°C, at which temperature the cold receptors are silent. Finally, there is a powerful burst of activity when the skin is abruptly cooled from 40°C.

These examples serve, without going into detail, to illustrate the capacity of the dorsal horn to handle the sensory inflow from the skin. Mention must be made, however, of the growing evidence for the complex interactions that can occur, involving some neurones on which many different kinds of afferent unit converge (Class 2 neurones) and of the large number of small interneurones in the substantia gelatinosa that have a modulating activity on the sensory output from the dorsal horn. Both aspects are fully covered in recent reviews (Willis and Coggeshall, 1978; Cervero and Iggo, 1980).

Ascending sensory pathways

The cutaneous sensory input continues its ascent to the sensorium along a number of parallel pathways. Some leave from the dorsal column nuclei and go to the ventrobasal thalamic nuclei (Brown and Gordon, 1977); others originate in the dorsal horn and travel either ipsilaterally in the

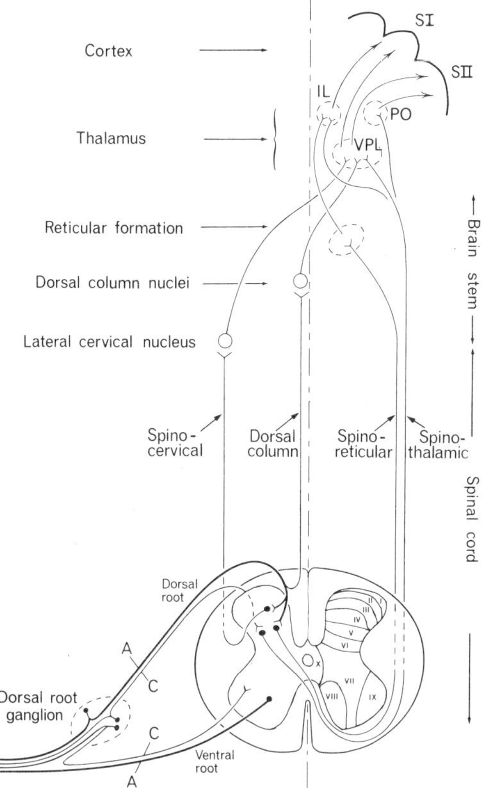

Figure 7 Diagram to illustrate the sensory pathways from cutaneous receptors, via the spinal roots and dorsal horn of the spinal cord to relay nuclei in the brain stem and thalamus to the somatosensory receiving areas (SI and SII) of the cerebral cortex. The spinal cord is shown in cross section, with the lamination of grey matter on one side and neuronal systems on the other.

spinocervical tract, or the dorsal column post-synaptic system or contralaterally in the ventral and lateral spinothalamic tracts, but all eventually reach the thalamus (Fig. 7). Within these various pathways can be found examples of all kinds of second-order neurones, with some evidence for segregation of various kinds into particular paths. Thus the thermosensory (Class 4) and the nociceptor-driven (Class 3) neurones tend to project into the spinothalamic tract. But this pathway also contains neurones with a convergent sensory input (from muscles and joints as well as skin). The existence of parallel pathways also adds to the difficulty of analysing the sensory role of any particular tract, as also does species variation in the development and extent of different routes (Webster, 1977).

Cerebral cortex

All the sensory pathways, by definition, go to the cerebral cortex, since conscious sensory experience in man depends on its presence. Electrophysiological analysis has amply confirmed the existence of special receiving areas in the cerebral cortex for cutaneous (as well as other somatic) sensory input. There is a well-ordered topographical map of the body in the parietal cortex (areas 1, 2 and 3 of Brodmann), but it is distorted so that those body regions with a large sensory nerve supply (such as the face) occupy a disproportionately large area of the cortex (Adrian, 1943). At its first appearance the sensory input retains both topographical and functional identity, but this is progressively blurred in the surrounding cortical areas in which a great deal of interactive processing occurs (Mountcastle, 1974), and which is possibly the site of the mysterious conversion of nerve impulses and membrane potentials into sensations.

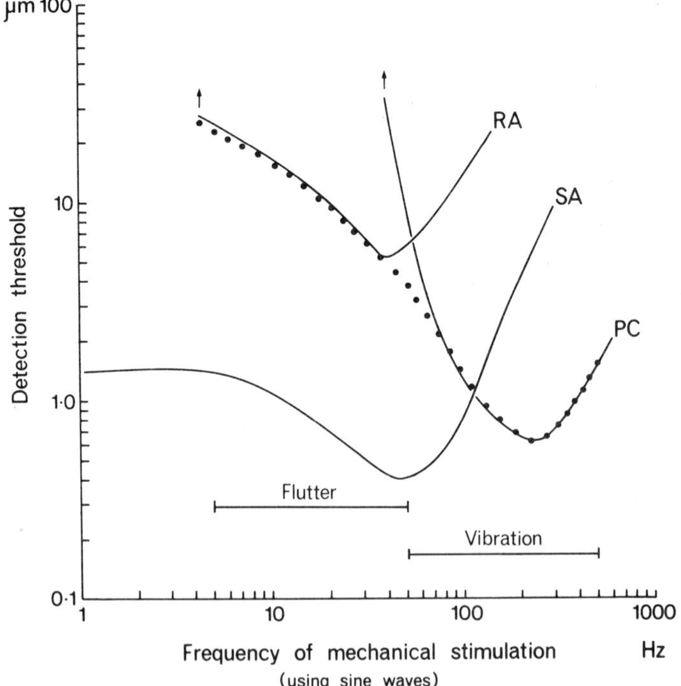

Figure 8 Threshold sensitivity curves for mechanical stimulation at various frequencies for three cutaneous receptors. RA (rapidly adapting, Meissner corpuscle and hair follicle Type G), SA (slowly adapting Type I) and PC (Pacinian corpuscle). The dotted curve corresponds to human sensory and monkey behavioural thresholds for similar stimuli. These are matched at low frequencies by the RA and at high frequencies by the PC receptors. Human sensations of flutter are mediated by RA and of vibration are mediated by PC receptors.

Sensory correlates of receptor activity

Finally, evidence is presented that speaks for a remarkable preservation of the identity of afferent input from specified receptors. In behavioural studies in monkeys and psychophysical experiments in man, Mountcastle and co-workers (reviewed in Mountcastle, 1974) have tested the hypothesis that specific kinds of cutaneous receptor mediate specific sensory inputs. They have correlated the behavioural and sensory responses to strictly-defined quantitatively controlled mechanical vibration of the skin with the discharge characteristics of the cutaneous afferent units recorded in the same subjects under identical conditions. The main points of the results are summarized in Fig. 8. The three solid curves show, for three categories of mechanoreceptor, the detection threshold amplitude for vibratory stimuli at the frequencies indicated on the abscissa. The three classes of receptor are RA, or rapidly-adapting (Meissner corpuscles in glabrous skin, hair follicle Type G in hairy skin); PC, Pacinian corpuscles, and SA, slowly-adapting SAI receptors. For each receptor class there is a characteristic curve of sensitivity. The dotted curve is the corresponding behavioural or sensory threshold tested in animals or conscious subjects with the actual sensory experience of flutter or vibration indicated by the bars There is a remarkably close match of the RA receptors and the threshold for flutter and of the PC receptors and the sense of vibration. At the same time there is no correlation of these sensory responses with the SA receptor curve.

These results are a first indication that in sensory processing, at least in primates, there is a significant preservation of the input in the first-order afferent units. They give added weight to the conclusion reached earlier in the paper about the specificity of cutaneous receptor systems.

REFERENCES

Adrian, E. D. (1943) Afferent areas in the brain of ungulates *Brain*, **66**, 89–103.

Andres, K. H. (1966) Über die Feinstruktur der Rezeptoren an Sinushaaren *Z. Zellforsch.*, **75**, 339–365.

Beck, P. W. and Handwerker, H. O. (1974) Bradykinin and serotonin effects on various types of cutaneous nerve fibres *Pflügers Archiv.*, **347**, 209–222.

Berkhoudt, H. (1976) The epidermal structure of the bill tip organ in ducks *Netherlands Journal of Zoology*, **25**, 561–566.

Bessou, P., Burgess, P. R., Perl, E. R. and Taylor, C. B. (1971) Dynamic properties of mechanoreceptors with unmyelinated (C) fibers *J. Neurophysiol.*, **34**, 116–131.

Blix, M. (1884) Experimentelle Beiträge zur Lösung der Frage über die specifische Energie der Hautnerven *Z. Biol.* München, **20**, 141–156.

Boman, K. K. A. (1958) Electrophysiologische Untersuchungen über die Thermoreceptoren der Gesichtshaut *Acta Physiol. Scand.*, **44**, 1–79.

Brown, A. G. and Gordon, G. (1977) Subcortical mechanisms concerned in somatic sensation *Brit. med. Bull.*, **33**, 121–128.

Brown, A. G. and Iggo, A. (1963) The structure and function of cutaneous "touch corpuscles" after nerve crush *J. Physiol.*, **165**, 28–29*P*.

Brown, A. G. and Iggo, A. (1967) A quantitative study of cutaneous receptors and afferent fibres in the cat and rabbit *J. Physiol.*, **193**, 707–733.

Brown, A. G., Rose, P. K. and Snow, P. J. (1977) The morphology of hair follicle afferent fibre collaterals in the spinal cord of the cat *J. Physiol.*, **272**, 779–797.

Brown, A. G., Fyffe, R. E. W., Noble, R., Rose, P. K. and Snow, P. J. (1980) The density, distribution and topographical organization of spinocervical tract neurones in the cat *J. Physiol.*, **300**, 409–428.

Burgess, P. R. and Perl, E. R. (1973) "Cutaneous mechanoreceptors and nociceptors" in *Handbook of Sensory Physiology, Vol. 2, Somatosensory System* (ed. Iggo, A.) Springer, Berlin, 29–78.

Burgess, P. R., English, K. B., Horch, K. W. and Stensaas, L. J. (1974) Patterning in the regeneration of Type I cutaneous receptors *J. Physiol.*, **236**, 57–82.

Cervero, F. and Iggo, A. (1978) Reciprocal sensory interaction in the spinal cord *J. Physiol.*, **284**, 84–85*P*.

Cervero, F. and Iggo, A. (1980) Substantia gelatinosa of the spinal cord—a critical review *Brain*, **103**, 717–772.

Cervero, F., Iggo, A. and Ogawa, H. (1976) Nociceptor-driven dorsal horn neurones in the lumbar spinal cord of the cat *Pain*, **2**, 5–24.

Chambers, Margaret R., Andres, K. H., von Duering, M. and Iggo, A. (1972) The structure and function of the slowly adapting type II mechanoreceptor in hairy skin *Q. Jl. exp. Physiol.*, **57**, 417–445.

Christensen, B. N. and Perl, E. R. (1970) Spinal neurons specifically excited by noxious or thermal stimuli: marginal zone of the dorsal horn *J. Neurophysiol.*, **33**, 293–307.

Clifton, G. L., Vance, W. H., Applebaum, M. L., Coggeshall, R. E. and Willis, W. D. (1974) Responses of unmyelinated afferents in the mammalian ventral root *Brain Res.*, **82**, 163–167.

Gottschaldt, K.-M. and Kräft, I. (1978) A new hypothesis about the receptor mechanisms in avian terminal cell receptors *J. Physiol.*, **284**, 67–68*P*.

Gottschaldt, K.-M. and Lausmann, S. (1974) The peripheral morphological basis of tactile sensibility in the beak of geese *Cell. Tiss. Res.*, **153**, 477–496.

Gottschaldt, K.-M., Iggo, A. and Young, D. W. (1973) Functional characteristics of mechanoreceptors in sinus hair follicles of the cat *J. Physiol.*, **235**, 287–315.

Gray, J. A. B. and Matthews, P. B. C. (1951) A comparison of the adaptation of the Pacinian corpuscle with the accommodation of its own axon *J. Physiol.*, **114**, 454–464.

Hensel, H. and Zotterman, Y. (1951) Quantitative Beziehungen zwischen der Entladung einzelner Kältefasern und der Temperatur *Acta physiol. scand.*, **23**, 291–319.

Hensel, H., Andres, K. H. and von Duering, M. (1974) Structure and function of cold receptors *Pflügers Archiv.*, **352**, 1–10.

Hunt, C. C. (1974) "The Pacinian corpuscle" in *The Peripheral Nervous System* (ed. Hubbard, John I.) Plenum Press, New York, 405–420.

Iggo, A. (1959) Cutaneous heat and cold receptors with slowly-conducting (C) afferent fibres *Q. Jl. exp. Physiol.*, **44**, 362–370.

Iggo, A. (1960) Cutaneous mechanoreceptors with afferent C fibres *J. Physiol.*, **152**, 337–353.

Iggo, A. (1969) Cutaneous thermoreceptors in primates and sub-primates *J. Physiol.*, **200**, 403–430.

Iggo, A. (1974) "Activation of cutaneous nociceptors and their actions on dorsal horn neurones" in *Advances in Neurology, Vol. 4* (ed. Bonica, J. J.) Raven Press, New York, 1–9.

Iggo, A. (1976) "Is the physiology of cutaneous receptors determined by morphology?" in *Progress in Brain Research, Vol. 43* (eds. Iggo, A., Ilyinsky, O. B.) Elsevier, Amsterdam, 15–31.

Iggo, A. and Gottschaldt, K.-M. (1974) "Cutaneous mechanoreceptors in simple and complex sensory structures" in *Mechanoreception* (ed. Schwartzkopff, J.) Westdeutscher Verlag, Opladen, 154–176.

Iggo, A. and Muir, A. R. (1969) The structure and function of a slowly-adapting touch corpuscle in hairy skin *J. Physiol.*, **200**, 763–796.

Iggo, A. and Ogawa, H. (1977) Correlative physiological and morphological studies of rapidly adapting mechanoreceptors in cat's glabrous skin *J. Physiol.*, **266**, 275–296.

Iggo, A. and Ramsey, R. L. (1976) "Thermosensory mechanisms in the spinal cord of monkeys" in *Sensory functions of the skin. Wenner-Gren Symp. Vol. 27* (ed. Zotterman, Y.) Pergamon Press, Oxford, 285–304.

Jänig, W. (1971) Morphology of rapidly and slowly adapting mechanoreceptors in the hairless skin of the cat's hind foot *Brain Res.*, **28**, 217–231.

Light, A. R. and Perl, E. R. (1979) Spinal termination of functionally identified primary afferent neurons with slowly conducting myelinated fibers *J. comp. Neurol.*, **186**, 133–150.

Merkel, F. (1875) Tastzellen und Tastkörperchen bei den Haustieren und beim Menschen *Arch. mikr. Anat.*, **11**, 636–652.

Mountcastle, V. B. (ed.) (1974) "Neural mechanism in somesthesia" in *Medical Physiology, 13th edition. Vol. I* Mosby, St. Louis, 307–347.

Müller, J. (ed.) (1844) *Handbuch der Physiologie des Menschen*, 1, p. 667 ff. Hölscher, Coblenz.

Pease, D. C. and Quilliam, T. A. (1957) Electron microscopy of the Pacinian corpuscle *J. biophys. biochem. Cytol.*, **3**, 331–343.

Perl, E. R. (1968) Myelinated afferent fibres innervating the primate skin and their response to noxious stimuli *J. Physiol.*, **197**, 593–615.

Quilliam, T. A. (1966) "Unit design and array patterns in receptor organs" in *Touch, Heat and Pain*, Ciba Foundation Symposium (eds. De Reuck, A. V. S., Knight, J.) J. & A. Churchill Ltd., London, 86–116.

Schmidberger, G. (1932) Über die Bedeutung der Schnurhaare bei Katzen *Z. vergl. Physiol.*, **17**, 387–407.

Schmidt, R. F. (1973) "Control of the access of afferent activity to somatosensory pathways" in *Handbook of Sensory Physiology, Vol. 2. Somatosensory System* (ed. Iggo, A.) Springer, Berlin, 151–206.

Snow, P. K., Rose, P. J. and Brown, A. G. (1976) Tracing axons and axon collaterals in spinal neurons using intracellular injection of horseradish peroxidase *Science*, **191**, 312–313.

Thunberg, T. (1902) Untersuchungen über die bei einer einzelnen momentanen Hautreizung auftretenden zwei stechenden Empfindungen *Skand. Arch. Physiol.*, **12**, 394–442.

Vincent, S. B. (1913) The tactile hair of the white rat *J. comp. Neurol.*, **23**, 1–34.

von Frey, M. (1895) Beiträge zur sinnesphysiologie der Haut, III *Ber. Verh. K. Saechs. Ges. Wiss. Leipzig* (*Math.-Phys. Kl.*), **47**, 166–184.

Webster, K. E. (1977) Somaesthetic pathways *Brit. med. Bull.*, **33**, 113–120.

Willis, W. D. and Coggeshall, R. E. (eds.) (1978) *Sensory Mechanisms of the Spinal Cord* John Wiley & Sons, New York.

Zotterman, Y. (1939) Touch, pain and tickling: an electrophysiological investigation on cutaneous sensory nerves *J. Physiol.*, **95**, 1–28.

CHAPTER EIGHTEEN

THE ORIENTATION OF BEES IN THE EARTH'S MAGNETIC FIELD

H. MARTIN AND M. LINDAUER

Reports on the perception of the earth's magnetic field by animals increase in number from year to year. The activities of *Volvox*, *Paramecium* and *Drosophila* are influenced by the magnetic field (Palmer, 1963; Ozhigova and Ozhigov, 1966; Tshernyshev and Danilevsky, 1966; Picton, 1966). Brown and co-workers (1964, 1966) found planarians and snails to orientate menotactically within the earth's magnetic field. According to Becker (1963, 1964, 1965, 1971) and Schneider (1961, 1963*a*, *b*), termites, flies, and cockchafers maintain a definite compass direction within the earth's magnetic field. In *Coptotermes amanii*, artificial changing of the direction of the magnetic field leads to a corresponding deviation of the compass direction in the nest galleries (Becker, 1971). Wiltschko *et al.* (1971, 1972) have found that European robins placed in a round cage show a migration preference to the north in spring, and a preference for the south in autumn. When the direction of the magnetic field is changed, the direction of migration undergoes a corresponding change. Homing pigeons are reported by Keeton to return to their base from an unknown area even if the sky is completely clouded. But if small magnets are fixed to their backs the orientation is disturbed (Keeton, 1969, 1971, 1974). The scepticism first shown towards these papers is easily understandable. Until now, no receptors have been established as possible transducers. On the other hand, the intensity of the natural magnetic field is too weak to explain a ferromagnetic effect. With respect to an induction by electromagnetic or paramagnetic effects, the strength of the field is appropriate. The magnetic energy per volume (E_m/vol) of a field with the intensity of 0.5 Oe which equals the earth's permanent magnetic field (EMF) is about 5×10^{-10} W sec/cm^3. The daily periodic variations of the EMF are between 10^{-13} and 10^{-14} W sec/cm^3. By comparison, the most sensitive range of the human ear (at 3200 Hz) may be stimulated by an energy of 8×10^{-18} W/sec, while the human eye requires an energy of 6×10^{-17} W/sec.

The biologist should bear in mind that for billions of years the earth's magnetic field has offered two important orientation cues to animals. Firstly, as total intensity and inclination are specific data for each geographical point, compass-directions can be fixed from it, and one can of course navigate by the aid of the magnetic field. Secondly, because of its periodic variations, observed for the solar as well as for the lunar day (whose effect is about $\frac{1}{10}$ that of the solar day), it offers a geophysical index of time which has some advantages over the principal *Zeitgeber*, such as alternation between light to dark, temperature variation, etc.

This report will provide evidence that bees are sensitive to a magnetic field of about the same intensity as the natural field, and that the natural field is actually used for orientation. A possible mechanism of perception will also be discussed.

Gravity orientation of bees is disturbed by the earth's magnetic field

In the tail-wagging dance, the angle between sun and goal is exactly correlated with gravity (von Frisch, 1965). However, there are small misdirections in these indications of direction, which show a typical diurnal course. It changes completely if the dancing place is turned by 90°, e.g. from a north–south position to east–west position. In this case, the stimulus from the gravity field would remain constant. The stimulus of the earth's *magnetic* field, however, will affect a dancing bee in a different way, because the angle between the wagging line and the lines of force is changed. If the comb is orientated in magnetic east–west position and the dancing place north–south, the wagging-line is affected only by the vertical component of the magnetic field; for a north–south position of the comb and the dancing place in east–west orientation, the magnetic inclination-line is effective. The misdirection completely disappears if the earth's magnetic field is compensated to 0–4 %. The dancers now orientate exclusively with respect to gravity (Lindauer and Martin, 1968; Martin and Lindauer, 1977; Kilbert, 1979). Furthermore, the daily curves of the misdirection are found to be correlated with the diurnal variations of the earth's magnetic field (Lindauer and Martin, 1972; Martin and Lindauer, 1973, 1977; Kilbert, 1979).

For each position of the comb, the dance is free of any misdirection in two situations (zero points). If the dancing place is in a "north"- or "south"-position the zero-points are marked at 0° and 180°, corresponding to the vertical component of the magnetic field. If the dancing place is directed to the east or west the wagging-line coincides with the plane of inclination: thus, for instance, in Würzburg, with inclination 65°, the zero points occur at 25° or 205° (east), or 155° and 335° (west). Generally, we can state that the zero-point can be registered when the inclination coincides with the sagittal plane of the dancing bee; i.e. when the magnetic field lines are parallel to the sagittal plane of the dancer—irrespective of whether the comb is oriented south–north or east–west, in vertical or slope position. When we bend the comb, the dancing bees follow this rule also, "hanging" on the underside of the comb.

We have checked our daily curves obtained in Morocco in 1967 and Gran Canaria in 1971 with respect to the rules set out above. For a magnetic inclination of 49° (Morocco), the zero-points were expected to be 41° and 221° (east) and 139° and 319° (west). For Gran Canaria, where the inclination is 42°, zero-points are 48° and 228° (east) and 132° and 312° (west). The experimental curves from Frankfurt, Würzburg, and Gran Canaria as well as those from Morocco were found to fit our calculations. Summing up all curves with the comb in vertical position, we may state that the directions of dancing deviate by only 0.2° from the expected values, taking into account all angles from 2° before and 2° after the calculated zero-point (standard deviation = $\pm 3.7°$, $n = 346$, e.g. 346 dances within the sector 2° before and 2° after the zero-point are included).

The correlation between misdirection (Mi) and the variations of the magnetic field can be described by the following two functions which depend on the prevailing variation of the earth's magnetic field (ΔF): these functions can vary within one day between

$$Mi = (eA_2 \pm eA_1) \cdot \lambda \text{ (anhysteresis) and}$$

$$Mi = (eA_2 \pm \frac{v}{2}(eA_2 - eA_1)^2 \cdot \lambda \text{ (hysteresis).}$$

where

Mi = misdirection = deviation of the dance angle

λ = scale factor

eA = effective magnetic work = $\log(\Delta F + 1)\mu \cdot \sin \alpha_m \cdot d\alpha$

ΔF = variation of EMF

μ = permeability (≈ 1)

α_m = "magnetic angle". $\alpha_m = 0°$ is the zero-point in the misdirection-curve.
($\alpha_m = \alpha_s$ (perpendicular line) in one position only, when the comb is orientated E–W. In all other positions, $\alpha_m \neq \alpha_s$).

$d\alpha$ = steps of degrees in the calculated dancing curve (without misdirection) to definite α_m and ΔF

v = Rayleigh constant (0.20–0.24) as confirmed by experimental data

Due to the normal fluctuation of ΔF, the hysteresis predominates.

A theory of magnetoreception

The mechanism of magnetoreception is still not known. Except in elasmobranch fishes which measure, by highly sensitive electroreceptors, the electric field generated when they move as "conductors" through a magnetic field, it is very improbable, especially in terrestrial animals, that specific magnetoreceptors exist. Our data on the *Missweisung* (*Mi*) in the wagging dance can best be interpreted in terms of paramagnetic effects.

Many organic molecules become paramagnetic by aligning the spins of their unpaired electrons with the external magnetic vectors. In all long-term experiments (where we recorded the *Missweisung* over one hour or longer) we could find a hysteresis effect, and the *Missweisung* itself is found to be temperature dependent. Given this background, and existing knowledge of the histological structure of the gravity receptors, we propose that bioradicals that might exist as paramagnetic "mono-crystals" in the allertic caps and/or in the microtubuli can be magnetized, even in very weak magnetic fields. In this way, the bioradicals, acting as dipoles are orientated circularly.

This process, together with the "contact-angle-hysteresis" process of Blake and Haynes (1973) whereby free bioradicals come into contact step by step with the substrate, should influence the structure of the membrane in the caps and in the microtubuli, and as a consequence influence the ion flux.

Another theory, which is favoured today by a number of eminent researchers (Walcott, Gould, Kirschvink, Wolfe, Deffeyes, Blakemore, Frankel) is based on the detection of magnetite crystals (Fe_2O_2) in bacteria, in the abdomen of the honeybee, in some tissues of the pigeon's head, and in chitons: it seems likely that these magnetite-crystals are involved in orientation in the magnetic field.

The mechanism can easily be understood in bacteria, where the whole organism, filled with crystals of magnetite, reacts as a single domain ferromagnet. However, if magnetite-crystals in higher animals like honey-bees and pigeons are diffusely localized in tissue, the nervous system cannot obtain information on the exact compass orientation of the whole organism, since to our knowledge no *Richtcharakteristik* (directional characteristic) can be provided by the alignment of the crystals. The phenomena of adaptation, temperature dependence and also the *Richt-charakteristik*, recorded in bees (Martin and Lindauer, 1977; Kilbert, 1979), cannot adequately be explained by the presence of magnetite. This theory therefore demands an exact localization of the ferromagnet domain, where it can transduce the aligned position of the crystals into an altered electrical impulse.

REFERENCES

Becker, G. (1963) Magnetfeldorientierung von Dipteren *Naturwissenschaften*, **50**, 664.

Becker, G. (1964) Reaktion von Insekten auf Magnetfelder, elektrische Felder und atmospherics *Z. ang. Entomologie*, **54**, 75–88.

Becker, G. (1965) Zur Magnetfeld-Orientierung von Dipteren *Z. vergl. Physiol.*, **51**, 135–150.

Becker, G. (1971) Magnetfeld-Einfluss auf die Galeriebau-Richtung bei Termiten *Naturwissenschaften*, **58**, 60.

Blake, T. D. and Haynes, I. M. (1973) "Contact-angle hysteresis" in *Progress in Surface and Membrane Science*, Vol. 6 (eds. Danielli, Y. F., Rosenberg, M. D., Cadenhead, D. A.) Academic Press, New York-London, 125–138.

Blakemore, R. (1975) Magnetotactic bacteria *Science*, **190**, 377–379.

Brown, F. A. Jr. (1966) Effects and after-effects on planarians of reversals of the horizontal magnetic vector *Nature*, **209**, 533–535.

Brown, F. A. Jr., Barnwell, F. H. and Webb, H. M. (1964) Adaptation of the magnetoreceptive mechanism of mud-snail to geomagnetic strength *Biol. Bull.*, **127**, 221–231.

Frankel, R. B., Blakemore, R. P. and Wolfe, R. S. (1979) Magnetite in freshwater magnetotactic bacteria *Science*, **203**, 1355–1356.

Gould, J. L., Kirschvink, J. L. and Deffeyes, K. S. (1978) Bees have magnetic resonance *Science*, **201**, 1026.

Keeton, W. T. (1969) Orientation by pigeon: Is the sun necessary? *Science*, **165**, 922–928.

Keeton, W. T. (1971) Magnets interfere with pigeon homing *Proc. Nat. Acad. Sci.*, **68**, 102–106.

Keeton, W. T. (1974) "The orientation and navigational basis of homing in birds" in *Advances on the Study of Behavior*, Vol. 5 (eds. Lehrman, D. S., Hinde, R., Shaw, E.) Academic Press, New York, 47–132.

Kilbert, K. (1979) Geräuschanalyse der Tanzlaute der Honigbiene (*Apis mellifera*) in unterschiedlichen magnetischen Feldsituationen *J. comp. Physiol.*, **132**, 11–25.

Lindauer, M. and Martin, H. (1968) Die Schwereorientierung der Bienen unter dem Einfluss des Erdmagnetfeldes *Z. vergl. Physiol.*, **60**, 219–243.

Lindauer, M. and Martin, H. (1972) "Magnetic effect on dancing bees" in *Animal Orientation and Navigation* (NASA SP 262) (eds. Galler, S. F., Schmidt-Koenig, K., Jacobs, G. J., Belleville, R. E.) U.S. Govt. Printing Office, Washington (D.C.), 559–567.

Martin, H. and Lindauer, M. (1973) Orientierung im Erdmagnetfeld *Fortschr. Zool.*, **21**, 211–228.

Martin, H. and Lindauer, M. (1977) Der Einfluss des Erdmagnetfeldes auf die Schwereorientierung der Honigbiene (*Apis mellifera*) *J. comp. Physiol.*, **122**, 145–187.

Ozhigova, A. P. and Ozhigov, J. E. (1966) Constant magnetic field effect on paramecium movement *Biofizika II*, 1026–1033 (in Russian).

Palmer, J. C. (1963) Organismic spatial orientation in very weak magnetic fields *Nature*, **198**, 1061–1062.

Picton, H. D. (1966) Some responses of *Drosophila* to weak magnetic and electrostatic fields *Nature*, **211**, 303–304.

Schneider, F. (1961) Beeinflussung der Aktivität des Maikäfers durch Veränderung der gegenseitigen Lage magnetischer und elektrischer Felder *Mitt. schweiz. entomol. Ges.*, **33**, 223–237.

Schneider, F. (1963*a*) Ultraoptische Orientierung des Maikäfers (*Melolontha vulgaris* F.) in künstlichen elektrischen und magnetischen Feldern *Erg. Biol.*, **26**, 147–157.

Schneider, F. (1963*b*) Systematische Variationen in der elektrischen, magnetischen und geographisch-ultraoptischen Orientierung des Maikäfers *Vjschr. naturforsch. Ges.* (Zürich), **108**, 373–416.

Tshernyshev, W. B. and Danilevsky, M. L. (1966) The effect of the alternative magnetic field on the activity of flies *Protophormia terrae-novae* R.D.J. *Obteschej Biol.* (Moscow), **27**, 496–498 (in Russian).

Walcott, C. (1977) Magnetic fields and the orientation of pigeons under sun *J. exp. Biol.*, **70**, 105–124.

Walcott, C., Gould, J. L., and Kirschvink, J. L. (1979) Pigeons have magnets *Science*, **205**, 1027–1028.

Wiltschko, W., Höck, H. and Merkel, F. W. (1971) Outdoor experiments with migrating European robins in artificial magnetic fields *Z. Tierpsychol.*, **29**, 409–415.

Wiltschko, W. and Wiltschko, R. (1972) Magnetic compass of European robins *Science*, **176**, 62–64.

CHAPTER NINETEEN
MAKING SENSE OF THE SENSES

RICHARD L. GREGORY

The sense of signals

The sense organs are transducers converting patterns of energy received from the external world into neural signals. Like any other signals, these must be in some kind of code, and must therefore be decoded so that sense can be read from them. It is clear from very many experiments in the perception of higher animals and man that the reading of sensory signals requires a vast store of background knowledge of the world. This is the contribution to perception of *cognitive*—knowledge-based—processes. This huge contribution of stored knowledge, and the power of heuristic procedures, make it difficult for the experimenter to judge the significance of recorded neural signals; for he may need to know the code, the relevant background stored knowledge, the situation of the organism, and the tasks it is set to perform, before he can read sense from his experiments. Perhaps for this daunting reason, the role of cognition tends to be minimized, and even ignored or rejected by physiologists. This by no means prevents excellent work; but it could hardly allow an adequate account or philosophy of how organisms make sense of sensory signals.

No doubt cognitive concepts become more important as we move from the peripheral to the central nervous system—for it is here that signals are read as representing objects or situations requiring predictive strategies. Perhaps only in simple reflexes, leading to a single response, can we ignore cognitive complexities.

In order to read any message, one alternative must be selected from many possibilities. This is the great lesson from the information theory of Norbert Weiner (1948), and Claude Shannon and Warren Weaver (1949). This is itself based on earlier work of H. Nyquist in America and K. Kumpfüller in Germany who independently stated, in 1924, that a given quantity of information is limited by bandwidth (frequency range) and duration. R. V. L. Hartley went further, in 1928, to *define* information as the successive selection of signs, or words, from a given list. For this definition *meaning* was rejected as subjective—for it is the physical activity, or patterns of signals, and not meanings (which seem mental) that are transmitted down engineers' information channels. It is also only signals that are transmitted in neural channels. Neural signals (in the form of action potentials) are subject to just the same limitations of bandwidth and disturbance by random activity ("noise"), and they must be more or less efficient according to the coding employed. There is potential for confusion here though, for Hartley and later writers continued to speak of "information", devoid of sense or meaning. This is a narrowing from common usage, and we have to explain how mere signals give meaning to organisms. For considering information in the narrow technical sense, we are concerned only with the statistical characteristics of physical events accepted as signals, and the bandwidth and noise level of the channel, and whether the code allows each symbol to be transmitted with appropriate relative frequencies so that they use up least time, on average, to transmit.

A fundamental contribution of information theory is that, to specify the amount of information in a transmitted message, we must know the size of the repertoire of possible messages from which selections are made. Hartley showed that a message of N distinguishable signs or symbols selected from a repertoire of S signs has S^N possibilities, and that (when the "quantity of information" is defined in logarithmic units to make it additive) information in this sense is quantified by:

$$H = N \log_2 S$$

Logarithms to the base 2 are used to conform to the useful convention of the elementary binary choice: hence, of course, the term "bit" for the unit of information.

Since the simplest choice is yes-or-no (or, on-or-off for a switch, or conducting-or-not-conducting for an all-or-none neurone) the information unit of a bit is uniquely useful. Norbert Weiner and Claude Shannon developed the Hartley approach by examining the statistical characteristics of signals, including the values of waves for analogue signals, and they reinterpreted Hartley's Law to define the average information of long sequences of N symbols as:

$$H_N = \sum_i - p_i \log p_i$$

The minus sign makes H_N positive, since it involves logarithms of p_i which are fractional.

The greatest quantity of information that can be transmitted through a channel with band width W over time T, in the presence of disturbing noise, was shown by Claude Shannon to be:

$$WT = \log_2\left(1 + \frac{P}{R}\right)\text{(bits)}$$

where P and R are mean signal and mean noise powers. This represents a definite limit which no channel can exceed. If the *coding* of the signals is non-optimal the information rate may be very much lower. For an example of this, consider the Morse code, which was invented by an American painter, Samuel Morse (1791–1872) and was first demonstrated in Washington Square, New York, on September 2nd 1837, over 1700 feet of wire. What is clever about Morse's code is the use of the smallest number of dots and dashes for the commonest letters. The uncommon letters take longer to transmit, and as they occur less frequently minimum time is lost on average, so this is an efficient code. We may expect corresponding strategies for sensory channels, but before we know the corresponding strategies we cannot measure the bit rate of neural channels with much accuracy, and we may easily over-estimate the neural bit rate by assuming optimal coding.

However this may be, a clear implication is that we cannot assess the information capacity of a channel, but only its possible upper limit, before we know the code in use and its appropriateness for the statistical character of the signals. But do we know these for any neural channels?

It is clearly also just as important to know whether the strategy for selecting between the available perceptions or actions is efficient. This should be like well-played "Twenty Questions". The N possibilities should be successively divided at each stage with equal probabilities by a binary choice. It is interesting how powerful this method can be, as we see by calculating the size of, say, a dictionary from which a given word can be found by successive binary choices following this strategy. (The items must however be ordered in some way, as dictionary words are by being alphabetically arranged, so that we can ask which are out and which may remain in after each choice.)

It is almost incredible that so few choices (see Table 1) can have such power to find a needle in a haystack—or to select memory or a perception or a course of action from brain-stored possibilities.

It should now be clear that there is something very odd about information as described by Shannon's theory, which is now almost universally accepted as the best and most useful account. Information described in these terms is quite different from anything else in the natural sciences as it depends not only on what *is*, but also on the set of what *might be*. This is so although information theory does not give any direct account of meaning. "What might be" can be the possibilities stored in or envisaged by an organism, so the greater its store of knowledge the more the information that may be transmitted by neural signals.

In trying to measure information rates we find two factors which are

Table 1

Binary decisions required	*Maximum word content of dictionary from which any word can be found*
1	2
2	4
4	16 = 1.6×10^{1}
8	256 = 2.6×10^{2}
16	65, 000 = 6.5×10^{4}
32	4, 300, 000, 000 = 4.3×10^{9}
64	19, 000, 000, 000, 000, 000, 000 = 1.9×10^{19}
128	340, 000, 000, 000, 000, 000, 000, 000, 000, 000, 000, 000, 000 = 3.4×10^{38}
256	160, 000, 000, 000, 000, 000, 000, 000, 000, 000, 000, 000, 000, 000, 000, 000, 000, 000, 000, 000, 000, 000, 000, 000, 000, 000 = 1.6×10^{77}

seldom if ever completely specified, so we can seldom if ever apply information theory rigorously to perception or behaviour. These factors are: (1) the size of the ensemble of possibilities N from which selections are drawn (or between which the signals discriminate), and (2) the relative frequencies (or the probabilities) of the stored alternatives. Without knowing these, we cannot determine information capacity, though we may be able to set some upper limits and arrive at reasonable estimates from measures of choice response times.

For human response time Edmund Hick (Hick, 1952) established the relation (Hick's Law):

$$t = K \log (N+1).$$

This relation was found by pressing finger keys controlling randomly arranged signal lights. The spatial relations between the lights and the keys had first to be learned. (It happens that I was the original subject for this experiment.) With each additional choice possibility (added alternative light), after familiarity with this change in N, the average choice time increases by just over 0.1 seconds (Hyman, 1953). This is interesting, for the increase is not due to the prevailing stimuli, but to the size of the set of *alternative* stimuli. So this finding represents no less than a direct refutation of stimulus-response accounts of behaviour. This conclusion is augmented by the obvious importance of prediction in skills, and most behaviour; for predictions are not signalled events or stimuli, but are assessments of what *might* happen. If what might happen is an important determinant of behaviour, as is clearly the case, obviously we cannot explain behaviour in terms limited to neurally signalled stimuli—however much "sense" is made of them!

In this connection, it is worth noting that even prolonged *absence* of channel activity can be a signal bearing useful information, so that it is not

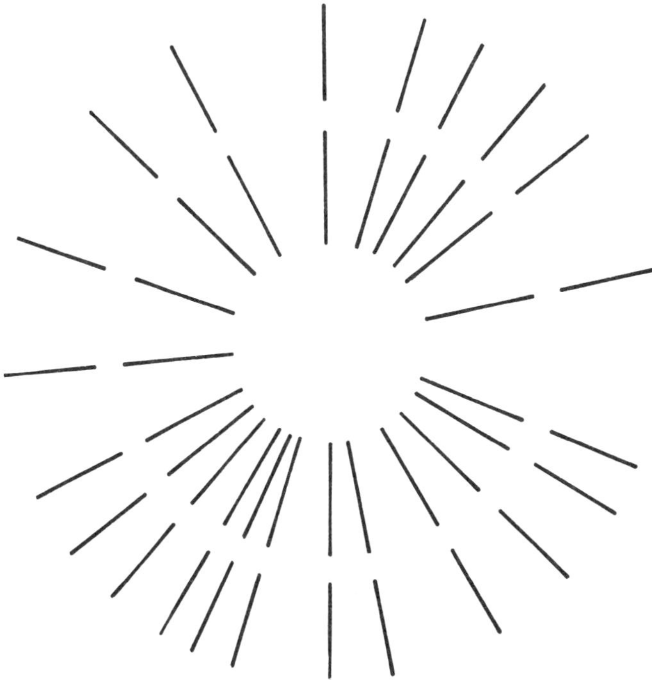

Figure 1 Illusory (cognitive) Contours, such as this bright ring and central disc, are produced whenever there are unlikely gaps forming probable objects. This appears to be a high level postulation, of masking or eclipsing objects. The contours are generated by surprising *absence* of stimulation, or signals. If so, it is not possible to equate perceived contours with peripheral neural activity.

possible to equate activity with signals, or with information. To give informal examples—a silence in a conversation can be as expressive as any outburst; and it was the fact that the dog did *not* bark in the night that led Sherlock Holmes to identify the villain who did mischief to the horse Silver Blaze. Again, surprising *absence* of stimulation evokes the phenomena of "Illusory Contours" (or "Cognitive Contours", Gregory, 1972). For an example see Fig. 1.

Subject to the kinds of hazards already mentioned, information rates have been measured for several human skills. The bit rate of even the most skilled human performance may seem surprisingly low—about 22 bits per second for an expert pianist, while speech does not exceed about 26 bits, and silent reading may reach 44 bits per second. These are very low in relation to the switching rates of electronic systems, for electronic components can change their states five or six orders of magnitude faster than neurones. A television channel has about 10^4 times greater band width than has a single optic nerve fibre, and this is nowhere near the limit for engineering channels. The effective band width of biological channels is, however, greatly increased by parallel paths. The vertebrate optic nerve is the extreme example, having a million parallel neural paths. On Rushton's (1961) estimate, a single nerve fibre (ideally free of noise) might in principle transmit up to 30 bits in a single time-discrimination interval of 0.1 seconds. This represents the capacity to select one out of a thousand million states; but this is far more than the number of intensity levels (about one hundred) which can be distinguished at a given level of adaptation by the eye, which is less than 5 bits. So something, perhaps the coding, is highly inefficient. This has the unfortunate consequence that we can hardly hope to use measures of peripheral nerve activity to test theories of perception before we know far more about the coding characteristics of neural channels.

It seems important to emphasize that high capacity channels can seldom, if ever, be adequate for monitoring the world—for objects are very often partly hidden by nearer objects, and are always oriented so that only some features are available for detection, identification and monitoring. So it seems clear that sophisticated inferences from limited available data are necessary for behaviour to be appropriate to the object world, even when sensory channels have high information capacity. Possibly this is why neuronal channels (and indeed sense organs) have not developed dramatically through evolution by comparison with the vast development of brains, with their vast store of knowledge derived from the past, which is applied to handle the present and predict the immediate future, as well as cope with entirely unsensed features of the world of known objects. It may further be suggested (Gregory, 1968) that the need to control behaviour from inferences based on inadequate, intermittent, unreliable, and arbitrarily selected sensory data is the principal evolutionary route along which intelligence has developed. This may in part explain why we are primarily "visual" animals, for vision requires a rich knowledge base and sophisticated mental references, leading far from the initiating stimuli, if it is to pay off in reliable predictive behaviour.

These considerations suggest two lines of thought: firstly, the evolutionary pressure towards parallel processing, giving transmission of information in channels with up to a million fibres, and secondly, the development of cognitive brain processes, involving rich data bases and subtle heuristic algorithms for generating predictive hypotheses from necessarily limited sensory data (which in any case can never give direct knowledge of the future) towards which behaviour must be directed to escape the absurdly limiting tyranny of reflexes.

It is the development of predictive perception, we may suppose, that gives us the power to imagine hypothetical possibilities, to be creative, and indeed to be scientists. We owe all this, I suggest, to the limited available information capacity of sensory channels, together with the survival value of generating possible futures to keep a step ahead of the competition and Nature. The generation and selection of possible futures is the basis of cognition and Mind. We shall discuss briefly these two central developments of neural functions.

The sense of developing parallel from serial processing in compound eyes

Scanning, which provides spatial information down a single time channel, although well-suited to television is highly inappropriate for the small bandwidths available for biological eyes. There is however a scanning eye in nature, which has but a single optic nerve fibre: the eye of the copepod *Copilia quadrata*. She (the male is dull by comparison) has a pair of scanning eyes, each having a large fixed anterior lens (Fig. 2), and deep in the body a smaller pear-shaped lens attached to a single photoreceptor (Gregory, Ross and Moray, 1964).

The optical elements of this eye are similar to the elements of a single ommatidium of the familiar compound eye, though the distance between the anterior and posterior lenses is enormously greater. Clearly, the curvature of the photoreceptor enables it to move laterally through the body fluids. *Copilia* is extremely transparent, and one can see the movements (which we take to be scanning) of the receptor and its

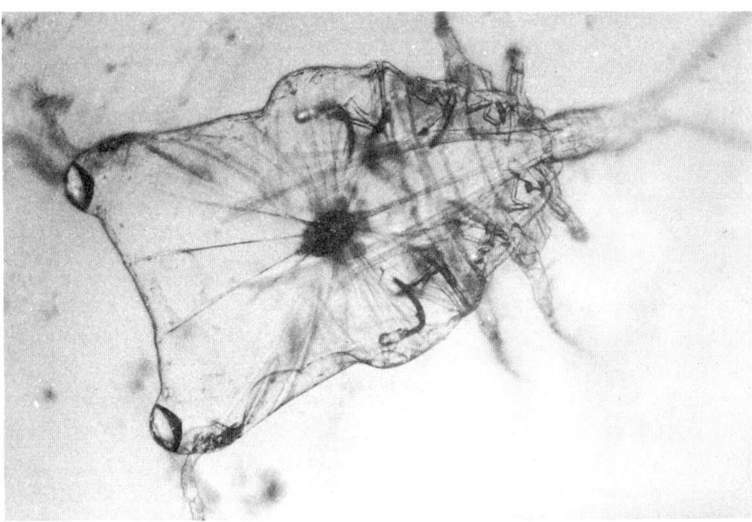

Figure 2 The single channel scanning eye of the copepod *Copilia quadrata*. The large anterior lenses and the posterior pear-shaped lenses can be seen, with their attached photoreceptors lying far back from the anterior lens of each eye. The optic nerve originates from the small bulge visible about halfway along the heavily pigmented curved "rod" receptor, for each of the two eyes, and enters the central "brain" or ganglion. In life, the posterior lenses and receptors move with a saw-tooth motion, exactly opposed to each other, across the image plane of the anterior lenses. The maximum scan rate, which is highly variable, is about two scans per second.

attached lens perfectly well in the living creature with a dissection microscope of 20–50× magnification. We have recorded the scanning movements, using videotape recording, and with an infrared-sensitive T.V. camera and IR source we have investigated whether scanning takes place in the dark: it does. Scanning is not continuous; and there is usually a burst of scanning before *Copilia* moves off from rest. At least in laboratory conditions, she may lie dormant for many minutes, apparently dead (there is no heart), and then suddenly start scanning away and leap into action. It is possible that her sole goal in life, at this final stage of her life-forms, is to seek a male. The males are larger, and appear more primitive, with far less well developed eyes. They are capable of glowing, quite brilliantly, from special regions; and it is possible that the female seeks the glowing and sometimes flashing lights of the male with her scanning eyes.

It is interesting to speculate on the evolutionary place of this single channel scanning eye. I have suggested (Gregory, 1968) that there is a hen-and-egg problem for the evolution of eyes, for eyes need elaborate analysing mechanisms to read the signals they provide. How then did the necessary computing neural mechanisms evolve before there were eyes, and how did eyes evolve before there was neural computing to make sense of visual signals? The point is that visual signals are far less directly related to significant events than touch or taste, which monitor features of the environment immediately important for survival. Vision is quite different, for visual features are indirectly related to the immediate necessities of survival—though once visual signals are read, they provide early warning of impending disaster or promising reward and so allow predictive strategic behaviour.

Possibly the first eyes took over existing touch neural mechanisms. These would develop without the hen-and-egg problem, for they are immediately useful in monitoring biologically important environmental variables. Now it is suggestive that there are two kinds of touch, involving very different touch analysing mechanisms: passive touch, and active or "haptic" touch. Passive touch works by *simultaneous* parallel processing from receptors lying on the body surface, while haptic touch works by *sequential* processing of signals, which may be from a single motile receptor exploring shapes in time. (Thus, one can recognize an English 50p coin, either by feeling its characteristic shape in the palm of the hand or by exploring it with a moving finger.) If the idea that eyes took over touch analysers is correct we may suggest that *simple* eyes took over passive skin touch, and *compound* eyes took over, or fed into, haptic touch mechanisms. We may suppose that the first compound eyes had only a single moving optic probe—as in *Copilia*. Information theory tells us that this could not compete with multi-pathway eyes, each pathway having the low bandwidth of afferent neurones. The pulse rate coding of neurones is no doubt, as suggested by William Rushton (Rushton, 1961), adopted to maintain signals by pulse restoration as in long distance telegraphy. The information transmission rate of nerve is surprisingly low; and as we have pointed out, adequate signalling is seldom if ever possible for direct control of sophisticated behaviour—and never for predictive behaviour. No doubt this is why the ancient peripheral nerve transmission system has not evolved into anything much more efficient; for real-time information from the world is simply not available for sophisticated and especially predictive behaviour: so development has gone into central mechanisms for augmenting sensory data with stored knowledge. Hence, we may suppose, the remarkable development of cognition in the higher animals and especially man (cf. Allman, 1977).

The sense of cognition

Cognition is the development and employment of knowledge for controlling behaviour and solving problems. We may identify three stages of cognitive perception. (1) The *signals* of the peripheral nervous system, derived from the transducer sense organs from received patterns of energy from the world, or from states of the organism; (2) the reading of the signals, essentially by decoding, to derive useful working data, which may require quite sophisticated processing; (3) the combining of sensory and stored data to produce the predictive hypotheses which are perceptions, and which control behaviour according to probable present or future states of the world (rather than directly from stimuli, which are essentially inadequate for controlling sophisticated and especially predictive behaviour).

It is now clear that information processing works both "upwards" from sensory signals, and also "downwards" from stored knowledge, which may be more or less general, of objects and states of affairs. The "bottom-up" and "top-down" procedures, although very different, are surprisingly difficult to separate experimentally by perceptual experiments; but fortunately phenomena of perceptual ambiguity can be applied to identify which is operating in given conditions. For example, when systematic changes of brightness, colour, or form take place, with, say, visual reversals of depth—when there is no change in the display or the sensory signals—then we know that "top-down" processes from the prevailing perceptual hypothesis are operating, for there are no changes of input signals to account for these perceptual changes, which may be dramatic (see Fig. 3). Since these occur, it is clearly impossible to give a full account of perception from recordings, however complete, of sensory signals: we must appreciate the contribution of stored knowledge, and how it is employed to augment and select and effectively modify sensory signals. At present this is beyond physiological understanding. We can however appreciate the importance and role of stored knowledge through attempts

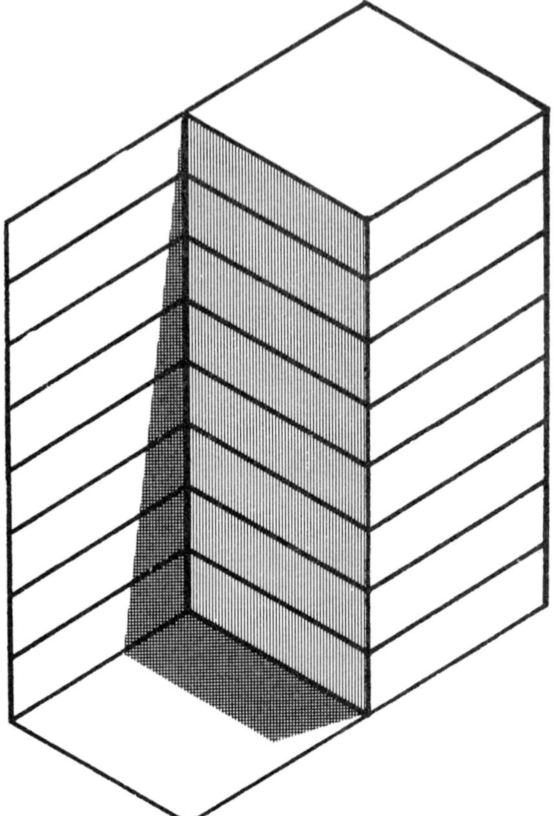

Figure 3 The shaded rectangle of this depth-ambiguous figure appears, for many observers, much lighter when it is a plausible shadow—as cast from an upper source—and darker when it is likely to be a mark or region of different albedo. We may think of the alternative depth perceptions as alternative hypotheses on the same signals and data. Each perceptual hypothesis of depth sets the brightness of this region according to its changed probable nature—shadow or a local difference in the albedo of the object.

to make artificial-intelligence machines recognize objects. Here of course the "physiology" is entirely different, but scene analysis and robot control through machine vision bring out some of the logical necessities for perception with clarity and detail.

It turns out that there are many useful restraints on the perceived shapes and properties of objects (Winston, 1977). These restraints are the limits to what is possible, or likely, which allow a small amount of information to control a great deal of behaviour. They allow machine (and no doubt organismic) perception to be far richer than may seem possible from the limited sensed data available. They are the basis of "sensory cues", from which the identity of objects can be inferred from sensory patterns of stimulation.

Some restraints are *logically* necessary (for example that only one object can be in a given place at a given time), and others are *contingent* (for example that shadows are usually cast from a source of illumination above objects; and that most objects have closed forms, with, in the case of man-made objects, many parallel lines and right-angular corners. Restraints on possible and probable object shapes are extremely important for object perception, for they allow the limited bandwidths of sensory channels to provide adequate information, by limiting the set of likely possibilities from which choices must be made.

The major point is that knowledge can only be applied, and visual cues for object recognition are only available, where there are restraints on what is possible or likely. This perhaps is most obviously so, and most interesting, in the case of perspective. To accept retinally converging lines as evidence of depth requires that retinal image convergence is generally associated and occurs with depth. This in turn requires that there are not too many objects which present converging lines when they are normal to the observer. Many distortion illusion figures (see Fig. 4) are of this form. It may be expected that such depth cue features as convergence can generate distortion when presented in atypical situations. We have found (Gregory and Harris, 1975) that these distortions do not occur when perspective is appropriate to the viewing position, and when the correct depth is seen. In short, then, when the sensory data and the prevailing perceptual hypothesis are appropriate, there are no marked distortions or illusions of this kind. The results of this experiment are shown in Fig. 5. It will be seen that the distortion of the Müller-Lyer arrows (perspective corners) is zero when seen (by stereoscopic projection) in depth and the viewing distance is also correct for the perspective angles of the figures. So

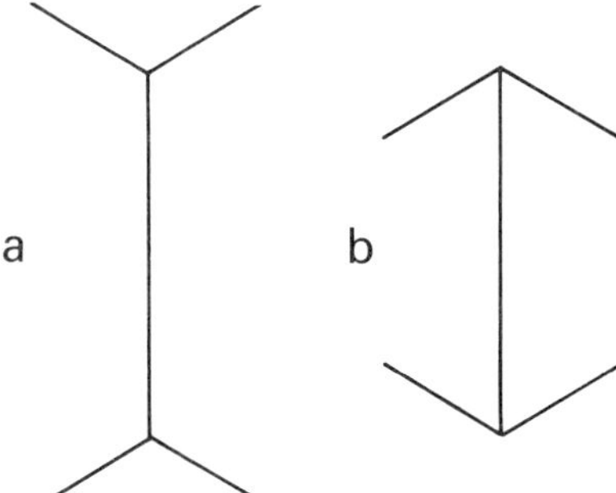

Figure 4 The Müller-Lyer illusion figure. (a) appears longer than (b). (a) is a perspective drawing of an inside corner; (b) of an outside corner. The question is whether the distortion is a visual channel signalling error, somehow induced by these angles; or whether these angles are providing inappropriate depth data, setting up distortion through cognitive processes of visual size scaling set by distance cues, normally to give invariance of size over a wide range of distances. This is clearly useful for object recognition and behaviour: though we may expect scaling to be upset in artificial conditions.

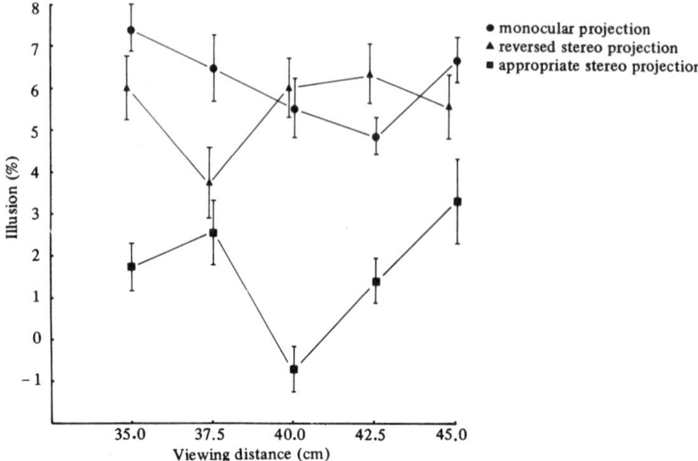

Figure 5 The curves show the extent of illusion (linear distortion) of the Müller-Lyer figure, presented at various viewing distances, so that the ingoing and outgoing "arrow heads" of the figures are correct perspective drawings of corners at the viewing distance of 40 cm only. It will be seen that (lower curve marked with square) the distortion is zero for this critical viewing distance. The upper curves show the return of the illusion, with (dots) reversed stereo and (triangles) no stereo depth—showing that the visual distortion occurs when either the perspective or the seen depth as signalled by perspective is inappropriate—even though the same angles are being signalled by the visual channel. The origin of this distortion thus appears to be cognitive, and not due to signalling distortion.

the usual distortion of lengths can hardly be due to signalling errors of the visual channel—but rather by reading the signals as depth data, when the figures are flat.

An essential point is that it is impossible for features such as convergence of lines or angles (such as the arrow fins of the Müller-Lyer illusion figures) to be read as depth information, and also to appear correctly when this reading is inappropriate—as it is for flat figures or objects having typical perspective shapes. Such illusion figures as these, and the conditions under which they do or do not create distortions, are powerful tools for establishing how sense is normally read (and sometimes misread) from neural signals.

To take another example, shadows are important for setting depth, but this depends on assuming that the light source is somewhere above the object. Most objects will reverse in depth when illuminated from below; but interestingly, this is not so for objects such as faces which are extremely unlikely to be reversed in depth, or be hollow. A hollow face—the mould of a face—refuses to appear hollow, as it is in fact, in spite of all visual cues except full stereoscopic vision (Fig. 6). I have indeed failed to produce stereo photographs which will reverse faces in depth with pseudoscopic viewing, or that with normal stereo will make hollow masks

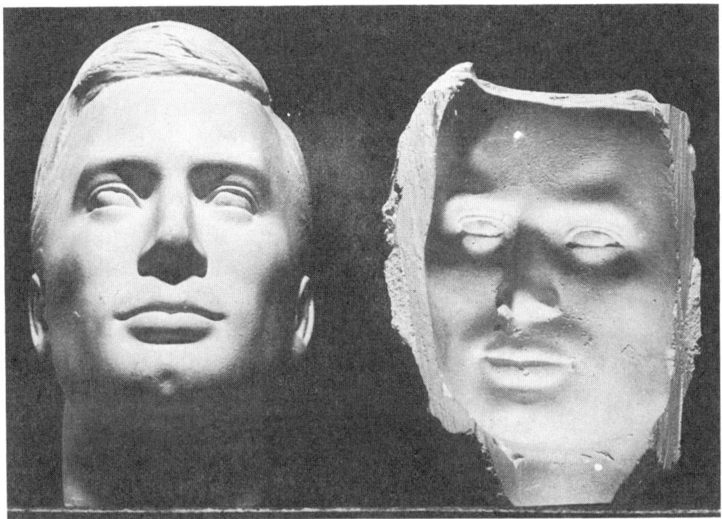

Figure 6 The left-hand face is normal; but the right-hand "face" is a hollow mask of the right-hand face. It appears as a face, and not hollow, even though the lighting is normal. Here the low probability of a face-like object being hollow sets the perception, against such strong visual cues as, even, stereoscopic signals.

appear hollow; so evidently very powerful probability biases from top-down processing set limits to the unusualness of what can be effectively displayed, and even to what can under any conditions be perceived.

The sense of meaning

We read meaning from the symbols of language, and more or less continually from the world of natural objects. How is meaning related to, or given by, information as defined in terms of mere selections? Is there so much more to meaning that analysis in terms of the narrow technical definition of information is virtually irrelevant—or indeed irreverent?

A key to how we might think of meaning in terms of information theory was suggested by Donald Mackay in a radio talk in 1960 (reprinted 1969 in *Information, Mechanism and Meaning*). Here it is suggested that the meaning of a message can be defined simply as its selective function on the range of the recipient's states of readiness for goal-directed activity. The meaning of a message for *you* is its selective function on *your* state of conditional readiness. This implies that meaning is not simply in the message (or in a perceived object) but rather, meaning is a relation between the message or perceived object and the recipient or perceiver. This certainly fits the well-established notion that with greater knowledge or understanding we can read more meaning into things.

All this seems to lead to the conclusion (which may be unacceptable to zoologists, physiologists, and even psychologists who may be less concerned with the physics of the nervous system) that to measure and appreciate the meaning of sensory information we need to know things which are very difficult to discover: coding efficiencies, and the repertoire of possibilities and conditional probabilities which are accepted by selective information and used for controlling behaviour and reading meaning from symbols and from the external world by perception.

What sort of answers can we suggest for the frankly philosophical question (or rather metaphysical, as we have no data-based repertoire of structured answers for selection by information): "How do we think, feel pains and pleasures, experience colours and shapes and weights, and the wonder of things? How indeed do we *experience* meaning?"

One might well say that there can be meaning without consciousness, or awareness (I use the terms interchangeably), but few will deny that music and pictures and jokes are "meaningful" in the full sense only through awareness or sensations which are special and private and not like anything we believe exists in the inanimate world of physics. Can physiology, psychology, or any other science make sense of the problem of consciousness?

A difficulty is the personal uniqueness of feelings of consciousness together with the at present insuperable experimental difficulty of establishing the physical basis of thought and of memory. Perhaps artificial intelligence offers some hope here, for computers can be test-beds for theories of thinking, and the fact that they are physically so different from brains helps in deciding whether thinking is essentially associated with protoplasm as a substance, or with processes or procedures which need not be uniquely carried out by brain mechanisms. I take the view that thought processes and memory can be simulated, and be made as real, in machines as in brains; but the basis of consciousness may still elude us, even when we have artificial-intelligence machines rivalling in mental capacities the higher organisms, including man (Gregory, 1980).

For consciousness, we may want to say that feeling and thinking could be represented by functional structures or processes not associated with protoplasm (in which case computers could be "conscious"); or we may prefer to believe that protoplasm as a substance *is* essential for awareness. Rushton (1961) suggests that the sole function of nerve is rapidly to secrete replicas of input concentrations of hormones to distant regions in the organism. He points out that the simplest animals have no nerves, and yet react with purpose—seeking and avoiding. Rushton says:

> Life for them presumably lies in their sensitivity to the chemical environment and the flow of protoplasm or thrash of flagella by which they can move in it, in the change of permeability with the mixing of cell ingredients, and in the secretion and removal of the hormones by which the activity is controlled.
>
> At the dawn of life, urges and efforts must have been chemical—have they ever been otherwise?

He then points out that nerves do not replace chemicals: they secrete them—instantly and precisely to distant locations. Without nerves, this would require (in large organisms) slow and imprecise diffusion. Darwin (1875, 1888) pointed out that some plants almost, if not quite, approach animal performance in responding selectively to specific stimuli, and we certainly find prediction in plants. But this hardly contradicts Rushton's account of the basic function of nerve, or indeed of his suggestion that we think and feel with our hormones. Rushton's account could also bear the interpretation that plants may have consciousness, which hardly seems acceptable.

We arrive at a situation where on the A.I. paradigm there is a danger, as we may see it, of attributing consciousness to machines; and on the chemical paradigm there is an equal danger of attributing awareness or consciousness to plants. So (most curiously) it seems that if we think about the problem at all, we decide the issue *politically*—by considering with whom or what we are prepared to share our awareness of the world and ourselves. If we ban computers and plants as acceptable companions, we are on our own, and we all know that such special cases fall outside the realm of science.

REFERENCES

Allman, J. (1977) Evolution of the visual system in early primates *Prog. Psychobiol. and Physiol. Psychol.*, **7**, 1–53.

Darwin, C. (1875) *Insectivorous Plants* John Murray.

Darwin, C. (1888) *The Movements of Climbing Plants* John Murray.

Gregory, R. L., Ross, H. E. and Moray, N. (1964) The curious eye of *Copilia Nature*, **201**,1166.

Gregory, R. L. (1968) "The evolution of eyes and brain—a hen-and-egg problem" in *The Neuro-psychology of Spatially Orientated Behaviour* (ed. Freedman, S. J.) University of Illinois Press, Urbana. (Reprinted in: Gregory, R. L. (1974) *Concepts and Mechanism of Perception* Duckworth.

Gregory, R. L. (1968) Perceptual illusions and brain models *Proc. Royal Soc.* "B", **171**, 279.

Gregory, R. L. (1972) Cognitive contours *Nature*, **238**, 51–52.

Gregory, R. L. (1980) "Regarding consciousness" in *Consciousness and the Physical World* (eds. Josephson, B. D., Ramachandran, V. S.) Pergamon Press, 31–47.

Gregory, R. L. and Harris, J. P. (1975) Illusion-destruction by appropriate scaling *Perception*, **4**, 203–220.

Hick, W. E. (1952) On the rate of gain of information *Quart. J. exp. Psychol.*, **4**, 11–26.

Hyman, R. (1953) Stimulus information as a determinant of reaction time *J. exp. Psychol.*, **45**, 188–196.

Mackay, D. M. (1969) *Information, Mechanism and Meaning* M.I.T. Press (Chap. 3).

Rushton, W. A. H. (1961) "Peripheral coding in the nervous system" in *Sensory Communication* (ed. Rosenblith, W. A.) M.I.T. Press, 169–181.

Shannon, C. E. and Weaver, W. (1949) *The Mathematical Theory of Communication* University of Illinois Press, Urbana.

Weiner, N. (1948) *Cybernetics* John Wiley, New York.

Winston, P. (1977) *Artificial Intelligence* Addison Wesley, Reading, Massachusetts.

CHAPTER TWENTY
UNUSUAL SENSES

FRANK A. BROWN, Jr.

Introduction

Does a novel perceptive domain in living creatures underlie those systems which have largely occupied the conventional biologist up to the present? Will we find in such a duplicity of domains the solutions to current biological mysteries such as the elusive timer for the well-recognized biological clock system, the extraordinary map-compass sense, the often reported apparent weather prediction, and the often suggested interactions among living things even after all known routes of communication are absent? This review introduces some results from critical investigations over more than 30 years which indicate that the answers to these questions are affirmative.

There is strong evidence that living substance itself possesses an inordinate degree of sensitivity to its environment. The investigations generating this evidence were not performed for the purpose of discovering new systems of perception with specific adaptive roles, but rather to establish fundamental phenomena involving subtle informational inputs and to describe some of their properties. Adaptive relevance, it is suggested, would gradually arise by selective evolution whenever a species stood to profit. In short, if an organism possesses a basic perceptive capacity and this capacity has potential usefulness it can be postulated that the species will somehow develop its practical use. The objections that have been directed at our explorations over the years, namely that the fields were too weak, the responses too small, or the noise too great, have not, in my judgment, been justified. We stand about where conventional sensory physiology was perhaps a century or two ago.

This account chiefly treats sensitivities to the electromagnetic spectrum beyond the infrared and ultraviolet, but does not deal with the recent exciting researches concerning infrasound, barometric pressure, gravitation, or pheromones. My concern is with the sensitivity of all living things to atmospheric electromagnetic fields that can provide information supplementing what is gained by the more conventional sensory systems. On the presumption that the evolution of special sensory cells and organs was anticipated by a more fundamental receptive capacity, and the special adaptive roles of the various recognized stimuli were preceded by more generalized receptivity, our objectives have entailed discovering statistically significant responses to very weak forces and then exploring through these responses the characteristics and properties of the response systems involved.

Also considered briefly are some of the kinds of information that, theoretically, can be derived by organisms from such informational inflow. The atmosphere reflects all the geophysical periods, the spatial organization of the planetary field, the movements of weather systems, and even the biofields projected from living creatures. Since the atmosphere is an integrated entity, the organisms are probably reading from the whole complex. Not knowing the information, we cannot know what noise it contains, but we have adequate reason to know that the noise in the organisms' measured responses can be enormous.

Organisms can be considered to be in a spatiotemporal continuum with their physical environment. Genome-guided differentiation results in the production of dynamic electromagnetic "islands", perhaps sophisticated bioelectronic ones, lying in an ocean of fluctuating electromagnetic atmosphere. We are concerned here with exploring the organisms' degrees and manners of dependence on their position in the vast continuum of weak, pervasive electromagnetic fields.

In brief, through a "common electromagnetic sense" the living system should possess, theoretically, almost endless potential for viewing indirectly virtually every aspect of its planetary environment, and even well beyond. Do the individual organisms, or instead, the organisms along with their physical environment, comprise complete functional units?

Organismic-environmental correlations

Whenever a statistically significant correlation exists, and persists, between a biological process and an environmental physical fluctuation in segment after segment of data, there must be a discoverable rational explanation. This is equally true whether or not there is any presently conceivable means by which the two series of concurrently fluctuating data may become related. To pass off casually the problem as a nonsense correlation is simply to avoid what can be a challenging investigation leading toward the description of novel complex linkages in chains of separately known events, or to the revelation of novel sensitivities of the living systems. When the problem is compounded by a careful screening of the organisms from fluctuations in every known factor to which they have been acceptably reported to be sensitive, only truly new findings can result.

In my laboratory in the late 1940's and early 1950's in studies of fluctuations in "constant conditions" of pigmentary system, O_2-consumption, and spontaneous activity in fiddler crabs, shell gaping in bivalve molluscs, and motor activity in the rat, we encountered correlations with motions of the sun and moon relative to the earth of such character and precision that the conventional wisdom was inadequate to explain them. These findings, together with many more casual ones from numerous other laboratories, clearly suggested that our knowledge of interactions between life and its ambience was only partially disclosed and that a rich reward might come to anyone who was willing to explore the subject patiently and critically.

Weather-factor correlations

We invented an automatically recording, barostatted respirometer with which living creatures, animal or plant, could be investigated over extended intervals in complete constancy of not only all the usual factors, but of ambient pressure and humidity as well. The organisms were hermetically sealed from all exchanges of materials with the outside environment for up to a week at a stretch and then only fleetingly exposed before other stretches. Many kinds of living things, including crabs, snails, potatoes, beans, salamanders and embryonated chicks were monitored to determine their hour by hour fluctuations in rates of O_2-consumption. Repeated mean solar-day, lunar-day, synodic monthly, and annual patterns were described using the averaged hourly means of a number of individuals.

That the systematic metabolic patterns were not wholly random, nor autonomous was confirmed from cross-correlations with the erratic weather-system factors, atmospheric pressure and temperature. It was quickly discovered that despite the screening of the organisms and their immediate ambient environment from the factors themselves, unambiguous cross-correlations occurred between respiratory rates of the organisms and the fluctuations in atmospheric pressure and temperature. Investigations with the potatoes, crabs, and chicks revealed a highly significant correlation between the mean rate of O_2-consumption (expressed as deviation from the mean for the day) for the interval 1600–1900 hours day by day and the total 1400–1800 h change in atmospheric pressure on the same days. Furthermore, both the 1600–1900 h metabolic rates, and the 1400–1800 h pressure changes were discovered to correlate highly significantly with the mean barometric pressure of the second day thereafter.

The clock hours of the correlating values for the pressure change and metabolism were highly specific. The studies with the potatoes and crabs disclosed that only one other time in the day could be found when a similar highly significant cross-correlation occurred, namely for the comparable morning hours. A further extensive search resulted in finding that the midnight to noon range of the day by day patterns of fluctuation of potatoes correlated positively with the mean daily outdoor temperatures near ground level at the same geographic site for temperatures below 14°C, but negatively for higher temperatures.

The potatoes, crabs, and chicks, while all showed a correlation with morning, evening, or both relationships, differed specifically from one another and with time. The potatoes and chicks whose mean daily cycles showed a maximum in the afternoon displayed an afternoon negative correlation with pressure change, the crabs with a minimum in the afternoon had a positive correlation. The form of an environmentally dependent mean daily cycle was apparently related to the sign of its response. The potato, which was investigated throughout the year, exhibited a fluctuating sign of its morning correlation over about three years of its observation, positive from April through October and negative during the remainder of the year.

The firm and persistent 24 h relationship of the times of correlation with atmospheric pressure implied that the organisms, though screened from every obvious cue to time of day, were in some manner apprised of the daily clock hours. Since barometric pressure reflects not only the passage of the random weather systems but also the solar-day tides of the atmosphere the organisms behaved as if they were steadily apprised of these tides as they were modulated by the weather. The mean daily patterns of the potatoes, which we followed for 11 years, were hence termed geophysically-dependent periodisms with the living systems thus incorporating the 24 h day into their very being. Also, following the well known annual modulation of the solar-day tides as they vary with photoperiod, the organisms appear to be intimately incorporated into the yearly cycles, similarly by obscure means. This yearly information was supplemented, of course, by the previously mentioned remarkable correlation with ground-level temperature from which the organisms were similarly shielded.

Geomagnetic correlation

Twenty-five mudsnails were monitored in our respirometers for a summer month and the mean daily rates of O_2-consumption were found, despite the constancy of every factor known to affect them, to vary irregularly through about a two-fold range from lowest to highest values. Searching for an environmental factor with which the pattern for the month might correlate, it was learned that by far the largest and most highly significant correlation occurred with the fluctuation in strength of the geomagnetic field with the snails in a 2-day lead relationship. Correlation with the same-day values lay very close to zero.

Sunspot correlation

A 4-month study of the day by day fluctuations in mean daily activity of a white rat led to the remarkable finding that the activity over about the first two months paralleled the fluctuation in sunspot number with surprising precision. Then, abruptly, the sign of the correlation changed and for the last two months the mean daily activities mirror-imaged the sunspot numbers. This inversion seemed to be related to the barometric pressure correlation since the time of inversion of the relationship between activity and sunspots corresponded very closely with time of inversion of sign of an ongoing correlation between the late afternoon activities and the afternoon pressure changes in the same rat. The derivations of the sunspot and barometric pressure correlations appeared to possess a common denominator. And, furthermore, since the organism could not view the sunspots, and the same specific pressure correlations persisted with other organisms in barostats, the mediating factor could be neither vision nor pressure.

Primary-cosmic-radiation correlations

It was discovered that animals and plants behaved as if they could sense primary cosmic radiation, a radiation from which they were thoroughly shielded by the earth's atmosphere. The primary radiation becomes completely transformed during penetration of the ionosphere and troposphere, so that the mean daily variation of ground-level radiation does not resemble that of the primary. Yet, inspection of mean daily and lunar-day patterns for 8 species of organisms over those 20 months for which simultaneous data were available disclosed that there was a tendency very far exceeding chance for the 30-day mean daily patterns either to parallel or to mirror-image the concurrent primary radiation ones. For example, fiddler-crab mean daily cycles mirror-imaged the radiation patterns; the sea-weed, *Fucus*, in its lunar day cycle paralleled the simultaneous radiation ones. Potatoes mirror-imaged the radiation for the first half day and paralleled it the second half. Crabs and potatoes both followed a major cycle alteration between corresponding months of 1954 and 1955. Despite the frequent sign reversals in the relationships, the organisms' fluctuations seemed steadily related to the primary radiation even over a two-year period during which an especially large change in the radiation patterns was noted by physicists. The inversional tendency could be noted even among the individual daily patterns of small populations of potatoes. The effects were independent of whether the organisms were simply in constant light and temperature, or sealed in the barostatted respirometers. The individual daily relationships in potatoes involved large amplitudes of change.

The similarities between the radiation and the biological patterns might be accountable if the organisms could perceive the small-amplitude changes steadily occurring in geomagnetism. The intensity of the radiation entering our atmosphere is well known to be inversely correlated with the strength of geomagnetism. The single-day potato correlations with the radiation suggested that small, natural geomagnetic fluctuations could produce relatively large changes in O_2-consumption in the potatoes. Was it possible that very weak geomagnetism had a strong biological influence? Did the inversional tendency reflect operation of a regulatory mechanism? Had the inversional tendency been responsible for failures of the many earlier attempts to demonstrate a significant biological influence of magnetism?

Whatever the mediating factors involved in these cosmic ray correlations, their strength did not exceed the atmospheric ones. Hence the ranges of variation in the factors were exceedingly small and the responses of the organisms relatively large.

Experiments on weak electromagnetic fields

The search for responsiveness of living things to very weak parameters of the ambient electromagnetic fields was made initially using mudsnails and planarian worms (Barnwell and Brown, 1964). Both these two widely different animals were remarkably sensitive to extremely small modifications in their ambient electromagnetic environment, but it very soon became apparent that the animal's response to an imposed field varied with geographic orientation of the experimental set-up and with time within the geophysical cycles of the solar day, lunar day, and synodic month. The responses were spatiotemporally modulated. Furthermore, an organism's response to a given experimental field could be modified by the simultaneous experimental alteration of another weak-field parameter. Since it was not possible to control all the known and unknown parameters, the response to a given parameter had to be sought not by the usual method of keeping all other factors constant, but rather by repeating the same test over and over again for months, or years, in order to randomize the other parameters. In short, the investigations were planned so as to reveal the effect of an experimental field-situation as functions of time and space, *other factors being equal.* Indeed, we felt that this was the best way to obtain a natural mean response to any imposed experimental field.

Magnetic field, time and space

In the light of the findings with primary cosmic rays, our first studies were directed at weak magnetism. Alnico permanent bar magnets were employed. Strengths were regulated by the distances from the magnets at right angles from their centres. The geographic directions of the fields were altered by turning a horizontal bar magnet to the various directions. We expected that the averaged effects would be quite small, and any results would depend upon statistical validation of their reality. The many experimental series that were performed upon the snails, planarians, and paramecia evolved a common picture. The planarians could distinguish the changing field directions with considerable mean precision. The effect of an experimental field varied, for a fixed time of day, with the direction of the field and time within the synodic monthly cycle. A lunar-day variation was occurring simultaneously with the solar-day one for all three species. Other findings were that the ability to resolve the direction of an experimental field was maximal when at the same strength as for the concurrent geophysical field, but that the organisms could accommodate over the course of about half an hour to an altered strength level.

That the magnetic responsiveness was in some manner related to biological rhythms correlated with the natural cycles, was evident from the discovery that an abrupt 180°-shift (N to S) in the geographic direction at which an experiment was being performed, or the equivalent reversal with a weak field from a bar magnet, reset instantly by 180° the monthly cycle the planarians were exhibiting. The planarians could read monthly time. And when one assayed the relative response of an organism to parallel and right-angle weak magnetic fields, it became evident that the receiving system within the organism behaved like a pair of directional antennae, one rotating with the period of the solar day and the other with the period of the lunar day. The organisms clearly possessed the capacity to "know" steadily the changing positions of the sun and moon though unable to see them directly.

In 1960 Jones, in New Zealand, discovered that several species of plants could distinguish between the two directions of uniform daily horizontal rotation. Growth was accelerated by counterclockwise rotation and slowed down by clockwise. More recently, in studies involving bean water uptake and planarian response to light, we have discovered this phenomenon to be the same in the northern hemisphere, and to be a consequence of rotation relative to the horizontal geomagnetic axis. Rotating an experimental magnetic field for stationary organisms is equivalent to the opposite direction of organismic rotation in the geomagnetic field.

We learned (Brown and Scow, 1978), when subjecting hamsters to a simultaneous 24 h light–dark schedule and square-wave 26 h cycle of higher and lower weak experimental magnetic fields, that cycles of both periods occurred in the animals. Helmholtz coils were used. Both horizontal and vertical experimental magnetic fields were studied. The average strengths were very close to the geomagnetic one. Four 26 h cyclic ranges lay between 8 and 260 milligauss. All magnetic cycles which were studied imposed a 26 h period on the hamsters. The magnet-induced cycle was quasi-sinusoidal instead of square-wave, indicating that the extremely weak magnetic cycles were entraining an intra-organismic complex of interrelated events to the 26 h period.

Electric field, time and space

To investigate the influence of electrical gradients upon a living system, other factors equal, the effect of an experimental horizontal gradient on snails and planarians was studied. The gradient was applied at right angles to the path of slowly moving animals and the effect recorded as the mean deviation in the path relative to the path in absence of the imposed gradient.

In all experiments the influence of a 2 volt cm^{-1} field in the air, produced by right and left copper or aluminium plates and a 45-volt B battery, was studied as the apparatus was turned in random order to each of 8 compass directions. The field for the animal in the water was of the order of 0.1 $\mu V\ cm^{-1}$. No difference between the response was noted for planarians whether the positive pole was to the right or left, and therefore the two values obtained each day were pooled. In experiments with planarians in the morning there was a systematic change in the effect of the field with compass direction. A maximum in right-turning response occurred when the path was southward, and maximum left-turning when the path was northward. There was a highly statistically significant compass directional relationship of the response. However, when observations were made in precisely the same manner in the afternoon the compass response pattern was roughly the mirror-image. There was a clear daily variation in the response to the electric gradient.

Not only were the planarians in water responsive to the air gradient of 2 volt cm^{-1}, which is near the average strength of the vertical gradient near the earth's surface resulting from the difference of about 300 000 volts between the ionosphere and the earth's surface, but the response varied systematically with geographic orientation and time of solar day.

The charge on the ionosphere varies with time of day with about a 40 % range and on universal time. The cycle is, therefore, described in Greenwich time. The gradient close to the earth's surface would vary with air conductivity, a highly variable factor. The horizontal gradient, used in the experiment, is also extremely variable, being influenced by weather systems and innumerable other factors in an organism's close environment.

High-energy radiation, time and space

We investigated the possibility that the living system might directly sense and respond to a high-energy background radiation. The experimental radiation source which was arbitrarily selected consisted of ^{137}Cs, an isotope with a half life of about 30 years and which emitted a very short-wave gamma radiation. The weak sources that were used permitted easy practical manipulation of strength with distance to produce fields on the organisms ranging up to 25 times the local background (bkgd) strength.

When sources were placed to right or left of northward creeping planarians with the field about 6 × bkgd the animals turned away from the source. A similar degree of turning away from the source was noted when the worms were creeping southward. However, when the planarians were creeping eastward or westward no response to the gamma field was evident. In another experimental series, it was found that when four strengths ranging from 1.5 to 25 × bkgd were used, northbound worms turned toward the source when the field was 1.5 × bkgd and increasingly strongly away from the source to fields of 6, 16, and 25 × bkgd. There was a linear relationship between the response of the worms and the common log of the radiation level over the range of the four strengths. This indicated a maximum in positive response to the gamma at some unidentified, very low, strength, below 1.5 × bkgd.

The response to the ^{137}Cs gamma radiation (6 × bkgd) exhibited a semimonthly periodism, northbound planarians turning away from a source maximally during 3 to 4 days prior to the syzygies and maximally toward it during 2 to 3 days following the syzygies. In still another series the responses to the gamma field displayed an annual pattern. To a 1.5 × bkgd field, the cycle was unimodal, the worms turning maximally away from the source in October and maximally toward it in July. To the strongest field, 9 × bkgd, the worms turned away from the source throughout the year with no systematic pattern evident, while to fields of 3 and 6 × bkgd there was suggestively a systematic bimodal cycle with maximum turning away from the source in April and August–September.

A three-summer investigation of responses of mudsnails to gamma radiation from ^{137}Cs disclosed that the response to a field of 6 × bkgd from right or left of moving snails varied systematically with geographic direction of the snail path, the time within the synodic monthly cycle, and with time of solar day. The response to fields from right and left differed between each other. The evidence suggested that response to background radiation of the snails, like planarians, was intricately integrated into the space-time continuum.

Mouse response to ^{137}Cs radiation was investigated. A white mouse in each of four actographs, two at each end of a wooden table, was monitored for hourly activity over about a three-month period in two levels of radiation. For three days two mice had a higher level (8 × bkgd) than the other two (1.5 × bkgd) and then the fields were reversed for three days. This was repeated 15 times. Thus, every mouse in its position on the table served as both "experiment" and "control". The difference between the mean daily activity patterns disclosed that the effect of the increased radiation included a 2% overall activity reduction and a 24 h pattern. There were three troughs of depression, at 0600 h, 1200 h, and 1800 h, with intervening peaks of augmentation. This daily pattern of stimulation and depression resembled closely the inverted form of the daily pattern of O_2-consumption in potatoes that was occurring simultaneously elsewhere in the same building in barostatted recording respirometers.

Biofields

Living things steadily generate spatiotemporally organized patterns which spread out into the ambient physical environment. Well-known special cases are electric fishes which not only pulse electromagnetic fields but can sense those that are broadcast by others and, indeed, appear to employ them in communication (see Szabo, this volume). Alternatively, they use them to explore the surrounding environment. It is also known that sharks can sense the fields generated by their prey, and utilize this information in food capture. Experiments by Becker (1977) have recently established that a similar ability to respond to fields of neighbouring organisms is seen in termites where construction of galleries is influenced. Evidence has been advanced from screening to support the conclusion that the foregoing interactions involve electric fields.

The species on which we have conducted a substantial amount of work is *Phaseolus vulgaris*, and the general behaviour is of a character that could be widespread, possibly universal. Seeds of this plant when placed in water slowly absorb the water, but at rates which steadily fluctuate from day to day. The rates do not vary randomly but appear in constant conditions of light and temperature to be a response to some unidentified pervasive atmospheric parameter or parameters. Clusters of closely packed seeds in separate, widely dispersed vessels display a highly significant positive correlation with one another in their water-uptake rates. Similar mean synodic monthly patterns have been described in widely scattered groups. Sometimes they are all quadrimodal and at other times, bimodal. It was found that beans absorbing water inside a ferric-metal lined room have patterns tending to mirror-image those of beans under exactly the same conditions of illumination and temperature, but outside the room.

A serendipitous finding was that when two clusters of beans in separate vessels were closely apposed, the two clusters exhibited a negative correlation with one another in rate of water uptake, but when the vessels were separated by some distance the correlation became positive. The beans in the closely adjacent vessels appear to be mutually induced to adopt opposite signs of response to the effective atmospheric fields producing the day to day fluctuations.

Further experiments disclosed that slow clockwise and counter-clockwise rotation also tended to induce opposite signs of the correlations between bean water uptake and the fluctuation of the atmospheric factor. Since a rotational effect has been learned to be a response to geomagnetism it was suggested that one field involved in the demonstration of interactions between clusters of bean seeds was geomagnetism.

To obtain more information concerning both fields that were involved, the biofields and atmospheric, beans were first assembled in a row of four copper Faraday cages, the successive cages being 35 cm from centre to centre. Correlating the beans in successive cages with one another gave a significantly more negative value than expectation, and correlating the alternate cages, a significantly more positive value. Since electric fields could no longer pass between the beans in different cages, it was presumed that both the fluctuating environmental field and the field effecting the interactions were magnetic. However, it was conceivable that the atmospheric field was a high-energy radiation.

The row of four Faraday cages was next supplemented by a second row of similar cages except that these were each lined by 0.014-in sheet mumetal which attenuated any outside static magnetic field to about 1 % and any static field passing from one cluster of beans to the next, to about 0.01 %. Now, correlating the beans in adjacent cages and those in alternate ones in exactly the same manner for each series over the succeeding $2\frac{1}{2}$ years, those in the Faraday cages displayed statistically significant long interval deviations from random, but altered between which were the more negative, adjacents or alternates. With lower amplitude, and without statistically significant deviations from randomness, the beans in the mumetal-lined cages mirror-imaged, over the duration of the observations, the fluctuating consecutive 30-day mean patterns displayed by the beans in the unlined cages. Since the correlations disclosed only bean interactions, this was interpreted to mean that the fluctuating environmental field to which all the beans were responding was, as in the aforementioned steel-shielded room, attenuated in the mumetal cages, but the biofield associating the groups could penetrate the screens readily. This strongly suggested the geomagnetic field to be the effective atmospheric force, and dynamic, or oscillating, biomagnetic ones to be effecting the interactions. The mumetal would be an ineffective barrier for the latter fields.

Another experiment cast further light on the phenomenon. The effect on interactions while the vessels occupied a specific pattern on slowly rotating tables, clockwise (CW) and counterclockwise (CCW), and a stationary one, was determined. CW and CCW rotation, over the course of two long experiments produced repeatable, differing effects on the patterns of interactions. The difference noted could be interpreted to result from different ranges of the interacting fields effected by the two directions of rotation. This explanation also suggested that the changes over time in the immediately preceding experiment was probably caused by changing levels of magnetic parameters in the atmospheric complex. Indeed, even the sudden disappearance of a phenomenon once of high statistical significance raises the obvious question of what happened to it.

Organismic behaviour and "unusual senses"

Space sense

Evidence has been advanced over the years that living things demonstrate abilities that indicate a "space sense" that still largely defies explanation in conventional terms. This is evident in the homing ability of such animals as birds, turtles, fishes, and insects that experiments have indicated still exist after every obvious cue has been eliminated. Homing pigeons, even when sealed in "constant conditions" and carried by a circuitous course to a new location even tens or hundreds of miles away, possess a means of knowing in what direction from home they have been displaced, can make their way there almost directly, and even when deprived of vision know when they have arrived. The living creature has a map sense of extraordinary precision. Many minor cues that can contribute to this phenomenon have been disclosed by experiments but a major residue remains. A small variation noted in the initial home heading has been shown to have a synodic monthly variation that inverts from time to time, suggesting that the mapsense is a component of a spatiotemporal mechanism of adjustment of the animal to its planetary field. The map-compass sense implies an operation enabled by the continuum of terrestrial and organismic fields.

Time sense

Living things also possess a sense of time within the natural geophysical cycles of the solar and lunar days, the synodic month, and the year that transcends every obvious cue to these cycles. We know that a family of biological rhythms approximating these periods is commonplace among organisms. Some adaptive daily rhythms are labile and may be manipulated by changing levels of constant light, by light–dark and temperature changes, and by numerous other factors such as feeding schedules, noise, and application of particular chemical substances. In constancy of all factors that can alter these rhythms, the rhythms commonly drift slowly over the day to progressively earlier or later hours. This latter behaviour has spawned the hypothesis that they are privately timed within each individual by clocks adaptively approximating the daily period. The drifting rhythms with their odd periods deviating slightly from the natural periods have been termed circadian, circatidal, circamonthly and circannual. The light and temperature cycles are postulated to keep the internal clocks accurate. However, beneath the drifting rhythms there still persist fluctuations reflecting all the major geophysical periods of the planet. There exists, for example, a solar-day periodism locked to the local-time clock hours of the day, and a mean lunar-day periodism locked to the local-time hours of the lunar day. Neither a view of the sun nor moon, or even consequent light changes are directly responsible for these relationships to local time. The well-known and frequent activities of subtle and pervasive atmospheric synchronizers, the great stability, and the near temperature- and drug-independence of the "circa" periods have produced an alternative hypothesis for their origin, namely an active cycle-by-cycle resetting of the rhythms from underlying geophysically dependent periodisms. This alternative hypothesis, unlike private timers, is testable and an experiment that could demonstrate a functional relationship between solar-day cycles derived by organismic-environmental interaction and the phase-labile will now be described.

If circadian rhythms, for example, are dependent on and indeed generated from the underlying exogenous solar-day cycles by a frequency transformation involving the normal phase-shifting machinery of the adaptable rhythms (a hypothetical process termed *autophasing*), then one would expect that a shortening of the external solar-day cycle would result in a shortening of any rhythmic period of the organism that depended on it, while lengthening of the external cycle would be accompanied by a lengthening of the organism's period. The external cycle would be shortened by a uniform rate of eastward motion and lengthened by similar westward motion. An experiment that we performed in 1955 with fiddler crabs suggested this approach. The crabs which were carried by aircraft from Boston to San Francisco in darkness to a darkroom there, were subjected, on the day of their flight, to an approximately 27 h environmental day, and the rhythm of colour change during the day of travel had become inexplicably phase-delayed by about 20 minutes. An essential repetition and extension of this result, effected by uniform travel throughout consecutive days, investigating a circadian rhythmic period in "constant light and temperature", on a ship cruising a few hundred miles a day eastward for 4 or 5 days, and then cruising westward at the same rate for an equal period of days, would be expected to yield a readily measurable, systematic respective shortening and lengthening of the circadian cycles. A positive result would indicate unambiguously that the clock timer was directly regulated by the environment. Any residual lag between the intraorganismic and environmental cycle would reflect inertia of the biological cycle. With the indications presented earlier that living things are integrated electromagnetically into the space-time continuum, the probability seems high that a positive result would be obtained in the experiment. A positive result would also simplify the compass sense of such animals as birds where there are two mechanisms, geomagnetism and clock-sun-compass to explain the compass sense. Both would have merged into the continuum.

Weather sense

Biometeorologists are involved primarily with the roles of such obvious weather factors as air pressure and temperature, light, humidity, etc. Yet we know that even with all these factors carefully controlled the organism continues to derive information from its ambient environment that can indicate the weather-associated changes in barometric pressure and in temperature. The day and daylight lengths are also conveyed by the annual alteration in atmospheric tides and, therefore, the time of year. This information gained from the atmospheric pervasive field is all useful to the organism in enabling a more intimately knit association with the physical environment. Organisms can anticipate and prepare for the substantial changes in the natural cycles in their environment. Indeed, we have seen one potential contributing explanation for the mysterious prediction by organisms of the weather by one to three days, as has often been claimed by naturalists. Rates of barometric pressure-change at specific hours, and geomagnetism, may both be involved though the pressure information is mediated by the electromagnetic continuum.

Biofield sense

The ability of bean seeds to interact through generated fields was surprising. The sensitivity of the bean seeds when placed in water to fields of other nearby absorbing seeds and their mutual responsivenesses is extraordinary, and may exemplify one kind of organizer within populations. One can speculate that this phenomenon is widespread and constitutes an essential element in the maintenance of uniformity in populations. Homeostasis would appear to involve, therefore, not only the individual but also interacting groups of living things with some adopting one phase, and others the opposite phase in their fluctuations in response to their pervasive environment. Indeed, members of closely paired groups can deviate very substantially from one another in constant conditions while maintaining a far more constant mean for the pair.

Modulation of conventional sensory activities

A prominent manner in which the foregoing unusual electromagnetic sensory capacity operates is in the modulation of the activities of the well-known sense organs and the behaviour in which they participate. What may appear, for example, to be a simple response to a specific experimental pattern of illumination can systematically change as one alters the experimental set-up to different geographic directions at any given time, or performs the experiment at a different time of day, month, or year. This is probably one important though unacknowledged reason why contemporary controls have long been an element in the experimental biological sciences. But as our knowledge of the unusual senses clearly indicates, an adequate control should not be performed at another time nor in a different place or orientation. As biologists insist on ever greater precision and longer-term experiments the importance of the steadily operating roles of the unusual senses will become more and more apparent.

General conclusions and summary

A substantial amount of work, especially over the past quarter of a century, by scientists seeking additional sensory capacities to enable plausible, scientific explanations of such phenomena as the map sense and the biological clock system has disclosed what was intuitively believed, namely that living creatures are not limited to the conventional senses, even when the hearing and visual spectra are extended as has recently been done. A specific electric sense has become firmly established for many fishes and a special magnetic-compass sense for a variety of such animals as insects, fishes, and birds. Concurrently it has been demonstrated that electric and magnetic senses are widespread, or possibly universal, but evidence is also appearing that suggests that the whole electromagnetic spectrum from the high-quantum-energy, gamma radiation to the extremely low-quantum-energy, essentially static electric and magnetic fields, can elicit measurable responses from living things. Normal responses to the non-optical electromagnetic spectrum obviously involve very weak fields of the strengths of the atmospheric ones and their fluctuations. This renders it quite improbable that the effect is any more thermal in nature than for the visual wavelengths.

As a consequence of sensing the atmospheric complex of electromagnetic fields the organism has potentially available an enormous amount of information. The field strength and direction fluctuates with position in space, with time in the geophysical cycles, with weather, and is modulated by the biofields of other organisms. Since organisms have undergone their whole evolution within the earth's atmosphere one can rationally postulate that they have succeeded in differentiating specific aspects that most reliably provide information of adaptive use to themselves. Optimal adaptation to their terrestrial environment would include recognition of their home niche and territory, sites of foods, and routes of migration through cues that would form a continuum with the remainder of their planetary field. We still do not know the specific parameters or complexes, but known transient disruptions by experimental electromagnetic fields suggest that they lie within the domain of such fields. Fluctuations of the same fields comprising geophysical cycles suggest that the same, or closely related parameters, contribute the clocks of life. The behaviour of life on this planet employs a spatiotemporal integration of sophisticated degree, and electromagnetism appears to be an essential element in the system. Possibly gravitational fields will eventually be proven to play roles as suggested recently by Schneider (1975) in Switzerland.

Another feature of the physical environment is its great variability due to the passage of weather systems. Since organisms hermetically separated, in unvarying conditions, from all obvious weather factors are nevertheless apprised of the ongoing outdoor temperatures, pressures and pressure changes, they are notified of favourable conditions for making their exits from protected sites and otherwise conducting their lives. In view of the existence of lead relationships of pervasive parameters to which they are sensitive they are theoretically able to prepare for some of the conditions to come.

The sensitivity to the fields of adjacent organisms that results in a mutuality of selection of positive and negative stances in their response to environmental fluctuations, is adaptive for populations. It enables the maintenance of a "mean state" within the population while simultaneously the extraordinarily sensitive individuals will fluctuate more widely, and it provides further reason for animal co-operation.

The apparent ease with which single organisms, or small groups of them, can shift from positive correlation with the effective parameters of the atmosphere to negative, and vice versa, has probably been responsible for one of the greatest difficulties for appreciating the roles of the unusual senses in the behaviour of organisms. While the use of averages may often yield insignificant findings whether for populations of individuals at any given moment, or for single individuals during repeated experiments, the use of variances will frequently disclose that two phases exist with one displaced 180° from the other, and even sometimes 90° as well. Although some insights into causes of the phase shifts have been uncovered—seasonal changes, slow clockwise vs. counterclockwise rotation, mutuality between adjacent organisms, etc.—the changes appear to be regulated in a still more complex way. Possibly these states are a consequence of a fundamental search for a stable equilibrium.

Inversions are known in response to both scalar and vector properties of environmental fields. It must be assumed that at least some degree of functional rectification of the responses of organisms occurs to permit the statistically demonstrable map and compass senses as well as the biological clocks.

The strange properties of the receptive mechanisms for these unusual senses, their fluidly labile and dynamic characteristics, and yet their stability, basic similarities, and omnipresence without regard to structural differentiations or phylogenetic status, suggest them to be rooted in the foundations of life itself. The senses seem to depend upon the dynamic steady state that differentiates living from nonliving. Such a poised, unstable equilibrium has been recently termed a bioplasma by Sedlak (1979) in Poland, who believes that biologists should extend the older concepts of classical corpuscular physics, which stresses chemistry and molecular biology, to include the newer concepts of wave physics. He believes that living things should be treated as integrated bioelectronic entities possessing metabolically energized semiconductors such as proteins, with piezo-, ferro-, and pyroelectric components and hypothetical biolasers, with magnetohydrodynamic interactions. The organism could be conceived as a microminiaturization of complex and dynamic electronic circuitry, a living, reproducing receiver-computer-responder thriving upon ambient electromagnetics. Such a revolution in our concept of the nature of life, alien as might seem to most modern biochemists, seems ultimately to be inevitable if biology is to incorporate the advances in modern physics in its attempts to account for such mysteries as consciousness, information transfer and storage, steady state, and unusual senses.

In brief, informational inflow through unusual senses can trigger relatively substantial effects upon the individual despite extremely low energies of the stimuli. The living system seems always sensitively poised to receive the messages. The physiologist and behaviourist have been able to progress despite ignoring these activities chiefly as a consequence of the statistical reduction of their mean effects and the dominance of conventional stimuli. But now no longer ignorable are the omnipresent geophysically correlated biological rhythms, and there should soon follow the biological alterations associated with time, place, and orientation, the subtle weather-induced alterations, and the effects of subtle organismic interactions.

SELECTED BIBLIOGRAPHY

Barnwell, F. H. and Brown, F. A. Jr. (1964) "Responses of planarians and snails" in *Biological Effects of Magnetic Fields* (ed. Barnothy, M.) Plenum Press, New York, 263–278.

Becker, G. (1977) Communication between termites by biofields *Cybernetics*, **26**, 41–44.

Brown, F. A. Jr. (1959) Living clocks *Science*, **130**, 1535–1544.

Brown, F. A. Jr. (1960) Response to pervasive geophysical fields and the biological clock problem *Symp. Quant. Biol., Cold Spring Harbor*, **25**, 57–71.

Brown, F. A. Jr. (1962) Extrinsic rhythmicality: a reference frame for biological rhythms under so-called constant conditions *Ann. N.Y. Acad. Sci.*, **98**, 775–787.

Brown, F. A. Jr. (1969) A hypothesis for extrinsic timing of circadian rhythms *Canad. J. Bot.*, **47**, 287–298.

Brown, F. A. Jr. (1971) Some orientational influences of non-visual, terrestrial electromagnetic fields *Ann. N.Y. Acad. Sci.*, **188**, 224–241.

Brown, F. A. Jr. (1972) The clocks timing biological rhythms *Amer. Sci.*, **60**, 756–766.

Brown, F. A. Jr. (1976) "Evidence for external timing of the biological clocks" in *An Introduction to Biological Rhythms* by J. D. Palmer, Acad. Press, New York, chap. 7.

Brown, F. A. Jr. (1979) Dynamic biomagnetism associates bean seeds *Experientia*, **35**, 468–470.

Brown, F. A. Jr. and Chow, C. S. (1975) Non-equivalence for beans of clockwise and counterclockwise magnetic motion: A novel terrestrial adaptation? *Biol. Bull.*, **148**, 370–379.

Brown, F. A. Jr. and Scow, K. M. (1978) Magnetic induction of a circadian cycle in hamsters *J. Interdisc. Cycle Res.*, **9**, 137–145.

Bryant, T. R. (1972) Gas exchange in dry seeds: circadian rhythmicity in absence of DNA replication, transcription and translation *Science*, **178**, 634–636.

Dubrov, A. P. (1978) *The Geomagnetic Field and Life. Geomagnetobiology* Plenum Press, New York.

Kreithen, M. L. (1978) "Sensory mechanisms for animal orientation—Can any new ones be discovered?" in *Animal Migration, Navigation, and Homing* (eds. Schmidt-Konig, K., Keeton, W. T.) Springer Verlag, Berlin-Heidelberg.

Jones, R. L. (1960) Response of growing plants to a uniform daily rotation *Nature*, **185**, 775.

Ossenkopp, K.-P. and Barbeito, R. (1978) Bird orientation and the geomagnetic field. A review *Neuroscience and Biobehavioral Rev.*, **2**, 255–270.

Presman, A. S. (1970) *Electromagnetic Fields and Life* Plenum Press, New York.

Rothen, A. (1974) Circadian activity of a nickel-coated glass slide used for carrying out immunologic reactions at a liquid-solid interface *Biophys. J.*, **14**, 987–988.

Schneider, F. (1975) Gibt es sinnesphysiologisch wirksam Gravitationswellen?—Ein Problem der ultraoptischen Orientierung *Vierteljahr. Naturforsch. Gesell. Zurich*, **120**, 33–79.

Sedlak, W. (1979) *Bioelektronika, 1967–1977* Instytut Wydawniczy Pax, Warsaw.

Webb, H. M. and Brown, F. A. Jr. (1959) Timing long-cycle physiological rhythms *Physiol. Rev.*, **39**, 127–161.

CHAPTER TWENTY-ONE

CODING AND INTEGRATION IN RECEPTORS AND CENTRAL AFFERENT SYSTEMS

Principles Illustrated by Electroreception and Other Modalities in Lower Vertebrates

THEODORE HOLMES BULLOCK

Introduction: encoding and integration in receptors

Instead of another review of all the details so far brought to light about electroreception, I have cast this contribution in the form of a review of some general principles of coding and integration in sensory systems, especially those that can be induced from our knowledge of electroreceptive and related octavolateral systems in fishes. Although the centre of gravity of this book is on the peripheral aspects, this chapter includes some principles pertaining to central afferent processing out of a conviction that we need to know the central destinations and the kind of information each is specialized for, in order to understand the sense organs properly.

The purpose of this section is to construct a framework of operating principles of peripheral sensory integration, that is to say, the encoding and integrative principles by which receptors signal stimuli to the central nervous system. The reason for choosing examples from octavolateral, especially electroreceptors, is that these receptors not only give a fresh view of what is essentially a restatement of elementary sensory physiology, but in many cases they offer the clearest evidence for a principle likely to be quite general.

The basic code for "what" and "where"

Considering single afferent axons, the basic code for "what and where" is the principle of labelled lines. This is a more modern name for the principle enunciated by Johannes Mueller and commonly called the Law of Specific Nerve Energies. It says that the central nervous system acts as though each axon had a label; i.e. that the c.n.s. "knows" or "assumes" that any signals arriving over a given afferent axon represent stimuli within a certain receptive field which is defined in terms of form of stimulus (modality, "what") and locus of stimulus on the sensory surface ("where"). The receptive fields are specified by probability statements, with respect both to modality and to locus. That is, the label is on the line and the c.n.s. assumption is that a signal in this line most probably represents the occurrence of a stimulus in a certain modality or submodality or, with somewhat less probability, an incident in another modality or submodality; likewise for topographic specification of the most probable and the less probable sites of occurrence of the stimulus on the sensory surface. Thus, there is a built-in ambiguity with respect to the forms of stimuli and the sites of stimuli, within these receptive fields. How wide or how narrow are the receptive fields is a primary variable among afferent axons; there is an important diversity among the axons coming from one sense organ or type of receptor.

A. Labels may be discrete

This assertion is the same as that of the Law of Specific Nerve Energies and represents the familiar situation that there can be unambiguous labels, for example comparing those of the optic nerve and the auditory nerve. In contrast, the wide variety of skin and body wall receptors is more debatable; some authors believe that somatosensory receptors are typically quite multimodal and ambiguous (see Iggo, this volume). Among the octavolateralis receptors of lower vertebrates are excellent examples of various degrees of ambiguity including some whose labels are quite discrete. These provide good precedent for the considerable variety of somatosensory receptors in higher vertebrates, often with rather sharply defined modality specificity. For example, the electroreceptors and the mechanoreceptors in gymnotiform electric fish probably have almost non-overlapping modality specificity. I would also cite the two classes of electroreceptors particularly in the so-called high frequency wave species (e.g. *Eigenmannia* and *Apteronotus*) whose constant electric organ discharge (hereafter EOD) has an accurately maintained rate of about 300 Hz in the former genus and 1000 Hz in the latter, differing among individuals within the species. The receptor classes are called *ampullary* and *tuberous* and have virtually non-overlapping ranges of frequency of alternating current sensitivity (Bullock, 1974). Ampullary units are most sensitive in the range of about 1–20 Hz (Peters and Buwalda, 1972; Akoev *et al.*, 1976*a*, *b*; Andrianov *et al.*, 1974), tuberous units in the ranges of about 300 to 1000 Hz, in the two genera named, matched in each individual fish to the resting EOD frequency of that individual. In other genera, particularly among the so-called pulse species of gymnotiform and mormyriform fishes, i.e. those whose EOD is a small fraction of the—usually irregular—interval between EOD's, tuberous units have best frequencies matched to the maximum of the power spectrum of the pulses, hence specific to the species and even the part of the body (Bastian, 1976*b*, 1977; Hopkins, pers. comm.).

B. Labels may partially overlap

Many receptors, or the afferent nerve fibres from them, exhibit a more or less extensive overlap either in the forms of stimuli which can excite them or in the topography of their receptive fields. This means a degree of ambiguity and a degree of redundancy. This is probably the principal form of redundancy in the nervous system. It is important to realize that the redundancy is incomplete and that therefore there is partial uniqueness for each unit. Examples of topographic overlap are (i) contiguous ampullary receptors and (ii) contiguous tuberous receptors that encode "where" information. Examples with respect to submodality or form of stimulus include "T" and "P" types of tuberous receptors in wave species. These are interesting because the adequate stimuli are the same or very nearly so. Some authors say that the T units are typically more sensitive (Scheich and Bullock, 1974; Hopkins, 1976) whereas Viancour (1977) states that only under certain conditions is there a bimodality of sensitivity. But to the natural stimulus the two types respond in different ways on a half dozen response criteria, with very little overlap according to the earlier authors, but according to the last named author nearly complete overlap (see also Feng and Bullock, 1977). In other gymnotiform species having a pulse-like EOD instead of the wave-like EOD, the conspicuous subclasses of tuberous electroreceptors are the "M" type (Type I of Szabo, see Heiligenberg, 1977) and the "B" type (Type II of Szabo). In some stimulus ranges and species these are virtually non-overlapping subclasses whereas in other species and ranges of stimuli they may significantly overlap. A different type of example is represented by the mechanoreceptors of the lateral line in elasmobranchs and those of the macula neglecta in the ear of carcharhinid sharks. The neuromasts of the former primarily respond to near-field turbulence and mass movement of water, perhaps in the frequency range up to some tens or 100 Hz; the hair cells of the macula neglecta are believed (Corwin, 1977*a*, *b*, 1978; Bullock and Corwin, 1977, 1979) to respond to very low amplitude displacement (velocity) waves from the far-field acoustic sources, with best frequencies of several hundred Hz.

Basic codes for "how much"

Considering single axons that signal to the central nervous system by nerve impulses, the main claim I want to make is that stimulus intensity is encoded not by one but by *several* different codes. This is an important conclusion, at variance with the usual textbook account that assumes "the" nerve impulse code is mean frequency of nerve impulses.

A. Frequency codes

It should be realized that frequency is the parameter for a class of codes and not the self-evident designation for a single code. There can be considerable difference depending on the epochs of time over which the frequency is averaged and upon the method of weighting. For instance it seems likely that commonly a moving average weights the most recent intervals most heavily; the decline of influence of a given spike with time defines an integrative time constant. Many examples could be cited from more familiar cases including more tonic and more phasic receptors. However, I choose two examples from the tuberous electroreceptors because they illustrate a special feature in which some frequency coders are different from others.

(i) The P units (probability coders) change in probability of following an AC current depending on its intensity, so that there is considerable structure in the impulse train. Intervals tend to be multiples of the minimum interval which is that of the stimulus and there is some, weak, autocorrelation, such that each interval is influenced by the preceding interval to a degree dependent upon the mean interval; hence the stimulus intensity.

(ii) B units (burst duration coders) code intensity by the addition or subtraction of spikes at the end of a burst that follows each stimulus pulse. The intervals are fixed and the latency is nearly fixed. The epoch of averaging the frequency, if it is relevant at all, must be shorter than the EOD interval since that interval is commanded by the brain. Rather than a continuous sliding average, the burst would be best read by a central device triggered at the beginning of each burst.

It seems clear that some impulse trains are treated as frequency-coded mainly because we can read them in terms of impulses per unit of time. The central analyser neurones may however read the train differently and measure a parameter not properly called frequency. Our classification of the code must be considered tentative until we know how the normal decoding is done.

B. Nonfrequency codes

Codes that do not involve change in frequency are of several kinds and have been summarized by Perkel and Bullock (1968). Illustrations are: (i) those that encode information by change in the interval variance (at the same mean frequency), for example by reducing the standard deviation of a quasi-random distribution of intervals; (ii) the closely related temporal microstructure code in which some fine grained temporal pattern may develop and convey information without changing the mean frequency (the simplest of these is the alternately short and long interval train that can develop from a train of uniform intervals) and (iii) a class of non-interval codes, well illustrated by the T units among tuberous electroreceptors, which can be called phase coders. The normal physiological stimulus (*Eigenmannia*) is a sine wave with some harmonics and the T units follow every cycle of the stimulus with an impulse, one for one. According to the intensity of the stimulus this impulse fires at an earlier or later phase in the cycle. This kind of code requires, of course, that some time reference be available to the central analyser that decodes the information. In that sense this is a multichannel code and these will be dealt with primarily in the section below on central afferent systems. It should be noted here also that some of the codes mentioned previously under Frequency Codes will in fact be more properly designated non-frequency codes when we understand the parameter that is influential to the decoder. Burst duration coders and even the probability coders may be read by the central analyser in a way which is not best described in terms of mean frequency. The important conclusion of this section is that there is not *a* nerve impulse code but at least several. Most of these are presumptive or candidate codes until it has been demonstrated that both the method of encoding and of decoding used under natural conditions conform to the presumed parameter used.

It should not be thought that the large volume of literature and the many sensory receptors whose physiology has been studied carefully have given us an adequate understanding even of the main coding types. Before we can even claim to have the broad picture in perspective it will be necessary to discover in a significant variety of receptors both the encoding parameters and the decoding parameters of the second order neurones (see Perkel and Bullock, 1968), if not the mechanistic explanation of these properties. I expect, more as a statement of faith than of insight, that rules will emerge about when and where nature uses different types of codes. Different codes may be in use simultaneously even in the single afferent axon signalling different kinds of information to different second order neurones.

Input-output functions

The main conclusion here is that input-output functions are of various types, both in the slope of the function and other parameters. Linear functions, log functions and power functions are found in different cases in particular ranges; none is general. Much remains to be learned about the incidence, correlates and biological meaning of different kinds of input-output functions.

A. Receptors are typically bandpass filters

With respect to the frequency domain of the stimulus, many receptors are most responsive in a certain range of frequency and fall in sensitivity on each side of this range, thus conforming to a broad definition of a bandpass filter. Examples from electroreceptors are (i) many ampullary units whose best frequency lies between 1–20 Hz, and (ii) tuberous units with best frequencies between 100–1000 Hz according to the species and to the individual. It has been found in the high frequency wave species, where the EOD is very steady and has a preferred resting value, characteristic of the individual, that the receptors have their best frequencies very close to their EOD frequency. The question remains open in these cases whether the match between the best frequency of the receptors and the normal stimulus frequency due to the pacemaker in the brain that drives the electric organ, is the result of plasticity of the one or the other. It is quite significant, in the light of the homologies of the octavolateralis system, that the electroreceptors—which are without any mechanical stage in stimulation—are extremely similar in sharpness of tuning to mammalian cochlear nerve fibres of the same best frequency. This would seem to support the idea of the so-called second filter—the non-mechanical, postbasilar membrane contribution to the tuning characteristic of cochlear nerve fibres (see Russell, this volume).

B. Sensitivity is not a unitary property measured by a single number

It is commonly asserted that for many sensory systems the absolute threshold approaches a theoretical limit based on the nature of the stimulus energy. Thus the quantum flux of light or the increment of acoustic energy above the thermal noise level are often considered to justify comparison with the physiological or behavioural thresholds of the sensory system. It is important however to realize that in view of the possibility of spatial summation there is not a necessary relationship between the threshold of the single receptor unit and that of the whole system. Although a photoreceptor cannot be stimulated with less than one quantum of light, the system may respond to a flux of light with far less than one quantum per receptor during the response time. This will depend upon circuit properties, on the statistical structure of the noise or spontaneous fluctuation of the elements, on the integration time, and on the sophistication of the analyser. For many mechanoreceptors the stimulus acting on a population of receptors has a property of congruence that helps to distinguish it from that part of the noise which is independent in each receptor. That is, the common vectorial influence can permit summation and the detection of signals whose individual effect upon the receptors is far less than the background noise in each unit. An example is represented by the hypothesized mode of action of the acoustic receptors in carcharhinid sharks, according to Corwin (1977*a*). Here the macula neglecta, with more than 300 000 hair cells, has 50 times more hair cells per nerve fibre than does the human cochlea, and may thereby be able to detect extremely small congruent motions of the displacement (velocity) wave from sound sources hundreds of metres away. The excursion of the water particles has been estimated to be 0.02 Ångstrom units (Myrberg *et al.*, 1969), which is about 20 times the estimate for the excursion of the basilar membrane of the human cochlea at threshold.

Increment sensitivity may be the more relevant measure in many cases than the absolute sensitivity, given by the threshold of first detection of stimulus above a nonstimulus background. Tuberous electroreceptors are good examples, since they normally receive a continual stimulus from the EOD of the same individual at an intensity far higher than the biologically significant *changes* in the electric field caused by objects in the environment that distort the field. Ampullary receptors in nonelectric fish have an ongoing background discharge in the absence of special stimuli and this spontaneous activity may achieve the equivalent of putting the receptor into the steep part of the input-output function.

Inevitably each of these considerations of the performance characteristics of peripheral receptors has led us into considerations of the performance of central analysers. One further example is the proposition that signal detection in the presence of noise or spontaneous firing may depend on prior "knowledge" of the structure of expected signals from normally encountered biological stimuli that the receptors and central analysers have evolved to detect. This idea has been embodied in applications to biological systems of optimal filter theory. Electroreceptors of both wave and pulse species of electric fish are good examples (Heiligenberg and Altes, 1978) and the same seems likely in other somatosensory modalities such as the infrared receptor system in rattlesnakes (Bullock, 1957).

Receptor mechanisms underlying these properties

The quantitative features of the receptor mechanism that account for the coding and input-output properties remain for the most part to be worked out. Among the specially relevant features surely will be the transfer functions between the graded receptor potentials and the postsynaptic potentials in the afferent axon terminals, including some that are not often examined. Among the latter I mention in particular the properties of any tendency to spontaneous subthreshold oscillation. "Spontaneous" here is used not in the sense of independence from environmental states and conditions but of the purely intrinsic timing of events in the receptor cell. The tendency to oscillate may be seen after single brief stimuli in some octavolateralis receptors, either in the subthreshold potentials themselves or in a succession of phases of the recovery cycle following an impulse or even a subthreshold stimulus. In tuberous electroreceptors there is such a succession of supernormal and subnormal phases and the period is matched to the electric organ discharge period of the individual fish (Viancour, 1977, 1979*a*, *b*). This example of a property of the receptor mechanism is potentially very influential in determining input-output properties. Aspects of oscillation such as the damping factor, the regularity or irregularity, and the electrotonic or other communication between sites of oscillation will all be influential in respect to the coding, the sensitivity as a function of frequency, the role of noise and the like.

One more lesson from electroreceptors may have wide applicability. It is clear at least in the wave species, with their steadily maintained quasi-sinusoidal EOD that the encoding leading to afferent fibre spikes occurs in the *time* domain and is not properly described in the frequency domain. There is a more critical part of the cycle, and other parts do not have anything like the same influence (Scheich, 1977*a*, *b*, *c*; Viancour, 1977, 1979*a*, *b*). We suspect that the cochlear processes leading to auditory input to the brain may likewise be insightfully described in the time domain.

Decoding and integration in central afferent systems

The purpose of this section is to illustrate some forms of series and parallel processing in the central nervous system leading to recognition of expected stimuli and control of behavioural commands. The properties of the sense organs only make sense in the context of the brain's interests, which are commonly multiple.

Aspects of stimuli separately analysed in afferent systems

Electroreception illustrates well the principle, which may be quite general, that central analysis proceeds in parallel in separate subsystems simultaneously extracting different aspects of the total stimulus configuration. Sequential, hierarchical, series processing is superimposed, more in some subsystems than in others. We are still in an early stage in unravelling the processing that occurs in different central structures and the interdependency, anatomical connections and physiological interactions between them. Nevertheless the following distinct forms of extraction of aspects of stimuli can already be documented to a greater or lesser degree.

A. Motion and its direction

In addition to the signature of motion and its direction contained in the time course of afferent axon activity due to the asymmetry of receptive field configuration, second or higher order units in the electroreceptive portion of the lateral lobe and in specific parts of the cerebellum are particularly sensitive to these features. They presumably receive converging input from a number of afferent axons and respond according to the sequence of activation arriving in these (Enger and Szabo, 1965; Szabo, 1974; Bastian, 1974, 1975, 1976*a*, *b*).

B. Edges and contours

Already in the lateral lobe some units are particularly sensitive to the leading edge of moving objects and respond in the same way to metallic and plastic objects—which have opposite effect on the receptors and first order afferent neurones (Enger and Szabo, 1965). Much remains to be done to understand properly the analysis of objects and to explain the available quantitative information on behavioural object detection (Heiligenberg, 1977). Bastian (1974, 1975, 1976*a*) and Behrend (1977) have provided considerable detail about the responses of cerebellar units in gymnotiform wave species to moving objects. Concentric receptive fields are typical, with an excitatory centre and an inhibitory surround. Converging input from other modalities is common, especially proprioceptive and visual.

C. Topographic position and orientation

Using a small electric dipole as the stimulus we can move it around a catfish (*Ictalurus*, Siluriformes) while recording in the electrosense areas of the brain. The position along the body and the orientation of the dipole are analysed and displayed in the mesencephalic torus semicircularis (homologue of the inferior colliculus). A systematic mapping has been discovered by Knudsen (1978). It should be emphasized that this is not simply a map of a sensory surface as in the more familiar cases of the visual, acoustic and somatosensory systems but instead must be a computed map of the near-field external space, based on the convergence of many units with extensively overlapping receptive fields. These foreshadow the central maps of acoustic space recently demonstrated by Knudsen and Konishi (1978) in the mesencephalon of birds, similarly based on computation from converging units representing both sides of the body. Units have been found, in the cerebellum, by Bastian, that have also preferred distance—not responding best to the closest stimulus source.

D. Stimulus frequency

Evoked potentials in the brain of elasmobranchs can exhibit a higher best frequency than would be expected from ampullary unit properties or from behaviour (Kalmijn, 1974; Bullock, 1977, 1979).

Best frequency appears to be crudely mapped in the torus semicircularis of siluroid catfish according to Knudsen (1976). These are ampullary units and cover about two octaves in the low frequency range (*c*. 5–20 Hz). Not enough is known with respect to the tuberous receptors but since they typically represent a much more limited range of best frequencies there may not be such mapping of high frequencies.

E. Difference frequency between the fish and its neighbour

In gymnotiform and gymnarchid wave species with highly regular quasi-sinusoidal discharge the difference frequency or beat frequency between a given fish and its neighbours is a very important quantity. In the range > 0, < 10 it determines the "jamming avoidance response", a form of easily quantified and consistently reproducible behaviour (e.g. non-habituating) that lends itself to analysis. The result is that a great deal is known about the crucial parameters for behaviour and the neuronal basis. In a specific lamina of the torus semicircularis of *Eigenmannia*, Scheich found neurones of at least the fourth order which are specifically sensitive to the difference frequency, called ΔF, and which, in agreement with the behavioural sensitivity, reach their maximum response at 3 or 4 Hz, being less sensitive on either side of this value. This type of unit moreover was the first in the sequence from primary afferent units to those of the lobus lateralis and earlier torus semicircularis units to give a response unequivocally indicative of the sign of the ΔF, that is whether the neighbouring fish is higher or lower in its EOD frequency than is the fish under study. Under Scheich's conditions, these "ΔF decoder units" are believed to play a role in the control of the jamming avoidance response by accelerating or inhibiting the pacemaker unit in the medulla that commands the electric organ discharge (Scheich, 1977*a*, *b*, *c*). Under these conditions of stimulation the fish is compelled to use clues in the asymmetry of the beat envelope, due to phase specific harmonics in the quasi-natural EOD mimic, and it successfully solves the problem of recognizing plus from minus ΔF. Under other conditions (Heiligenberg *et al*., 1978; Heiligenberg and Bastian, 1980; Heiligenberg, 1980) it is compelled to use other clues in the unequal distribution over its body of the simulated neighbouring fish's EOD field—and it successfully solves the problem. This second method may be the more important naturally, when both kinds of clues are normally available. It depends on the convergence of two receptor classes, those encoding the amplitude changes during a beat cycle (P units) and those accurately signalling the fractional millisecond shifts in phase (equivalent to EOD zero-crossing time; *c*. 300 times per sec. in one direction) during each beat cycle. Direction of change sensitive central neurones compare different patches of skin to give the significance "my own EOD" to one of the rhythms (without having to make any such decision), and the significance $+\Delta F$ when amplitude is increasing while phase is advancing. Most of the necessary neurones have been found. An important part of the processing has not been directly observed as yet although it is inferred from the consequence, namely, smoothing. The EOD shows no sign of the beat or amplitude modulation that strongly affects the primary afferent input. Also there is no sign of the jitter of intervals which would be expected from observation of the P-type of afferent unit and corresponding second and third order central units; these are poorly phase-locked with respect to the EOD cycle. Presumably many units converge on the pacemaker, firing at different phases, both of the EOD cycle and of the beat cycle. It is worthy of note that we are in the presence of a time domain analysis of small differences in wave form of the stimulus, rather than of a frequency domain or a Fourier analysis.

F. Social signals

Electric fish belonging to the numerous genera of gymnotiforms and mormyriforms, including gymnarchids, are known to have an important repertoire of social signals. For example, EOD signs have been shown to signify aggression, submission, reproductive state, and generalized excitement. These are frequency modulations of the ongoing electric discharge rate. Their central analysis has not been much studied; however the tuberous electroreceptors have been found to project to certain parts of the telencephalon. It seems quite likely that the centres of specific analysis of socially significant frequency modulation will be found in this structure if not earlier.

Integration of converging modalities

Some analysis and control of behaviour requires that the interpretation of electroreceptive input be contingent on the simultaneous evaluation of input from other receptors, including tail position, visual and vestibular receptors.

A. Posture

Electric fish maintain posture relative to the angle of an electrically opaque substratum hidden by an electrically transparent false bottom. They tend to hold the transverse and the long axis parallel to the plane of the dielectric. We can infer that a computation of this plane is made from converging electroreceptors and that this is integrated with relevant input from vestibular and visual systems to govern the commands to the fins that maintain steady tilt. There is some evidence that the vestibular gravity reflex and the feeble dorsal light reflex are integrated in the mesencephalon but that the electroreceptive ventral substrate response requires the telencephalon (Meyer *et al.*, 1976, 1977; Feng, 1977).

B. Objects

Interpretation of the electric field distortion due to objects, obstacles, cavities, and other fish involves relative motion, and the evaluation of the position of the body, especially of the bending of the tail. In some species, such as *Apteronotus*, that spend a great deal of time in tilted and bizarre postures, the position of the body relative to gravity must also be important. There is some evidence (Bastian, 1975) that cerebellar units specialized for the detection of moving objects via electroreceptive input may also be influenced by proprioceptive input from bending the tail and by visual input, with a definite receptive field congruent with the tuberous receptive field. This will be favourable material for analysis of inter-modality integrations.

C. Control of EOD command

The electric organ discharge is commanded from a pacemaker centre in the medulla. This is physiologically a single unit, consisting of a number of nerve cells connected electrotonically. These project to relay cells and these in turn to the electromotor neurones in the spinal cord. While the command centre is a true pacemaker in manifesting an intrinsic rhythm with pacemaker potentials between output spikes, it is subject to accelerating and inhibiting inputs that differ according to the species. In some, like *Gymnotus*, visual, mechanical, chemical, as well as electric receptor input can alter the EOD rate. Each of these influences makes some biological sense, in the light of the ethology of the species. In some others, such as *Apteronotus*, there is extremely little influence from mechanoreceptors, chemoreceptors, visual and even electroreceptors except to specific social and jamming signals. The large nucleus of electrically coupled cells forming the physiological pacemaker unit is also an integrator in the sense that it smooths out irregularities in its input. Inputs from other parts of the brain, including the effective sensory modalities, need not be distributed uniformly through the cells of the nucleus since the electrotonic connections among them provide an integration that probably assures, in the usual case, that all descending output shares the same degree of influence from a given input. Besides integrating input in these senses, the pacemaker-command nucleus can be regarded as a simple pattern generator. Social signals can be brief, large accelerations of EOD rate ("chirps"), slower transient increases in rate, transient silence or large changes in interval variance (e.g. from regular to irregular).

Summary

Recent work on octavolateralis receptors, especially electroreceptors in electric and in other fishes, is used to illustrate a set of general principles widely applicable to sensory systems. Encoding in receptors and some of the associated forms of integration are set forth. Codes for "what" and "where", lines with discrete labels and lines with partially overlapping, partially ambiguous labels, codes for intensity including frequency- and nonfrequency codes, input-output functions such as bandpass filtering and the spatial summation of parallel channels are exemplified. Receptor oscillation as an active, tuned "ringing" is believed to play an important role. Decoding and integration in central afferent centres are surveyed to illustrate some forms of processing leading toward recognition of expected stimuli. Several aspects of stimuli are separately analysed in afferent centres, including motion and its direction, edges and contours, position, orientation, frequency, difference frequency (of steady frequency electric fish), and social sign stimuli. Converging modalities contribute to the recognition of the plane of the substratum, objects, obstacles and passages and to the control of the electric organ discharge.

Acknowledgements

Original research described herein was aided by grants from the National Science Foundation and National Institutes of Health.

REFERENCES

Akoev, G. N., Ilyinsky, O. B. and Zadan, P. M. (1976*a*) Physiological properties of electroreceptors of marine skates *Comp. Biochem. Physiol.*, **53A**, 201–209.

Akoev, G. N., Ilyinsky, O. B. and Zadan, P. M. (1976*b*) Responses of electroreceptors (ampullae of Lorenzini) of skates to electric and magnetic fields *J. comp. Physiol.*, **106**, 127–136.

Andrianov, G. N., Brown, H. R. and Ilyinsky, O. B. (1974) Responses of central neurons to electrical and magnetic stimuli of the ampullae of Lorenzini in the Black Sea skate *J. comp. Physiol.*, **93**, 287–299.

Bastian, J. (1974) Electrosensory input to the corpus cerebelli of the high frequency electric fish *Eigenmannia virescens J. comp. Physiol.*, **90**, 1–24.

Bastian, J. (1975) Receptive fields of cerebellar cells receiving exteroceptive input in a gymnotid fish *J. Neurophysiol.*, **38**, 285–300.

Bastian, J. (1976*a*) The range of electrolocation: A comparison of electroreceptor responses and the responses of cerebellar neurons *J. comp. Physiol.*, **108**, 193–210.

Bastian, J. (1976*b*) Frequency response characteristics of electroreceptors in weakly electric fish (Gymnotoidei) with a pulse discharge *J. comp. Physiol.*, **112**, 165–180.

Bastian, J. (1977) Variations in the frequency response of electroreceptors dependent on receptor location in weakly electric fish (Gymnotoidei) with a pulse discharge *J. comp. Physiol.*, **121**, 53–64.

Behrend, K. (1977) Processing information carried in a high frequency wave: Properties of cerebellar units in the high frequency electric fish *J. comp. Physiol.*, **118**, 357–371.

Bullock, T. H. (1957) "Neuronal integrative mechanisms" in *Recent Advances in Invertebrate Physiology* (ed. Scheer, B. T.) University of Oregon Press, Eugene, 1–20.

Bullock, T. H. (1974) "Specialized receptors in lower vertebrates. Introduction. An essay on the discovery of sensory receptors and the assignment of their functions together with an introduction to electroreceptors" in *Handbook of Sensory Physiology, Vol. III/3: Electroreceptors and Other Specialized Receptors in Lower Vertebrates* (ed. Fessard, A.) Springer-Verlag, New York, 1–12.

Bullock, T. H. (1977) Evoked potentials in the brain in elasmobranchs and siluroids to physiological stimulation of electroreceptors *Neuroscience Abstracts*, **3**(1166), 363.

Bullock, T. H. (1979) Processing of ampullary input in the brain: Comparison of sensitivity and evoked responses among elasmobranch and siluriform fishes *J. Physiol.*, **75**, 397–407.

Bullock, T. H. and Corwin, J. T. (1977) Central auditory physiology of sharks *Proc. XXVII Congress Internat. Union Physiol. Sciences, Paris*, 13: 107 (Abs.).

Bullock, T. H. and Corwin, J. T. (1979) Acoustic evoked activity in the brain in sharks *J. comp. Physiol.*, **129**, 223–234.

Corwin, J. T. (1977*a*) Morphology of the macula neglecta in sharks of the genus *Carcharhinus*. *J. Morph.*, **152**, 341–361.

Corwin, J. T. (1977*b*) Ongoing hair cell production, maturation, and degeneration in the shark ear *Neuroscience Abstracts*, **3**(8), 4.

Corwin, J. T. (1978) The relation of inner ear structure to feeding behavior in sharks and rays *Scanning Electron Microscopy/1978*, **2**, 1105–1112.

Enger, P. S. and Szabo, T. (1965) Activity of central neurons involved in electroreception in some weakly electric fish (Gymnotidae) *J. Neurophysiol.*, **28**, 800–818.

Feng, A. S. (1977) The role of the electrosensory system in postural control in the weakly electric fish *Eigenmannia virescens J. Neurobiol.*, **8**, 429–437.

Feng, A. S. and Bullock, T. H. (1977) Neuronal mechanisms for object discrimination in the weakly electric fish *Eigenmannia virescens J. exp. Biol.*, **66**, 141–158.

Heiligenberg, W. (1977) "Principles of electrolocation and jamming avoidance in electric fish. A neuroethological approach" in *Studies of Brain Function*, Vol. **I** (eds. Braitenberg, V., Barlow, H. B., Florey, E., Grüsser, O.-J., Van der Loos, H.) Springer Verlag, New York, 1–84.

Heiligenberg, W. (1980) The jamming avoidance response in the weakly electric fish *Eigenmannia.* A behavior controlled by distributed evaluation of electroreceptive afferences. (submitted).

Heiligenberg, W. and Altes, R. (1978) Phase-sensitivity in electroreception *Science*, **199**, 1001–1004.

Heiligenberg, W. and Bastian, J. (1980) The control of *Eigenmannia*'s pacemaker by distributed evaluation of electroreceptive afferences *J. comp. Physiol.*, **136**, 113–133.

Heiligenberg, W., Baker, C. and Matsubara, J. (1978) The jamming avoidance response in *Eigenmannia* revisited: The structure of a neuronal democracy *J. comp. Physiol.*, **127**, 267–286.

Hopkins, C. D. (1976) Stimulus filtering and electroreception: tuberous electroreceptors in three species of gymnotid fish *J. comp. Physiol.*, **111**, 171–207.

Kalmijn, A. J. (1974) "The detection of electric fields from inanimate and animate sources other than electric fields" in *Handbook of Sensory Physiology, Vol. III/3: Electroreceptors and Other Specialized Receptors in Lower Vertebrates* (ed. Fessard, A.) Springer-Verlag, New York, 147–200.

Knudsen, E. I. (1976) Midbrain responses to electroreceptive input in catfish: evidence of orientation preferences and somatotopic organization *J. comp. Physiol.*, **106**, 51–67.

Knudsen, E. I. (1978) Functional organization in the electroreceptive midbrain of the catfish *J. Neurophysiol.*, **41**, 350–364.

Knudsen, E. I. and Konishi, M. (1978) A neural map of auditory space in the owl *Science*, **200**, 795–797.

Meyer, D. L., Becker, R. and Graf, W. (1977) Ventral substrate response of fishes *J. comp. Physiol.*, **117**, 209–217.

Meyer, D. L., Heiligenberg, W. and Bullock, T. H. (1976) The ventral substrate response. A new postural control mechanism in fishes *J. comp. Physiol.*, **109**, 59–68.

Myrberg, A. A., Banner, A. and Richard, J. D. (1969) Shark attraction using a video acoustic system *Marine Biol.*, **2**, 264–276.

Perkel, D. H. and Bullock, T. H. (1968) "Neural coding" in *Neurosciences Research Program Bulletin*, **6**, 221–348.

Peters, R. C. and Buwalda, R. J. A. (1972) Frequency response of the electroreceptors ("Small Pit Organ") of the catfish, *Ictalurus nebulosus* LeS *J. comp. Physiol.*, **79**, 29–38.

Scheich, H. (1977*a*) Neural basis of communication in the, high frequency electric fish *Eigenmannia virescens* (jamming avoidance response). I. Open loop experiments and the time domain concept of a signal analysis *J. comp. Physiol.*, **113**, 181–206.

Scheich, H. (1977*b*) Neural basis of communication in the high frequency electric fish *Eigenmannia virescens* (jamming avoidance response). II. Jammed electroreceptor neurons in the lateral line nerve *J. comp. Physiol.*, **113**, 207–227.

Scheich, H. (1977*c*) Neural basis of communication in the high frequency electric fish *Eigenmannia virescens* (jamming avoidance response). III. Central integration in the sensory pathway and control of the pacemaker *J. comp. Physiol.*, **113**, 229–255.

Scheich, H. and Bullock, T. H. (1974) "The detection of electric fields from electric organs" in *Handbook of Sensory Physiology III/3: Electroreceptors and Other Specialized Receptors in Lower Vertebrates* (ed. Fessard, A.) Springer Verlag, New York, 201–256.

Szabo, T. (1974) "Anatomy of the specialized lateral line organs of electroreception" in *Handbook of Sensory Physiology III/3: Electroreceptors and Other Specialized Receptors in Lower Vertebrates* (ed. Fessard, A.) Springer Verlag, New York, 13–58.

Viancour, T. A. (1977) Mechanisms of frequency tuning: tuberous electroreceptors of *Eigenmannia virescens Proc. XXVII Congress Internat. Union Physiol. Sciences*, Paris, **13**, 788 (Abs.).

Viancour, T. A. (1979*a*) Electroreceptors of a weakly electric fish. I. Characterization of tuberous receptor organ tuning *J. comp. Physiol.*, **133**, 317–327.

Viancour, T. A. (1979*b*) Electroreceptors of a weakly electric fish. II. Individually tuned receptor oscillations *J. comp. Physiol.*, **133**, 328–339.

CHAPTER TWENTY-TWO

EPILOGUE

O. LOWENSTEIN

There are various ways of approaching the perplexing problems set for the biological investigator who is exploring the ways and means of interchange of information between the extra- and intrasomatic sources of potentially stimulating energy, and the organ systems saddled with the task of processing this information and of elaborating the organism's response, thereby ensuring its individually or phylogenetically successful survival and evolutionary future.

One category of problem which has been figuring in textbooks of zoology is posed by structures which, by dint of their position in the body and of their innervation, appear to be receptors of some kind—without, however, offering any obvious suggestions concerning the modality they subserve or their mode of functioning. Although such questions are becoming rarer, they are still with us. There are many types of sensillum, especially in the invertebrates, in need of such definitive characterization. The accounts of the exploration of the sensilla of the aphid antenna or of those found in a blind cave beetle may be recalled in this context. The lyriform organs of arachnids are another example, whose receptor role is now also better understood.

Receptor organs which have a well-known structure, receptive range and general mode of functioning still offer problems, such as the role played by their various auxiliary structures or ultrastructural components. The hair cell of the vertebrate inner ear continues to provide ample scope for experimental analysis on a number of levels. What is, for instance, the significance of the topographic patterns of distribution within the various sensory epithelia with respect to directional hearing in fishes? How should the different relationships between hair cells and overlying covering structures be functionally interpreted? We have discussed the functional role of this receptor cell's hair processes (i.e., kinocilia and stereocilia in the transduction of mechanical displacement or deformation, and the way in which these mechanical effects bring about the depolarization of the cell membrane at synaptic sites at some distance from the apical end of the cell) and it is clear that some progress in our understanding may be claimed to have been achieved by means of intracellular recordings, which for a long time were thought to be technically intractable. Problems are still posed by the ultrastructural differences between vestibular and cochlear hair cells on the one hand, and (within the cochlea) between inner and outer hair cells on the other, especially in relation to their different types of innervation. Here we are confronted with a call for a radical reappraisal of some functional assumptions. Yesterday's impossibilities are the stuff of which today's triumphs are made.

One striking feature of research into stimulus transduction in several kinds of receptor organs is the emergence of important evidence for a fundamental role of the calcium ion in the regulation of membrane permeability and stability. A clarification of the role of photon-catching and "auxiliary" pigments in visual organs is demonstrated for the vertebrate retina and for the retina of the arthropod compound eye, and there is report of some spectacular methodological advances, as in the case of the chemical characterization of pigment by combined histological, laser, and spectrographic localization of chemical entities within the photoreceptor. The use of a non-invasive technique in a study of pigment migration, which manifests itself in the appearance of the so-called pupillary responses in the insect eye, and the utilization of autofluorescence of rhabdomes combined with intracellular recordings are yielding important additional information on the distribution and mapping of various "spectral" types of receptors in the retinae of insect eyes. Our knowledge of colour vision in insects is also enhanced by the use of mutants of *Drosophila* in visual training experiments employing the aversive stimulus of shaking for conditioning.

Electrophysiologists have become increasingly aware of the dangers inherent in "single-unit" exploration of sensory afference, despite its intrinsic and overriding importance for quantification of stimulus-response relationships and for the tracing of pathways. In the latter context, one must direct attention to the decisive evidence furnished by the application of various dye-marking techniques and the way in which they aid the study of the configuration of receptor fields in sensory systems.

The complex multifactorial nature of the stimuli encountered in the study of chemoreception, especially of olfaction, directs attention to the importance of pattern recognition, i.e. the central processing involved when the organism itself (as opposed to the investigator) has to interpret the influx of sensory information. Here we come up against the problem of the relationship between reception, perception, and sensation, and face-to-face with the barrier of the inaccessibility of private experience. The way out of this impasse, successfully taken in research, is to study behavioural responses either in isolated effector systems or in the whole animal. Such responses may either be "spontaneous" or obtained by conditioning. Both methods have contributed to a deeper understanding, not only of sensory process as such, but also of specific adaptive relationships between types of animals and their individual physical and living environments. An assessment of the "meaningfulness" of certain stimulus situations is reminiscent of observational or introspective psycho-physical analysis in man, and leads to the recognition of species-specifically structured "images" or "models" of environments.

An account of some of the complexities of the human visual system forcefully draws attention to the fallacy of John Locke's concept of the *tabula rasa* with respect to the individual's build-up of *Umwelt* appreciation, and to the related assertion of Thomas Hobbes that

> there is no conception in Man's mind which hath not at first totally or in parts been begotten upon the organs of sense.

It must now be accepted that organisms are to a considerable extent genetically pre-programmed, not only obviously for the reception and transduction of physico-chemical events in the specific environments to which they have become adapted, but also especially pre-programmed for the selection and utilization of sensory information. The way in which the world is mirrored in the individual organism is as much a function of the structure of the mirror as of the nature of the energy flow acting upon it.

Reference was made in the introduction to an effective continuum of material reality and to the blurring of the boundaries between organism and environment by mutual interaction. This idea emerges in the context of recent advances in the study of animal responses to magnetic, electric, or electro-magnetic fields and to major geophysical cycles related to such fields. Although it must be conceded that we are still unable to pinpoint specific receptor systems in a number of these responses, the repeatable registration of them must be considered to be an established fact. Here, even more than elsewhere, the organism is seen to be embedded in the cosmic continuum, and a search for specific receptor structures may well be beside the point.

Index

C

D

E

I

J

K

L

M

N

O

P

Q

R

S